Vitamin D in 2020

Vitamin D in 2020: Stop or Not Yet?

Editors

Marie Courbebaisse
Etienne Cavalier

MDPI • Basel • Beijing • Wuhan • Barcelona • Belgrade • Manchester • Tokyo • Cluj • Tianjin

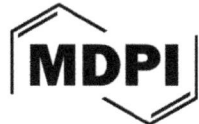

Editors
Marie Courbebaisse
Université Paris Descartes
France

Etienne Cavalier
University of Liège
Belgium

Editorial Office
MDPI
St. Alban-Anlage 66
4052 Basel, Switzerland

This is a reprint of articles from the Special Issue published online in the open access journal *Nutrients* (ISSN 2072-6643) (available at: https://www.mdpi.com/journal/nutrients/special_issues/vitamin_D_2020).

For citation purposes, cite each article independently as indicated on the article page online and as indicated below:

LastName, A.A.; LastName, B.B.; LastName, C.C. Article Title. *Journal Name* **Year**, *Volume Number*, Page Range.

ISBN 978-3-03943-867-9 (Hbk)
ISBN 978-3-03943-868-6 (PDF)

© 2020 by the authors. Articles in this book are Open Access and distributed under the Creative Commons Attribution (CC BY) license, which allows users to download, copy and build upon published articles, as long as the author and publisher are properly credited, which ensures maximum dissemination and a wider impact of our publications.

The book as a whole is distributed by MDPI under the terms and conditions of the Creative Commons license CC BY-NC-ND.

Contents

About the Editors vii

Marie Courbebaisse and Etienne Cavalier
Vitamin D in 2020: An Old Pro-Hormone with Potential Effects beyond Mineral Metabolism
Reprinted from: *Nutrients* 2020, 12, 3378, doi:10.3390/nu12113378 1

Nurul Nadiah Shahudin, Mohd Jamil Sameeha, Arimi Fitri Mat Ludin, Zahara Abdul Manaf, Kok-Yong Chin and Nor Aini Jamil
Barriers towards Sun Exposure and Strategies to Overcome These Barriers in Female Indoor Workers with Insufficient Vitamin D: A Qualitative Approach
Reprinted from: *Nutrients* 2020, 12, 2994, doi:10.3390/nu12102994 5

Thawinee Kamronrithisorn, Jittima Manonai, Sakda Arj-Ong Vallibhakara, Areepan Sophonsritsuk and Orawin Vallibhakara
Effect of Vitamin D Supplement on Vulvovaginal Atrophy of the Menopause
Reprinted from: *Nutrients* 2020, 12, 2876, doi:10.3390/nu12092876 21

Sarah Hakeem, Nuno Mendonca, Terry Aspray, Andrew Kingston, Carmen Ruiz-Martin, Carol Jagger, John C. Mathers, Rachel Duncan and Tom R. Hill
The Association between 25-Hydroxyvitamin D Concentration and Disability Trajectories in Very Old Adults: The Newcastle 85+ Study
Reprinted from: *Nutrients* 2020, 12, 2742, doi:10.3390/nu12092742 33

Mirela Ibrahimovic, Elizabeth Franzmann, Alison M. Mondul, Katherine M. Weh, Connor Howard, Jennifer J. Hu, W. Jarrard Goodwin and Laura A. Kresty
Disparities in Head and Neck Cancer: A Case for Chemoprevention with Vitamin D
Reprinted from: *Nutrients* 2020, 12, 2638, doi:10.3390/nu12092638 47

Joanna Milart, Aneta Lewicka, Katarzyna Jobs, Agata Wawrzyniak, Małgorzata Majder-Łopatka and Bolesław Kalicki
Effect of Vitamin D Treatment on Dynamics of Stones Formation in the Urinary Tract and Bone Density in Children with Idiopathic Hypercalciuria
Reprinted from: *Nutrients* 2020, 12, 2521, doi:10.3390/nu12092521 67

Jennifer Gjerde, Marian Kjellevold, Lisbeth Dahl, Torill Berg, Annbjørg Bøkevoll and Maria Wik Markhus
Validation and Determination of 25(OH) Vitamin D and 3-Epi25(OH)D3 in Breastmilk and Maternal- and Infant Plasma during Breastfeeding
Reprinted from: *Nutrients* 2020, 12, 2271, doi:10.3390/nu12082271 79

Agnieszka Kempinska-Podhorodecka, Monika Adamowicz, Mateusz Chmielarz, Maciej K. Janik, Piotr Milkiewicz and Malgorzata Milkiewicz
Vitamin-D Receptor-Gene Polymorphisms Affect Quality of Life in Patients with Autoimmune Liver Diseases
Reprinted from: *Nutrients* 2020, 12, 2244, doi:10.3390/nu12082244 97

Jenna R. Chalcraft, Linda M. Cardinal, Perry J. Wechsler, Bruce W. Hollis, Kenneth G. Gerow, Brenda M. Alexander, Jill F. Keith and D. Enette Larson-Meyer
Vitamin D Synthesis Following a Single Bout of Sun Exposure in Older and Younger Men and Women
Reprinted from: *Nutrients* 2020, 12, 2237, doi:10.3390/nu12082237 109

Maša Hribar, Hristo Hristov, Matej Gregorič, Urška Blaznik, Katja Zaletel, Adrijana Oblak, Joško Osredkar, Anita Kušar, Katja Žmitek, Irena Rogelj and Igor Pravst
Nutrihealth Study: Seasonal Variation in Vitamin D Status Among the Slovenian Adult and Elderly Population
Reprinted from: *Nutrients* **2020**, *12*, 1838, doi:10.3390/nu12061838 . . . . **125**

Michał Brzeziński, Agnieszka Jankowska, Magdalena Słomińska-Frączek, Paulina Metelska, Piotr Wiśniewski, Piotr Socha and Agnieszka Szlagatys-Sidorkiewicz
Long-Term Effects of Vitamin D Supplementation in Obese Children During Integrated Weight–Loss Programme—A Double Blind Randomized Placebo–Controlled Trial
Reprinted from: *Nutrients* **2020**, *12*, 1093, doi:10.3390/nu12041093 . . . . **141**

About the Editors

Marie Courbebaisse, MD, Ph.D., is a nephrologist who specializes in renal physiology and mineral metabolism. She is involved in clinical trials investigating the effects of vitamin D on skeletal and extra –skeletal health, such as the VITALE study (VITamine D Supplementation in RenAL Transplant Recipients) and the FEDEP study (Vitamin D and Preeclampsia).

Etienne Cavalier, Ph.D. and European Specialist of Laboratory Medicine (EuSpLM), is Professor of Clinical Chemistry at the University of Liège and Head of the Department of Clinical Chemistry at the CHU of Liège. He is the current President of the Royal Belgian Society of Laboratory Medicine and the Chairman of the IFCC-IOF Committee for bone markers. He is also a member of the Board of the European Society for Clinical and Economic Aspects of Osteoporosis, Osteoarthritis and Muskuloskeletal Diseases (ESCEO) and member of the Belgian Bone Club. He is a member of the scientific advisory board of the International Osteoporosis Foundation (IOF) and ESCEO, as well as a member of various societies of Clinical Chemistry, Nephrology and Endocrinology. Professor Cavalier has published more than 300 scientific papers in peer-reviewed journals indexed in Pubmed and has written 8 books or chapters.

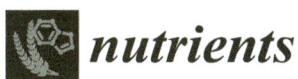

Editorial

Vitamin D in 2020: An Old Pro-Hormone with Potential Effects beyond Mineral Metabolism

Marie Courbebaisse [1,2,3,*] and Etienne Cavalier [4]

1. Faculty of Medicine of Paris Descartes, Paris University, 75006 Paris, France
2. Physiology Department, European Georges-Pompidou Hospital, AP-HP, 75015 Paris, France
3. INSERM U1151, 75015 Paris, France
4. Department of Clinical Chemistry, University of Liège, B-4000 Liège, Belgium; etienne.cavalier@chuliege.be
* Correspondence: marie.courbebaisse@aphp.fr

Received: 22 October 2020; Accepted: 30 October 2020; Published: 3 November 2020

Vitamin D is not a vitamin but a pro-hormone. It can be found as two forms, either vitamin D_2, which is the form found in plants, and vitamin D_3, which can be found in food (mainly fatty fish) but which is also produced by the cutaneous conversion of 7-dehydrocholesterol under the action of UVB. In human diets, vitamin D_2 is rarely found and vitamin D_3 represents the major part of vitamin D intakes. Both forms can also be found as supplements. Vitamin D, either from food, supplements or produced by the skin undergoes a first hydroxylation in the liver on carbon 25 under the effect of CYP2R1, a 25-hydroxylase, leading to the production of 25-hydroxy vitamin D (25OHD). 25OHD then undergoes a second hydroxylation on carbon 1 under the effect of a 1α-hydroxylase (CYP27B1) expressed in the proximal tubular cells of the kidney and is thus converted into 1,25 dihydroxyvitamin D or calcitriol, the active form of vitamin D, a steroid hormone with actions on mineral metabolism [1]. 25OHD is also a substrate for the 1α-hydroxylase expressed in several extra-renal tissues. These extra-renal tissues are dependent on adequate levels of 25OHD to ensure adequate local calcitriol production, which is responsible for the extra skeletal autocrine and paracrine actions of vitamin D, such as the modulation of renin and insulin synthesis, regulation of cell proliferation and apoptosis, and of innate and adaptative immunity [2].

The assessment of vitamin D status is based on the measurement of the serum concentration of 25OHD. Although there is a consensus to define severe vitamin D deficiency as a serum 25OHD concentration below 12 ng/mL (30 nmol/L), the definition of vitamin D adequate level is less consensual. Whereas the US Institute of Medicine considers that serum 25OHD concentrations between 20 and 50 ng/mL (50–125 nmol/L) [3] are adequate for the general population, the Endocrine Society considers 25OHD levels below 30 ng/mL (75 nmol/L) as insufficient [4], at least in some groups of patients (patients with osteoporosis or at risk of osteoporosis, patients with chronic kidney disease, patients with intestinal malabsorption and elderly at high risk of falling).

In addition to its protective effect against rickets and osteomalacia, vitamin D sufficiency has been associated with a reduced risk of many diseases, including type 2 diabetes mellitus, major cardiovascular events, cancers, infectious diseases and chronic kidney disease [5]. Of note, high 25OHD concentrations (above 40 ng/mL) have also been associated with an increased risk of cardiovascular events [6,7], potentially attributable to the increase in vascular and valvular calcifications. Randomized trials and meta-analyzes of randomized trials show that vitamin D supplementation reduces total fractures in elderly people, falls in frail elderly people, respiratory infections in the general population, blood pressure in hypertensive patients with vitamin D deficiency, and all causes of death [5].

However, the results of two recent large-scale US randomized controlled trials showed no effect of high doses of vitamin D on cardiovascular events and cancer incidence in the general population [8] or on diabetes incidence among persons at high risk of type 2 diabetes [9].

How should we thus position ourselves in 2020? Should we say "*stop*" or "*yet*"? Indeed, the aging of the population, but also new challenges and discoveries, are still triggering our interest for vitamin D. In this Special Issue of Nutrients entitled "Vitamin D in 2020: Stop or yet?", international experts, researchers and authors have been invited to submit their latest research ranging from epidemiological studies to interventional trials.

This Special Issue presents a compendium of excellent observational and interventional clinical studies regarding vitamin D. The high frequency of vitamin D insufficiency or deficiency among adults and the elderly [10], but also among mothers and their infants and in breastmilk [11], are underlined. Although vitamin D_3 production decreases with age, the significant role of outdoor sun exposure to increase serum vitamin D_3 concentrations in vivo in younger and older adults is demonstrated [12], and the barriers towards sun exposure and the potential improvement strategies to promote safe sun exposure to produce an optimal level of vitamin D are discussed [13]. Regarding 25OHD assessment, it is specified that the detection of 3-Epi25(OH)D_3 using liquid chromatography-tandem mass spectrometry prevents the overestimation of 25OHD and misclassification of vitamin D status [11]. Interventional studies showed no effect of cholecalciferol on body weight reduction in obese children participating in a weight management program [14], or on bone mineral density in children with hypercalciuria [15]. This last study emphasizes the safety of vitamin D treatment (400–800 IU/day) on calciuria and on the evolution of stones in the urinary tract in these children [15]. In post-menopausal women, ergocalciferol 40,000 IU/week did not change vulvovaginal atrophy compared to placebo, but improved vaginal pH and visual analog scale of vulvovaginal atrophy symptoms between baseline and 12 weeks in the vitamin D group [16]. In very old adults, 25OHD concentrations below 25 nmol/L were associated with moderate and severe disability trajectories, even after adjustment for sex, living in an institution, season, cognitive status, body mass index and vitamin D supplementation [17]. Of note, this association disappeared after further adjustment for physical activity [17]. Interestingly, vitamin D receptor polymorphisms are reported to influence individual susceptibility to develop chronic autoimmune liver disease and affect quality of life of these patients [18]. Finally, an in vitro study shows that treatment of head and neck cancer cell lines with vitamin D alters multiple cancer pathways at genes and proteins levels, supporting a potential role for vitamin D in cancer inhibition [19].

In conclusion, this Special Issue reinforces the high prevalence of vitamin D deficiency and insufficiency in the general population and the safety of this low cost molecule and open new perspectives regarding extra skeletal effects of vitamin D. We thank all the authors for their contributions to this Special Issue dedicated to an old pro-hormone whose potential interests beyond mineral metabolism are still being investigated.

Funding: This research received no external funding.

Conflicts of Interest: The authors declare no conflict of interest.

References

1. Holick, M.F. Vitamin D Deficiency. *N. Engl. J. Med.* **2007**, *357*, 266–281. [CrossRef] [PubMed]
2. Courbebaisse, M.; Souberbielle, J.-C.; Thervet, E. Potential Nonclassical Effects of Vitamin D in Transplant Recipients. *Transplantation* **2010**, *89*, 131–137. [CrossRef] [PubMed]
3. Rosen, C.J.; Abrams, S.A.; Aloia, J.F.; Brannon, P.M.; Clinton, S.K.; Durazo-Arvizu, R.A.; Gallagher, J.C.; Gallo, R.L.; Jones, G.; Kovacs, C.S.; et al. IOM Committee Members Respond to Endocrine Society Vitamin D Guideline. *J. Clin. Endocrinol. Metab.* **2012**, *97*, 1146–1152. [CrossRef] [PubMed]
4. Holick, M.F.; Binkley, N.C.; Bischoff-Ferrari, H.A.; Gordon, C.M.; Hanley, D.A.; Heaney, R.P.; Murad, M.H.; Weaver, C.M.; Endocrine Society. Evaluation, Treatment, and Prevention of Vitamin D Deficiency: An Endocrine Society Clinical Practice Guideline. *J. Clin. Endocrinol. Metab.* **2011**, *96*, 1911–1930. [CrossRef] [PubMed]
5. Bouillon, R.; Marcocci, C.; Carmeliet, G.; Bikle, D.; White, J.H.; Dawson-Hughes, B.; Lips, P.; Munns, C.F.; Lazaretti-Castro, M.; Giustina, A.; et al. Skeletal and Extraskeletal Actions of Vitamin D: Current Evidence and Outstanding Questions. *Endocr. Rev.* **2019**, *40*, 1109–1151. [CrossRef] [PubMed]

6. Durup, D.; Jørgensen, H.L.; Christensen, J.; Schwarz, P.; Heegaard, A.M.; Lind, B. A Reverse J-Shaped Association of All-Cause Mortality with Serum 25-Hydroxyvitamin D in General Practice: The CopD Study. *J. Clin. Endocrinol. Metab.* **2012**, *97*, 2644–2652. [CrossRef] [PubMed]
7. Dror, Y.; Giveon, S.M.; Hoshen, M.; Feldhamer, I.; Balicer, R.D.; Feldman, B.S. Vitamin D Levels for Preventing Acute Coronary Syndrome and Mortality: Evidence of a Nonlinear Association. *J. Clin. Endocrinol. Metab.* **2013**, *98*, 2160–2167. [CrossRef] [PubMed]
8. Manson, J.E.; Cook, N.R.; Lee, I.-M.; Christen, W.; Bassuk, S.S.; Mora, S.; Gibson, H.; Gordon, D.; Copeland, T.; D'Agostino, D.; et al. Vitamin D Supplements and Prevention of Cancer and Cardiovascular Disease. *N. Engl. J. Med.* **2019**, *380*, 33–44. [CrossRef] [PubMed]
9. Pittas, A.G.; Dawson-Hughes, B.; Sheehan, P.; Ware, J.H.; Knowler, W.C.; Aroda, V.R.; Brodsky, I.; Ceglia, L.; Chadha, C.; Chatterjee, R.; et al. Vitamin D Supplementation and Prevention of Type 2 Diabetes. *N. Engl. J. Med.* **2019**, *381*, 520–530. [CrossRef] [PubMed]
10. Hribar, M.; Hristov, H.; Gregorič, M.; Blaznik, U.; Zaletel, K.; Oblak, A.; Osredkar, J.; Kušar, A.; Žmitek, K.; Rogelj, I.; et al. Nutrihealth Study: Seasonal Variation in Vitamin D Status Among the Slovenian Adult and Elderly Population. *Nutrients* **2020**, *12*, 1838. [CrossRef] [PubMed]
11. Gjerde, J.; Kjellevold, M.; Dahl, L.; Berg, T.; Bøkevoll, A.; Markhus, M.W. Validation and Determination of 25(OH) Vitamin D and 3-Epi25(OH)D3 in Breastmilk and Maternal- and Infant Plasma during Breastfeeding. *Nutrients* **2020**, *12*, 2271. [CrossRef] [PubMed]
12. Chalcraft, J.R.; Cardinal, L.M.; Wechsler, P.J.; Hollis, B.W.; Gerow, K.G.; Alexander, B.M.; Keith, J.F.; Larson-Meyer, D.E. Vitamin D Synthesis Following a Single Bout of Sun Exposure in Older and Younger Men and Women. *Nutrients* **2020**, *12*, 2237. [CrossRef] [PubMed]
13. Shahudin, N.N.; Sameeha, M.J.; Mat Ludin, A.F.; Manaf, Z.A.; Chin, K.-Y.; Jamil, N.A. Barriers towards Sun Exposure and Strategies to Overcome These Barriers in Female Indoor Workers with Insufficient Vitamin D: A Qualitative Approach. *Nutrients* **2020**, *12*, 2994. [CrossRef] [PubMed]
14. Brzeziński, M.; Jankowska, A.; Słomińska-Frączek, M.; Metelska, P.; Wiśniewski, P.; Socha, P.; Szlagatys-Sidorkiewicz, A. Long-Term Effects of Vitamin D Supplementation in Obese Children During Integrated Weight-Loss Programme-A Double Blind Randomized Placebo-Controlled Trial. *Nutrients* **2020**, *12*, 1093. [CrossRef] [PubMed]
15. Milart, J.; Lewicka, A.; Jobs, K.; Wawrzyniak, A.; Majder-Łopatka, M.; Kalicki, B. Effect of Vitamin D Treatment on Dynamics of Stones Formation in the Urinary Tract and Bone Density in Children with Idiopathic Hypercalciuria. *Nutrients* **2020**, *12*, 2521. [CrossRef] [PubMed]
16. Kamronrithisorn, T.; Manonai, J.; Vallibhakara, S.A.-O.; Sophonsritsuk, A.; Vallibhakara, O. Effect of Vitamin D Supplement on Vulvovaginal Atrophy of the Menopause. *Nutrients* **2020**, *12*, 2876. [CrossRef] [PubMed]
17. Hakeem, S.; Mendonca, N.; Aspray, T.; Kingston, A.; Ruiz-Martin, C.; Jagger, C.; Mathers, J.C.; Duncan, R.; Hill, T.R. The Association between 25-Hydroxyvitamin D Concentration and Disability Trajectories in Very Old Adults: The Newcastle 85+ Study. *Nutrients* **2020**, *12*, 2742. [CrossRef] [PubMed]
18. Kempinska-Podhorodecka, A.; Adamowicz, M.; Chmielarz, M.; Janik, M.K.; Milkiewicz, P.; Milkiewicz, M. Vitamin-D Receptor-Gene Polymorphisms Affect Quality of Life in Patients with Autoimmune Liver Diseases. *Nutrients* **2020**, *12*, 2244. [CrossRef] [PubMed]
19. Ibrahimovic, M.; Franzmann, E.; Mondul, A.M.; Weh, K.M.; Howard, C.; Hu, J.J.; Goodwin, W.J.; Kresty, L.A. Disparities in Head and Neck Cancer: A Case for Chemoprevention with Vitamin D. *Nutrients* **2020**, *12*, 2638. [CrossRef] [PubMed]

Publisher's Note: MDPI stays neutral with regard to jurisdictional claims in published maps and institutional affiliations.

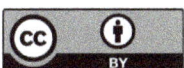

© 2020 by the authors. Licensee MDPI, Basel, Switzerland. This article is an open access article distributed under the terms and conditions of the Creative Commons Attribution (CC BY) license (http://creativecommons.org/licenses/by/4.0/).

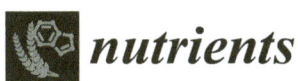

Article

Barriers towards Sun Exposure and Strategies to Overcome These Barriers in Female Indoor Workers with Insufficient Vitamin D: A Qualitative Approach

Nurul Nadiah Shahudin [1,2], Mohd Jamil Sameeha [2], Arimi Fitri Mat Ludin [3], Zahara Abdul Manaf [3], Kok-Yong Chin [4] and Nor Aini Jamil [2,*]

1. Faculty of Sports Sciences & Recreation, Universiti Teknologi MARA (UiTM) Cawangan Pahang (Kampus Jengka), Pahang 26400, Malaysia; p97542@siswa.ukm.edu.my
2. Centre for Community Health Studies (ReaCH), Faculty of Health Sciences, Universiti Kebangsaan Malaysia, Kuala Lumpur 50300, Malaysia; sameeha@ukm.edu.my
3. Centre for Healthy Ageing and Wellness (H-CARE), Faculty of Health Sciences, Universiti Kebangsaan Malaysia, Kuala Lumpur 50300, Malaysia; arimifitri@ukm.edu.my (A.F.M.L.); zaharamanaf@ukm.edu.my (Z.A.M.)
4. Department of Pharmacology, Faculty of Medicine, Universiti Kebangsaan Malaysia, Cheras 56000, Malaysia; gabrielchinky@gmail.com
* Correspondence: ainijamil@ukm.edu.my

Received: 14 July 2020; Accepted: 4 September 2020; Published: 30 September 2020

Abstract: The prevalence of vitamin D insufficiency is significant even in tropical countries such as Malaysia. Sun exposure is the primary source of vitamin D for most people due to limited intakes of food containing vitamin D and supplements. This study explored the perception of barriers towards sun exposure and strategies to overcome these barriers among vitamin D insufficient women workers in Kuala Lumpur, Malaysia. Twenty-five female indoor workers with serum 25-hydroxyvitamin D < 50 nmol/L participated in seven focus group discussions (FGDs). Barriers towards sun exposure were lack of accurate knowledge of vitamin D, health concern towards sun exposure, time constraints, desire to have fair and beautiful skin, sedentary lifestyle, indoor workplace, weather, lack of social support, living arrangement, safety concerns, and religious or cultural practices. The improvement strategies were classified into lifestyle changes and workplace opportunity for sun exposure. Public education on safe sun exposure to produce an optimal level of vitamin D is necessary. Future studies should evaluate the effectiveness of sunlight exposure program at workplace for the high-risk vitamin D deficiency group.

Keywords: vitamin D; sunlight exposure; barriers; indoor workers; female; focus group discussion

1. Introduction

Vitamin D insufficiency remains to be a concerning health issue worldwide due to its high prevalence among populations from various countries, cultural backgrounds and age groups [1], including tropical countries receiving substantial amount of sun exposure throughout the year [2]. However, the significant health impact of low vitamin D status remains unclear. Although incidence of rickets and osteomalacia are increasing in certain places, these conditions remain relatively rare worldwide [3,4]. The clinical evidence of vitamin D deficiency and nonskeletal health is not yet validated [5]. In countries where dietary vitamin D food intake and supplements are limited [6], and fortification of food with vitamin D is not compulsory, sunlight exposure is the primary source of vitamin D among the populations [6,7]. Government bodies often establish sun exposure guidelines to ensure a balance between the beneficial and harmful effects of sunlight [7]. However, it is almost impossible to provide guidance that fulfils all aspects because several factors can influence the cutaneous synthesis of vitamin D such as the zenith angle and latitude, different times of the day, air pollution, skin pigmentation, body surface area exposed when outdoors and age [8,9]. Currently, there are no sun exposure guidelines in Malaysia [10].

Previous studies around the world suggest that vitamin D deficiency is attributed to limited sun exposure, lack of dietary vitamin D food intake [11,12], urbanization [12], air pollution [13], obesity [14] and sedentary lifestyle [15]. It has been speculated that the excess body fat retains vitamin D in the body fat compartments resulting in decreased bioavailability of vitamin D among the obese individuals. This could also explain the lower vitamin D status among females compared to males as a result of higher body fat mass in females [16]. The limited sun exposure, especially in tropical countries, such as Malaysia, Thailand, Saudi Arabia and Iran, is mainly due to sun avoidance practice that is influenced by cultural, racial and religious backgrounds [2,6,8,9]. Malaysia is a unique multi-racial country, which is mainly composed of Malays, Chinese and Indians with various skin types. The high-risk groups of vitamin D insufficiency in Malaysia are children [17], adolescents [18,19], females [19–21], urban population [17,21], indoor workers [6,21], obese [17,18] and Indian and Malay ethnicities due to higher skin pigmentation and clothing styles (especially among Malay women wearing full-body garments) [2,6,17,19].

Cutaneous synthesis of vitamin D through outdoor activities and sun-bathing is widely practice by the westerners [9,11,22]. However, this practice was not popular among the vast majority of the Asian populations [23–25]. Sun-bathing and outdoor activities for sports and recreation are uncommon and not part of Asian culture [26,27]. Incidental sun exposure might occur while commuting to and from destinations, especially amongst those using public transportation. However, due to urbanization, most Asians are passive commuters and indoor workers [23,27].

A recent study on knowledge, attitude and practice conducted among high-risk female office workers in Kuala Lumpur, Malaysia suggested that further investigation into the factors contributing to vitamin D deficiency is essential as they have a moderate attitude and practice towards sunlight exposure and dietary intake of vitamin D [10]. This information that could be garnered from such studies would provide practical recommendations to the public and health agencies to prevent vitamin D deficiency among the Malaysian population. The current study is an extension of the previous study [10], which aimed to explore the perceived barriers towards sun exposure and strategies to overcome these barriers among indoor women workers with insufficient vitamin D status in Kuala Lumpur, Malaysia.

2. Materials and Methods

2.1. Study Participants

The participants from this study were derived from a recent study conducted among women office workers working in a medical university and teaching hospital in Kuala Lumpur, Malaysia [10]. In brief, they were indoor women workers with insufficient vitamin D level (serum 25-hydroxyvitamin D (25OHD) concentration <50 nmol/L) [28] and aged between 18 and 59 years. Indoor workers are defined as those working in an indoor setting for at least four days a week. Purposive sampling technique was used to ensure participants were recruited from four groups: (i) administrative staff (clerical staff, administrative staff assistants and lab technicians); (ii) executive (officers and top management employees); (iii) academicians (lecturers, senior lecturers and professors); and (iv) clinicians (medical assistants, nurses and doctors). Pregnant, lactating, or menopause women were excluded from this study. This study was approved by the Research Ethics Committees of Universiti Kebangsaan Malaysia (approval code: UKM PPI/111/8/JEP-2019-116).

2.2. Focus Group Discussion (FGD)

The FGDs were conducted in Bahasa Malaysia between October and November 2019 in a meeting room. All participants answered basic questionnaires and had given their written informed consent prior to participating in the FGD. Each FGD was led by a trained moderator (NNS), monitored by an experienced qualitative researcher (MJS) and observed by a research assistant. The moderator audiotaped all sessions using a video recorder (Sony, ICD-UX560F, Japan), while the research assistant was tasked with taking notes and recording descriptions of the participants' non-verbal behaviors. These notes offered as a backup to resolve any issues regarding audio clarity and to monitor participants' body language during the session.

The moderator first explained the purpose of the discussion, rules and regulations of FGD, followed by asking a series of specific, predetermined questions (Table 1). Two main topics were discussed, namely (i) barriers to receiving adequate sun exposure to synthesise vitamin D; and (ii) strategies to improve their vitamin D insufficiency. All participants were encouraged to share their ideas and opinions, and suitable probes were used to obtain in-depth findings. Recruitment was stopped when no new relevant information emerged due to data saturation.

Table 1. Focus Group Discussion Questions.

Topic	Questions
Barriers	(1) Internally, what do you think leads to your vitamin D insufficiency? (2) Externally, what do you think contributes to your vitamin D insufficiency? (3) What prevents or restricts you from sun exposure on weekdays? (4) What prevents or constraints you from sun exposure on weekends?
Improvement Strategy	(1) Do you want to improve your vitamin D status? (2) What are you going to do to improve your vitamin D level? (3) What type of activities do you want your employer to do to promote workplace sun exposure? (4) Can you suggest a suitable workplace intervention program? (frequency, intensity, type and time)

2.3. Data Coding and Analysis

The Consolidated Criteria for Reporting Qualitative Research (COREQ) framework [29] was used to guide the reporting of the findings. Audio recordings were transcribed verbatim. The transcripts were thematically analyzed using NVivo version 12 [30]. Each transcript was reviewed line-by-line and codes were categorized concurrently by three coders (NNS, NAJ and MJS). The identified codes were either single words (e.g., hot, beauty) or short phrases (e.g., sunscreen usage) that captured the essence of the excerpts [31]. Subsequently, the codes were grouped under broad domains of the discussion guide and theoretical constructs (e.g., time constraints). The discrepancies in coding were discussed with the research team (NNS, NAJ, MJS, AFML and ZAM) until a mutual agreement was achieved for the final nodes as described by Hadi and Closs [32]. As all researchers had expertise in nutrition and exercise health, they attempted to suspend their perspectives to avoid biases and focused on participants' statements that described their perceptions and experiences during the FGD.

2.4. Trustworthiness

To ensure the quality and trustworthiness of this study, multiple approaches were used. Prolonged engagement with study participants helped to gain their trust and establish rapport [32], as the researcher worked with the same participants during the preliminary study in February to May 2019 [10], until the FGD session conducted in October 2019. An audit trail was used to improve the quality of the instrument [32]. The lead researcher (NNS) met with supervisors (NAJ & MJS) after the first two FGDs to discuss possible questions to be revised and checked on probes improvement. Furthermore, peer debriefing was applied where the weekly meetings were conducted between NAJ, MJS and NNS to discuss on data analysis and interpretations continuously throughout the research process. Lastly, thick description of this study was presented in the methodology section to obtain external validity to ensure that this study could be transferable to other settings, situations and populations [32].

3. Results

Twenty-five female indoor workers took part in seven FGDs. Each group contained three to five participants and ranged from 45 min to 1 h in duration. Table 2 shows the participants' characteristics. Majority of the participants were between 30 and 39 years old (64%), married (64%), had a diploma or a higher education background (80%) and worked as an administrative staff (76%). Most of them had low to middle household-income (92%).

Table 2. Participants' Characteristics.

Variable	n	(%)	Mean	SD
Age				
18–29 years	3	12%		
30–39 years	16	64%	35.6	5.8
40–49 years	6	24%		
Marital Status				
Single	6	24%		
Married	16	64%		
Divorced/widowed	3	12%		
Education				
Secondary school	5	20%		
Diploma	10	40%		
Bachelor or higher	10	40%		
Occupation				
Administrative staff	19	76%		
Executive	1	4%		
Academician	3	12%		
Clinician	2	8%		
Household Monthly Income (MYR *)				
Low (<3860)	12	48%		
Middle (3860–8319)	11	44%		
High (>8319)	2	8%		

* MYR: Malaysia Ringgit.

3.1. Barriers towards Sun Exposure

A total of eleven perceived barriers towards sun exposure for adequate vitamin D status were identified and categorized into internal and external factors (Table 3). Five themes were recognized from the internal factor, including lack of knowledge due to misinformation about how vitamin D is synthesized upon exposure to sunlight or ultraviolet B (UVB) irradiation. Health concern was another barrier towards sun exposure, which was further classified into pre-existing medical conditions and risks for skin cancer. Other internal barriers towards sun exposure were time constraints associated with family and work commitments, desires to have fair and beautiful skin and sedentary lifestyles.

Table 3. Themes for barriers towards sunlight exposure.

Factor	Themes	Quotes
Internal factor	Lack of knowledge	"I got my vitamin D synthesized when I was driving. The sun rays were felt through the windscreen of my car," (33 years old, clinician). "Vitamin D sun is the morning sun. The afternoon and evening sun do not help to produce vitamin D, right?" (27 years old, administrative staff).
	Health concern	"If we are exposed under the sun, will it cause skin cancer? That is why I prefer to stay indoors" (49 years old, administrative staff). "I have this stigma that sunlight can make me fall sick, get fever or headache, regardless whether it is in the morning, afternoon or evening's sunlight," (41 years old, administrative staff). "I can't stand with the hot sun these days. It is so much different compared to younger days, and the heat was unbearable. I believe the sun rays these days is harmful and can cause cancer. It is because of the thinning ozone," (32 years old, administrative staff). "I am a patient of cardiovascular disease. I had a minor stroke two years ago. That is why I didn't go out much these days. Whenever I walk, I tend to get tired quickly, thus making me feel lazy (to walk)," (44 years old, administrative staff). "I am very much an indoor person because my health doesn't permit (me to exercise). I must be cautious whenever (I'm) outside because my respiratory system is very sensitive. For example, if I were to go out at the park, it needs to be somewhere dust-free and less polluted because I can get sick quickly and (it) may cause prolonged cough for months," (34 years old, executive).
	Time constraints	"I don't have enough time to go out after work. There are times when I would only reach home at 7.00 p.m. due to heavy traffic," (34 years old, administrative staff). "I don't have time to do any activities before or after work because I stay far from the office, approximately 30 km away. I usually reach home in an hour. Sometimes, I have to travel for 2 h," (32 years old, administrative staff). "No time to go out on weekdays. Once I reach home, I need to cook and do all the house chores. As for the weekends, I will do major cleaning, cooking and spend some family time at home. Plus, my husband works on the weekends. Most of the time, I just let the kids play at the car porch (covered) instead of going out," (35 years old, administrative staff). "I don't have time to do any outdoor activities on the weekends because I have part-time work commitment as a phlebotomist," (33 years old, administrative staff).
	Desire to have fair and beautiful skin	"I wear long sleeves whenever I'm out because it's hot and I'm afraid of becoming dark," (37 years old, clinician). "I used to have a lot of freckles. My beautician said the UV rays could cause freckles. That is why I avoid sun exposure," (35 years old, administrative staff). "I think because of ageing, I have been consistently using SPF moisturizer for the past three years to keep hydrated. So, I can avoid wrinkles and dry skin," (42 years old, administrative staff).
	Sedentary lifestyle	"I don't do any outdoor activities. The most I would do on the weekends is to hang out at eateries," (33 years old, administrative staff). "I often spend time at home on the weekend watching television," (24 years old, administrative staff). "I don't know why, but even when I had the chance (to go outdoor), I prefer to stay at home or indoor activity," (42 years old, administrative staff).

Table 3. *Cont.*

Factor	Themes	Quotes
External factor	Indoor workplace	"I am confined indoors during work from 8.00 a.m. to 5.00 p.m. So, sun exposure is limited during the weekdays. I normally take my lunch in the office or cafe, which is in the same building. So, there is no reason for me to go out," (41 years old, administrative staff). "I work in a diagnostic lab that is in the basement. I don't see the sun during working hours," (32 years old, clinician).
	Weather	"Malaysia's weather is so hot. So, I prefer to stay indoors," (33 years old, clinician). "Our weather is so unpredictable, especially during the rainy season. I skip being outdoors and choose to spend the time at my favorite eateries instead," (37 years old, administrative staff).
	Lack of social support	"My husband works during the weekends. Normally, I would wait for his off days to go for an outing. Otherwise, I just spend time with my son at home," (35 years old, administrative staff). "I am single and don't have a lot of friends. I will only go out to the park if my nephews or nieces come over to visit me. I wish to go out more often, but I don't have anyone to go with," (37 years old, academician). "My husband is not an outdoor person. He loves to go shopping and eat at the mall. So, I have no choice but to follow him as we normally go there at least twice a week," (32 years old, executive).
	Living arrangement	"I stay in a high-rise apartment, and there is no direct sunlight coming in. I don't get sunlight because my apartment doesn't come with a balcony. I even have to dry my clothes inside," (32 years old, administrative staff). "I stay at an apartment on the fourth floor, and I don't go out often even during the weekends, just too lazy to go down," (31 years old, clinician). "I stayed in a sub-urban landed property. I don't get direct sunlight in my house compound. There are a lot of big trees surrounding my house," (44 years old, administrative staff).
	Safety concern	"I prefer indoor activities instead of outdoors because of safety reasons. For example, if you were to go out during the early mornings at the park, it tends to be too quiet. I am scared to go there alone," (38 years old, administrative staff).
	Culture and religious practices	"I enjoy outdoor activities, but I don't like it when men are staring at me (in public)," (32 years old, executive). "I am particular in covering my aurah (part of the body that is prohibited from being revealed to other men for Muslim women). I was active before, doing workout and even join an aerobic class. However, I will make sure that I follow the rules (only exposing the face and both hands up to the wrists)," (42 years old, administrative staff).

For the external factor, six themes emerged including indoor workplaces, hot weather and unpredictable climate change. Lack of social support from the spouse, family members or friends to do outdoor activity together reduced the participants' interest to be exposed to the sun. Limited direct access to the sun at home as a result of living arrangement, house design and location of the house situated in the city were also mentioned. Finally, safety concerns and cultural and religious practices among Muslim women were also barriers towards sunlight exposure.

3.2. Strategy to Overcome the Barrier towards Sun Exposure

The discussion on the strategies to overcome the barrier towards sun exposure was classified into two factors (Table 4). The first is focusing on the personal improvement strategies that the participants were willing to perform on their own by changing their sun exposure behaviors to improve their vitamin D status. Suggestions included increasing outdoor activities during the weekends, practicing appropriate sunscreen usage, clothing adjustments that increase body surface area (BSA) exposed to sunlight, and improving their time management. The second part of the discussion is followed by suggestions for a suitable intervention program to be conducted by employers. The recommendations were categorized based on themes which include types, frequency, intensity and time that can be done based on workplace settings. Figure 1 summarizes the factors of barriers towards sun exposure and improvement strategies as identified by the indoor female workers in this study.

Table 4. Themes for strategies to overcome the barrier.

Factor	Themes	Quotes
Personal Improvement	Increase outdoor activity	"I am unsure whether I can do it on weekdays, but I will do more outdoor activities on the weekends. Maybe later in the afternoons after I am done with household chores," (35 years old, executive). "I need to make some changes, for example, do outdoor activities," (42 years old, administrative staff). "Outdoor outing with the family, for example a trip to the National Zoo. Not only we get to expose under the sun, but also (we) can spend quality time with the family," (31 years old, administrative staff).
	Practice appropriate sunscreen usage	"The least I can do is to reduce my sunscreen usage, not to apply too thick, especially in the mornings," (27 years old, administrative staff).
	Clothing adjustment	"I think I need to wear short-sleeved clothing instead of long-sleeved when I do my exercise so that I absorb more (sunlight)," (37 years old, clinician). "Just open (rolled up her sleeves) and expose it," (49 years old, administrative staff).
	Time management	"I will do house chores at night. So, I can go out during the day," (32 years old, administrative staff).
Intervention Program at Workplace	Type of activity	"Walking around the campus. For example, aim for the daily 10,000 steps," (37 years old, academician). "Maybe just stay out, like sun-bathing with clothes on," (32 years old, administrative staff). "Group activity such as treasure hunt around the campus," (32 years old, administrative staff). "I guess an outdoor aerobic such as Zumba is the most suitable activity and we have done it before," (33 years old, clinician). "I think leisure activities like 'tele-match' and family day is suitable," (42 years old, administrative staff). "Maybe organize a run (paused) like the fun run. If it is conducted on weekends, we can include our family members too," (33 years old, administrative staff). "If we take a look at the current surrounding, I think outdoor cleaning activity is suitable as one of the methods to obtain sunlight," (33 years old, administrative staff). "Maybe the employer can provide an outdoor workstation that allows the staff to bring their laptop and do their work outdoors. Apart from the lab work which needs to be done indoors, I can do report writing and administrative related work outdoors," (41 years old, administrative staff).
	Frequency	"I think once a week is fine. If it's more than that, two or three times a week, that's a bit too frequent. It will disrupt my work, and I believe my employer will not approve it," (37 years old, administrative staff). "Twice a week is sufficient," (24 years old, administrative staff). "I think once a week is not sufficient, maybe around two to three times a week," (32 years old, administrative staff).

Table 4. *Cont.*

Factor	Themes	Quotes
	Intensity	"I prefer to do light exercise. I don't want to be drenched in sweat in the morning and I need to do work after that," (37 years old, academician). "The exercise intensity should be moderate. So, we can maintain our fitness apart from getting sun exposure. I think it can be boring if it's too slow and relaxed," (34 years old, administrative staff). "I prefer low intensity, more relax," (32 years old, administrative staff). "I prefer moderate (intensity) and gradually increase the intensity. Not only we get the benefit of sun exposure, but also at the same time (we) can improve our cardiovascular fitness," (38 years old, administrative staff).
	Duration and time of the day	"I think the best time to do the program is between 8.00 a.m. to 9.00 a.m. before we start work. It is inconvenient to work, stop for exercise, then work again," (42 years old, administrative staff). "Evening session is suitable, about 5.30 p.m. It is more relaxing to do exercise once the work is done," (33 years old, administrative staff). "10.30 a.m. onwards is suitable as normally we are less occupied around that time," (32 years old, administrative staff). "The first two hours between 8.00 a.m.–10.00 a.m. is fine to me," (33 years old, administrative staff). "I think I can spare 15 min for that (intervention)." (24 years old, administrative staff) "Half an hour is workable for me," (34 years old, administrative staff). "30 min is not enough, at least one hour per session," (34 years old, administrative staff).

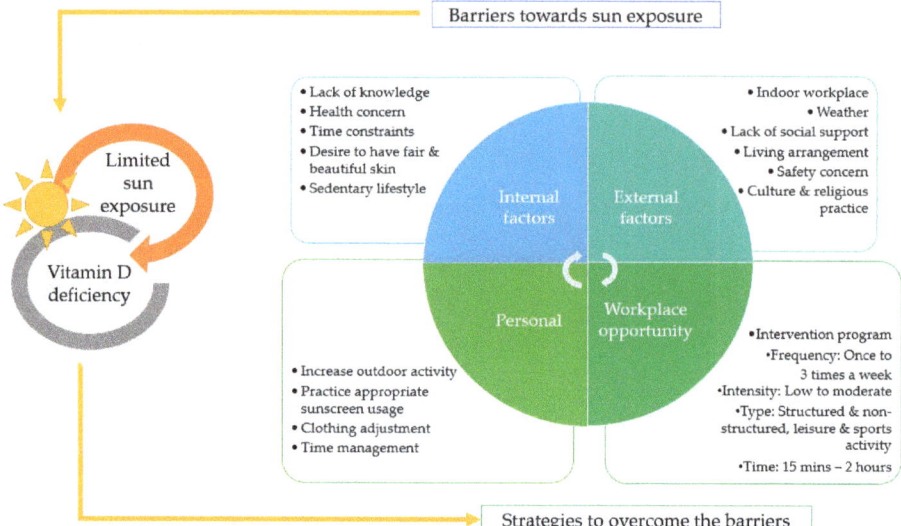

Figure 1. Barriers and improvement strategies to improve sun exposure for vitamin D.

4. Discussion

This study used a qualitative method of FGD to explore the barriers and improvement strategies towards sun exposure among women working indoors in the capital city of Malaysia with insufficient vitamin D status. The study provides new knowledge in this area, with practical messages that can be applied to the population at risk of vitamin D deficiency with a similar demographic background.

Lack of knowledge is on the top of the list for barriers towards sun exposure. We found that most of the participants had a misconception on the metabolism of vitamin D including how vitamin D is synthesized, and the differences between ultraviolet A (UVA) and UVB radiation. UVB is the sources of cutaneous synthesis of vitamin D and it cannot penetrate glass [11]. The participants assumed that the UVA they are exposed to while driving in the car and sitting by office window (with glasses) might provide them with vitamin D. A previous study done in a Malaysian sub-urban setting among post-menopausal Malay women found that poor knowledge on vitamin D influenced their sun exposure behavior [33]. The similarity of the findings could be owing to the lack of knowledge regarding vitamin D health benefits compared to other groups of vitamins among both urban and sub-urban females in Malaysia [1,6,33].

Health concerns to sun exposure, particularly increased risk of skin cancer, were mentioned in the FGD. According to the Global Cancer Observatory 2018 report, skin cancer was the 30th most common cancer in Malaysia and is not as prevalent as other cancers [34]. Most participants believed that they are susceptible to skin cancer due to the thinning of the ozone layer. They were not aware that skin cancer is not prevalent among Malaysians, especially the Malays. Our participants practiced poor sun protection behaviors, such as inappropriate amount and timing of sunblock application. They usually apply sunblock once in the morning together with their makeup before going to work. This finding is consistent with a previous study of skin cancer prevention practice among 400 university students in Kuala Lumpur, with the majority of the subjects being Malay women [35]. The study found that only 43.5% of the participants used sunblock, often applying them inadequately and forgetting to reapply after swimming, sweating, or other activities after the sunblock is degraded or washes-off [35]. A cross-sectional study in Queensland, Australia where the highest rate of skin cancer in the world reported that participants from low-income household tend to have uncertainty and concern about vitamin D and sun exposure [36]. Both studies suggested that sun protection education is needed in these populations to address the misunderstanding about skin cancer risk and improve the skin protection practice [25,35]. Some participants in our study also perceived that dizziness and fever were direct results of sun exposure, despite the lack of scientific evidence. This assumption also led to sunlight avoidance among our study participants.

Time constraint was frequently mentioned by the participants that caused limited sun exposure. All of the subjects in this study were working women in the urban area, who thrive to balance between work and family. This finding is consistent with a recent study among employees in Kuala Lumpur, who associated 'lack of time' with being busy with work, house chores and other family commitments [37]. A recent review highlighted that limited time spent outdoors among the urban population was due to their working nature, increased screen time and less manual work undertaken outdoor compared to rural population [12]. The majority of our participants drove to work. A typical driving scenario in the urban area encompasses a mixture of standstill traffic and slow traffic, depending on the route and time of the day [38]. Our participants spent on average around 1 to 1.5 h to commute daily to work. Once they reached home, they were bound to do house chores, further limiting their sunlight exposure time. Similar experiences were shared by women in eight European countries, whereby gender inequality and expectations of married working women, especially mothers, are higher in balancing work-family commitments compared to their counterparts [39].

The subjects of this study also expressed aesthetic concerns about sunlight exposure. This finding echoed previous reports among Asians, whereby a fair skin tone is often associated with beauty [25,40]. Common remarks such as fear of becoming dark, having freckles, sunburn and makeup usage, influenced sun avoidance behavior, especially among women [25]. Apart from sun protection cream, most moisturizers, foundation cream and compact powder these days, come with an added sun protection factor (SPF). The subjects surveyed also indicated a preference to stay indoors. A sedentary lifestyle has long been associated with vitamin D deficiency, physical inactivity, and health-related problems such as obesity and diabetes [2,19,20]. While the mechanism underlying the association between vitamin D and obesity is still uncertain, the low vitamin D status in obese individuals could be due to their sedentary lifestyle and low outdoor activity, vitamin D sequestration in adipose tissue, or simply a volumetric dilution effect [14]. A population study in Malaysia reported that only 14% of adults in Malaysia ever exercised and the majority spent 74% of the day being sedentary such as watching television, lying down, or hanging out to have drinks [41]. These factors are also correlated with our participants' social support given by their spouse, friends and employers [42]. It was previously reported that single individuals preferred to stay at home when there was no company while married couples with kids mainly adhered to their family commitments [37].

Being bounded indoors at their workplace as well as living arrangements are among the external factors leading to a lack of sunlight exposure. On average, indoor workers spend eight hours a day at the office for five days a week during the day. A similar investigation in Singapore found that indoor workers were among the high-risk group for vitamin D deficiency, probably because UVB is filtered by the glass window of the office [43]. Similar to other densely populated cities like Hong Kong and Singapore, the majority of the populations in Kuala Lumpur live in high-rise buildings [44], due to higher land costs. Low-income groups typically reside in a flat unit or a low-cost apartment with basic facilities, whereas the middle- and high-income groups may opt to live in a condominium with full facilities such as a playground, in-house park for jogging or walking, tennis court and swimming pool. The majority of our participants who lived in high-rise buildings mentioned that they either did not receive direct sunlight from their unit, or did not have sports or recreational facilities from their surrounding vicinity to encourage them to go out. A study among Saudi women attributed the lack of sun exposure to the modern house designs. Currently, the house design in Saudi has changed towards closed and high rise buildings built without a balcony, thus, limiting their sun exposure compared to living in a home with older designs that often incorporate a courtyard that allows sun ray to enter the house [45]. Apart from geographical reasons, the external barrier was influenced by cultural and religious practices similar to those of Muslims in our study. The Malays in Malaysia are generally

Muslims. As a Muslim woman, specific clothing guidelines commonly observed based on Quranic teachings allows only the face and hands to be exposed when in public [45,46]. Our participants further highlighted that religious restrictions that affect their actions and activities in public also limit their sun exposure.

Outdoor safety is an emerging barrier towards sun exposure among our subjects. The rising cost of living in Kuala Lumpur has given rise to an increased crime rate in the vicinity. Based on the criminal index in Malaysia from the year 2009 to 2015, 16,034 street crime investigations were carried on snatch thefts, robberies and similar offences [47]. These crimes were almost exclusively targeted on women walking alone in open areas [47]. Our participants mentioned that they too felt worried and insecure about being outdoors, even in public parks.

Strategies to tackle the barriers to sun exposure were mentioned by the participants through two factors: personal improvement and workplace opportunity. First and foremost, most of the participants agreed that they need to change their lifestyle to improve their vitamin D status. An educational program is essential for the promotion and enhancement of personal improvements to sunlight exposure. Besides, participants also believed that employers could play an essential role in promoting sun exposure at the workplace. Activities such as Zumba, aerobics and light exercise may be suitable to be conducted at workplace to promote both sunlight exposure and physical activity. Various timing and frequency proposed by the participants, ranging from 15 min to 2 h, once to three times a week. Besides, employers could also provide outdoor workstations that allow for sun exposure while being at work whenever necessary. These suggestions, however, would be subject to approval by the employer and improvements in existing organizational policies. A structured program of gradual increment from low to high intensity activities for 30–60 min was suggested in previous study among desk-based employees in Kuala Lumpur, Malaysia [37]. However, dietary vitamin D intake and supplements may be recommended to make up the shortfall from sunlight exposure, especially among those who have limited sunlight exposure, for whatever reasons they may have. A recent data showed a positive association between adherence to the Mediterranean diet and vitamin D status that could be explained by the synergistic anti-inflammatory and antioxidant effects of its high consumption of whole grain and plant-based food and moderate intake of fish, white meat, and eggs [48].

This study provides insight into the barriers towards sun exposure among vitamin D insufficiency women. However, several limitations were noted in this study. Firstly, it was conducted in one institution, with an uneven representatives from four target groups; administrators, executives, academicians and clinicians, due to time and work commitment constraints. Therefore, the findings in this study mainly reflect the perceptions of the administrator group. This study was also conducted among the Malay women population only, thus, it does not reflect the perception of other ethnic groups in Malaysia. Future studies should explore the barriers towards sun exposure among other at-risk groups, such as shift workers in Malaysia to understand their perspective on this matter. Furthermore, an intervention study should be performed to assess the effectiveness of sunlight exposure program in the workplace in improving vitamin D status of female indoor workers in Malaysia.

5. Conclusions

The Malay female indoor workers with insufficient vitamin D level reported that the barriers to sun exposure were influenced by both internal and external factors, such as work commitments, environment, and social factors. An educational program should be mooted in spreading accurate information on the importance of sun exposure and the best practice for optimal level of vitamin D. Working women should also take the initiative to maximize their sun exposure during the weekends. Apart from lifestyle changes, employers also can play an active role in promoting positive sun exposure at the workplace by organizing outdoor activities. Regardless, further evaluation on the effectiveness of sunlight exposure program among female indoor workers remains necessary.

Author Contributions: Conceptualization, N.N.S., M.J.S., A.F.M.L. and N.A.J.; formal analysis, N.N.S. and M.J.S.; funding acquisition, N.A.J.; investigation, N.N.S.; methodology, N.N.S., M.J.S. and N.A.J.; software, N.N.S., M.J.S. and N.A.J.; supervision, M.J.S. and N.A.J.; validation, M.J.S., A.F.M.L., Z.A.M. and N.A.J.; writing—original draft, N.N.S.; writing—review and editing, M.J.S., A.F.M.L., Z.A.M., K.-Y.C. and N.A.J. All authors have read and agreed to the published version of the manuscript.

Funding: This work was supported by a research grant from the Universiti Kebangsaan Malaysia (Project Code: GGPM-2017-098). The Universiti Kebangsaan Malaysia had no role in the design, analysis or writing of this article.

Acknowledgments: We would like to thank all the study participants for their contributions in this study. Thanks are also extended to Nur Syazwani binti Mastor and Nurul Nabila binti Md Yusuf who assisted with the logistics and preparation.

Conflicts of Interest: The authors declare no conflict of interest.

References

1. Scott, D.; Ebeling, P.R. Vitamin D and public health. *Int. J. Environ. Res. Public Health* **2019**, *16*, 848. [CrossRef]
2. Shafinaz, I.S.; Moy, F.M. Vitamin D level and its association with adiposity among multi-ethnic adults in Kuala Lumpur, Malaysia: A cross sectional study. *BMC Public Health* **2016**, *16*, 232. [CrossRef] [PubMed]
3. Creo, A.L.; Thacher, T.D.; Pettifor, J.M.; Strand, M.A.; Fischer, P.R. Nutritional rickets around the world: An update. *Paediatr. Int. Child Health* **2016**, *37*, 84–98. [CrossRef] [PubMed]
4. Bouillon, R.; Antonio, L. Nutritional rickets: Historic overview and plan for worldwide eradication. *J. Steroid Biochem. Mol. Biol.* **2020**, *198*, 105563. [CrossRef] [PubMed]
5. Rosen, C.J.; Adams, J.S.; Bikle, D.D.; Black, D.M.; Demay, M.B.; Manson, J.E.; Murad, M.H.; Kovacs, C.S. The nonskeletal effects of vitamin D: An Endocrine Society scientific statement. *Endocr. Rev.* **2012**, *33*, 456–492. [CrossRef] [PubMed]
6. Abd Aziz, N.H.; Yazid, N.A.; Abd Rahman, R.; Abd Rashid, N.; Wong, S.K.; Mohamad, N.V.; Lim, P.S.; Chin, K.-Y. Is first trimester maternal 25-hydroxyvitamin D level related to adverse maternal and neonatal pregnancy outcomes? A prospective cohort study among Malaysian Women. *Int. J. Environ. Res. Public Health* **2020**, *17*, 3291. [CrossRef]
7. Bonevski, B.; Bryant, J.; Lambert, S.; Brozek, I.; Rock, V. The ABC of vitamin D: A qualitative study of the knowledge and attitudes regarding vitamin D deficiency amongst selected population groups. *Nutrients* **2013**, *5*, 915–927. [CrossRef]
8. Farrar, M.D.; Webb, A.R.; Kift, R.; Durkin, M.T.; Allan, D.; Herbert, A.; Berry, J.L.; Rhodes, L.E. Efficacy of a dose range of simulated sunlight exposures in raising vitamin D status in South Asian adults: Implications for targeted guidance on sun exposure. *Am. J. Clin. Nutr.* **2013**, *97*, 1210–1216. [CrossRef]
9. Wacker, M.; Holick, M.F. Sunlight and vitamin D: A global perspective for health. *Derm. Endocrinol.* **2013**, *5*, 51–108. [CrossRef]
10. Jamil, N.A.; Shahudin, N.N.; Abdul Aziz, N.S.; Chew, J.Q.; Wan Aminuddin, W.A.A.; Mat Ludin, A.F.; Chin, K.Y.; Abdul Manaf, Z.; Mat Daud, N. Knowledge, attitude and practice related to vitamin D and its relationship with vitamin D status among Malay female office workers. *Int. J. Environ. Res. Public Health* **2019**, *16*, 4735. [CrossRef]
11. Holick, M.F. Vitamin D deficiency. *N. Engl. J. Med.* **2007**, *357*, 266–281. [CrossRef] [PubMed]
12. Mendes, M.M.; Darling, A.L.; Hart, K.H.; Morse, S.; Murphy, R.J.; Lanham-New, S.A. Impact of high latitude, urban living and ethnicity on 25-hydroxyvitamin D status: A need for multidisciplinary action? *J. Steroid Biochem. Mol. Biol.* **2019**, *188*, 95–102. [CrossRef] [PubMed]
13. Barrea, L.; Savastano, S.; Di Somma, C.; Savanelli, M.C.; Nappi, F.; Albanese, L.; Colao, A. Low serum vitamin D-status, air pollution and obesity: A dangerous liaison. *Rev. Endocr. Metab. Disord.* **2017**, *18*, 207–214. [CrossRef] [PubMed]
14. Savastano, S.; Barrea, L.; Savanelli, M.C.; Nappi, F.; Somma, C.D.; Orio, F.; Colao, A. Low vitamin D status and obesity: Role of nutritionist. *Rev. Endocr. Metab. Disord.* **2017**, *18*, 215–225. [CrossRef]
15. Awad, A.B.; Alappat, L.; Valerio, M. Vitamin D and metabolic syndrome risk factors: Evidence and mechanisms. *Crit. Rev. Food Sci. Nutr.* **2012**, *52*, 103–112. [CrossRef]
16. Muscogiuri, G.; Barrea, L.; Somma, C.D.; Laudisio, D.; Salzano, C.; Pugliese, G.; Alteriis, G.D.; Colao, A.; Savastan, S. Sex differences of vitamin D status across BMI classes: An observational prospective cohort study. *Nutrients* **2019**, *11*, 3034. [CrossRef]

17. Poh, B.K.; Rojroongwasinkul, N.; Nguyen, B.K.L.; Sandjaja; Ruzita, A.T.; Yamborisut, U.; Hong, T.N.; Ernawati, F.; Deurenberg, P.; Parikh, P. 25-hydroxy-vitamin D demography and the risk of vitamin D insufficiency in the South East Asian Nutrition Surveys (SEANUTS). *Asia Pac. J. Clin. Nutr.* **2016**, *25*, 538–548. [PubMed]
18. Khor, G.L.; Chee, W.S.S.; Shariff, Z.M.; Poh, B.K.; Arumugam, M.; Rahman, J.A.; Theobald, H.E. High prevalence of vitamin D insufficiency and its association with BMI-for-age among primary school children in Kuala Lumpur, Malaysia. *BMC Public Health* **2011**, *11*, 95. [CrossRef] [PubMed]
19. Quah, S.W.; Abdul Majid, H.; Al-Saddat, N.; Yahya, A.; Su, T.T.; Jalaludin, M.Y. Risk factors of vitamin D deficiency among 15-year-old adolescents participating in the Malaysian Health and Adolescents Longitudinal Research Team Study (MyHeARTs). *PLoS ONE* **2018**, *13*, e0200736. [CrossRef]
20. Moy, F.M. Vitamin D status and its associated factors of free-living Malay adults in a tropical country, Malaysia. *J. Photochem. Photobiol.* **2011**, *104*, 444–448. [CrossRef]
21. Nurbazlin, M.; Chee, W.S.S.; Rokiah, P.; Tan, A.T.B.; Chew, Y.Y.; Siti Nusaibah, A.R.; Chan, S.P. Effects of sun exposure on 25(OH) vitamin D concentration in urban and rural women in Malaysia. *Asia Pac. J. Clin. Nutr.* **2013**, *22*, 391–399. [PubMed]
22. Gilchrest, B.A. Sun exposure and vitamin D sufficiency. *Am. J. Clin. Nutr.* **2008**, *88*, 570S–577S. [CrossRef] [PubMed]
23. Nimitphong, H.; Holick, M.F. Vitamin D status and sun exposure in southeast Asia. *Derm. Endocrinol.* **2013**, *5*, 34–37. [CrossRef]
24. Man, R.E.K.; Li, L.J.; Cheng, C.Y.; Wong, T.Y.; Lamoureux, E.; Sabanayagam, C. Prevalence and determinants of suboptimal vitamin D levels in a multiethnic Asian population. *Nutrients* **2017**, *9*, 313. [CrossRef] [PubMed]
25. Jang, H.; Koo, F.K.; Ke, L.; Clemson, L.; Cant, R.; Fraser, D.R.; Seibel, M.J.; Tseng, M.; Mpofu, E.; Mason, R.S.; et al. Culture and sun exposure in immigrant East Asian women living in Australia. *Women Health* **2013**, *53*, 504–518. [CrossRef] [PubMed]
26. Aman, M.S.; Fauzee, M.S.O.; Mohamed, M. The understanding of meaning and cultural significance of leisure, recreation and sport in Malaysia towards capitalizing human resources. *J. Glob. Bus.* **2007**, *3*, 129–135.
27. Nguyen, H.T.T.; von Schoultz, B.; Nguyen, T.V.; Dzung, D.N.; Duc, P.T.M.; Thuy, V.T.; Hirschberg, A.L. Vitamin D deficiency in northern Vietnam: Prevalence, risk factors and associations with bone mineral density. *Bone* **2012**, *51*, 1029–1034. [CrossRef]
28. Ross, A.C.; Manson, J.E.; Abrams, S.A.; Aloia, J.F.; Brannon, P.M.; Clinton, S.K.; Durazo-Arvizu, R.A.; Gallagher, J.C.; Gallo, R.L.; Jones, G.; et al. The 2011 report on dietary reference intakes for calcium and vitamin D from the Institute of Medicine: What clinicians need to know. *J. Clin. Endocrinol. Metab.* **2011**, *96*, 53–58. [CrossRef]
29. Tong, A.; Sainsbury, P.; Craig, J. Consolidated criteria for reporting qualitative research (COREQ): A 32-item checklist for interviews and focus groups. *Int. J. Qual. Health Care* **2007**, *19*, 349–357. [CrossRef]
30. *NVivo Qualitative Data Analysis Software*, version 12; QSR International (UK) Limited: Cheshire, UK, 2019.
31. Fereday, J.; Muir-Cochrane, E. Demonstrating rigor using thematic analysis: A hybrid approach of inductive and deductive coding and theme development. *Int. J. Qual. Methods* **2006**, *5*, 80–92. [CrossRef]
32. Hadi, M.A.; Closs, S.J. Ensuring rigour and trustworthiness of qualitative research in clinical pharmacy. *Int. J. Clin. Pharm.* **2016**, *38*, 641–646. [CrossRef]
33. Istiany, A.; Rahman, S.A.; Kasim, Z.K.; Swee, W.C.S.; Yassin, Z.; Parid, A.M. Effect of nutrition education and sun exposure on vitamin D Status among post-menopausal Malay women. *Int. J. Sci. Eng. Investig.* **2012**, *1*, 91–97.
34. World Health Organization. Cancer Today Population Fact Sheet (Malaysia). 2019. Available online: https://gco.iarc.fr/today/data/factsheets/populations/458-malaysia-fact-sheets.pdf (accessed on 10 April 2020).
35. Al-Naggar, R.A.; Bobryshev, Y.V. Practice of skin cancer prevention among young Malaysian. *Community Med. Health Educ.* **2012**, *2*, 2. [CrossRef]
36. Youl, P.H.; Janda, M.; Kimlin, M. Vitamin D and sun protection: The impact of mixed public health messages in Australia. *Int. J. Cancer* **2008**, *124*, 1963–1970. [CrossRef]
37. Zahara, A.M.; Abdul Hadi, R.; Arimi Fitri, M.L.; Siti Munirah, A.B. Motivations, barriers and preferences to exercise among overweight and obese desk-based employees. *Int. J. Sport Exerc. Psychol.* **2020**, 1–15. [CrossRef]

38. Abas, M.A.; Rajoo, S.; Zainal Abidin, S.F. Development of Malaysian urban drive cycle using vehicle and engine parameters. *Transp. Res. Part D Transp. Environ.* **2018**, *63*, 388–403. [CrossRef]
39. Beham, B.; Drobnič, S.; Präg, P.; Baierl, A.; Lewis, S. Work-to-family enrichment and gender inequalities in eight European countries. *Int. J. Hum. Resour. Manag.* **2020**, *31*, 589–610. [CrossRef]
40. Blebil, A.Q.; Dujaili, J.A.; Teoh, E.; Wong, P.S.; Bhuvan, K.C. Assessment of awareness, knowledge, attitude, and the practice of vitamin D among the general public in Malaysia. *J. Karnali Acad. Health Sci.* **2019**, *2*, 171–180. [CrossRef]
41. Poh, B.K.; Safiah, M.Y.; Tahir, A.; Siti Haslinda, M.D.; Siti Norazlin, N.; Norimah, A.K.; Wan Manan, W.M.; Mirnalini, K.; Zalilah, M.S.; Azmi, M.Y.; et al. Physical activity pattern and energy expenditure of Malaysian adults: Findings from the Malaysian Adult Nutrition Survey (MANS). *Mal. J. Nutr.* **2010**, *16*, 13–37.
42. Waters, C.N.; Ling, E.P.; Chu, A.H.Y.; Ng, S.H.X.; Chia, A.; Lim, Y.W.; Müller-Riemenschneider, F. Assessing and understanding sedentary behaviour in office-based working adults: A mixed-method approach. *BMC Public Health* **2016**, *16*, 360. [CrossRef]
43. Divakar, U.; Sathish, T.; Soljak, M.; Bajpai, R.; Dunleavy, G.; Visvalingam, N.; Nazeha, N.; Soh, C.K.; Christopoulos, G.; Car, J. Prevalence of vitamin D deficiency and its associated work-related factors among indoor workers in a multi-ethnic southeast Asian country. *Int. J. Environ. Res. Public Health* **2020**, *17*, 164. [CrossRef] [PubMed]
44. Wahab, S.R.H.A.; Ani, A.I.C.; Sairi, A.; Tawil, N.M.; Razak, M.Z.A. Classification of high-rise residential building facilities: A descriptive survey on 170 housing scheme in Klang Valley. *MATEC Web Conf.* **2016**, *66*, 00103. [CrossRef]
45. Aljefree, N.; Lee, P.; Ahmed, F. Exploring knowledge and attitudes about vitamin D among adults in Saudi Arabia: A qualitative study. *Healthcare* **2017**, *5*, 76. [CrossRef] [PubMed]
46. Jamil, N.A.; Yew, M.H.; Noor Hafizah, Y.; Gray, S.R.; Poh, B.K.; Macdonald, H.M. Estimated vitamin D synthesis and dietary vitamin D intake among Asians in two distinct geographical locations (Kuala Lumpur, 3°N v. Aberdeen, 57°N) and climates. *Public Health Nutr.* **2018**, *21*, 3118–3124. [CrossRef] [PubMed]
47. Latimaha, R.; Bahari, Z.; Ismail, N.A. Examining the linkages between street crime and selected state economic variables in Malaysia: A panel data analysis. *J. Ekon. Malays.* **2019**, *53*, 59–72.
48. Barrea, L.; Muscogiuri, G.; Laudisio, D.; Pugliese, G.; de Alteriis, G.; Colao, A.; Savastano, S. Influence of the Mediterranean Diet on 25-hydroxyvitamin D levels in adults. *Nutrients* **2020**, *12*, 1439. [CrossRef]

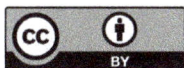

© 2020 by the authors. Licensee MDPI, Basel, Switzerland. This article is an open access article distributed under the terms and conditions of the Creative Commons Attribution (CC BY) license (http://creativecommons.org/licenses/by/4.0/).

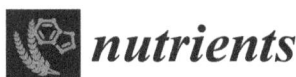

Article

Effect of Vitamin D Supplement on Vulvovaginal Atrophy of the Menopause

Thawinee Kamronrithisorn [1], Jittima Manonai [2], Sakda Arj-Ong Vallibhakara [3,4], Areepan Sophonsritsuk [5] and Orawin Vallibhakara [5,*]

1. Department of Obstetrics and Gynaecology, Faculty of Medicine, Ramathibodi Hospital, Mahidol University, Bangkok 10400, Thailand; giftgizz83@gmail.com
2. Female Pelvic Medicine and Reconstructive Surgery Unit, Department of Obstetrics & Gynaecology, Faculty of Medicine, Ramathibodi Hospital, Mahidol University, Bangkok 10400, Thailand; jittimabartlett@gmail.com
3. ASEAN Institute for Health Development, Mahidol University, Nakhon Pathom 73170, Thailand; dr.sakda@gmail.com
4. Department of Clinical Epidemiology and Biostatics, Faculty of Medicine, Ramathibodi Hospital, Mahidol University, Bangkok 10400, Thailand
5. Reproductive Endocrinology and Infertility Unit, Department of Obstetrics and Gynaecology, Faculty of Medicine, Ramathibodi Hospital, Mahidol University, Bangkok 10400, Thailand; areepan.sop@mahidol.ac.th
* Correspondence: orawinra38@gmail.com

Received: 25 July 2020; Accepted: 14 September 2020; Published: 21 September 2020

Abstract: The effects of oral vitamin D supplements on vaginal health in postmenopausal women with vulvovaginal atrophy (VVA) was evaluated. A double-blinded, randomized placebo-controlled trial was conducted for 12 weeks to investigate changes on vaginal maturation index (VMI), vaginal pH, and the visual analog scale (VAS) of VVA symptoms. The vitamin D group received oral ergocalciferol, at 40,000 IU per week, while the placebo group received an identical placebo capsule. Eighty postmenopausal women were enrolled. There were no significant differences in baseline characteristics between both groups. In an intention-to-treat analysis, VMI, vaginal pH, and VAS of VVA symptoms showed no significant differences between both groups at the six and 12 weeks. However, the mean difference of VMI in the vitamin D group between baseline and at six weeks showed significant improvement (5.5 + 16.27, $p<0.05$). Moreover, the mean vaginal pH and VAS of VVA patients in the vitamin D group were significantly improved at both six and 12 weeks compared to baseline. The oral vitamin D supplementation for 12 weeks potentially improves vaginal health outcomes in postmenopausal women with VVA symptoms, demonstrated by the improved mean VMI, vaginal pH, and VAS at six and 12 weeks between baseline, however, no significant differences were observed from the placebo treatment.

Keywords: vulvovaginal atrophy; VVA; vaginal maturation index; VMI; vaginal health; vitamin D; ergocalciferol; vitamin D supplement

---

1. Introduction

Vulvovaginal atrophy (VVA) is common, however, many postmenopausal women are not aware of this problem. This condition results from the changes in the female reproductive system during menopause, after cesstion of ovulation and the accompanying reduction in estrogen levels. VVA symptoms are a component of Genitourinary Syndrome of Menopause (GSM), a new terminology defined by the International Society for the Study of Women's Sexual Health and the North American Menopause Society in 2014. Symptoms include dryness, burning sensation, and irritation of the vulvovagina, as well as, sexual problems such as insufficient lubrication, and dyspareunia (pain during sexual intercourse). Lower urinary tract symptoms are also part of GSM and include frequency, recurrence of urinary tract infections, urinary urgency, and stress urinary incontinence. Signs of VVA from physical examination are thinning, drying, and the pallor of the vaginal epithelium due to the decreased ratio of superficial cells to parabasal cells. In addition, a reduction of lactic acid production associates with increased susceptibility to bacterial vaginosis infection [1–3]. The vaginal microbiota among postmenopausal women is typically shifted from predominantly *Lactobacillus* species to the higher proportions of anaerobic organisms, including *Mobiluncus* species and *Atopobium vaginae*. These changes in the vaginal bacterial community are associated with the severity of the VVA symptoms [4]. The prevalence of VVA was reported to be as high as 45% among postmenopausal women. The most common complaints were vaginal dryness (55–75%) and pain during intercourse (40–44%) [5–7]. However, the majority of patients do not mention their VVA symptoms to health care providers. The European Vulvovaginal Epidemiology Survey of 2160 postmenopausal women reported that using questionnaires indicated a prevalence of severe symptoms of vaginal atrophy, and vulvar atrophy of 66% and 30%, respectively. In contrast, the physical examination confirmed VVA symptoms in as high as 90% in the participants [8]. Under-reporting and subsequent under-treatment of VVA result in more severe and progressive symptoms. This is, especially the case in the Eastern countries where the reported prevalence of VVA was very low, varying from 6-80% among studies conducted in Japan, Sri Lanka, Singapore, and India. However, other data from these studies indicate that the VVA prevalence may be much higher. These surveys report a very high prevalence of "avoiding intimacy" (54–77%) and "loss of interest in sex" (71–91%) among postmenopausal women [9]. VVA not only affects on the quality of life, sexual health, and couple relations, but is also associated with increased risk of depression and anxiety among postmenopausal women [10].

The standard treatment for VVA is hormonal therapy, which can be administered as systemic menopausal hormone therapy (MHT), local estrogen therapy, as well as through other promising novel hormonal regimens such as ospemifene and vaginal DHEA [2,3,11,12]. However, both ospemifene and vaginal DHEA are not yet available in Thailand. Moreover, the study of Women Initiative Study in the systemic MHT study revealed a significantly increased risk of coronary heart disease, invasive breast cancer, and stroke among patients that received conjugated equine estrogen combined with medroxyprogesterone acetate [13]. The announcement of the WHI studies in 2002 resulted in the declining use of systemic MHT by more than 50% and caused a reluctant presumption in both physicians and women worldwide [14]. Although, vaginal estrogen is the most effective treatment for VVA, the examination of the effectiveness and endometrial safety of this therapy has been limited with the longest study period of only one year. Moreover, the only vaginal estrogen available in Thailand is the estriol-lactobacilli combination [15,16]. Non-hormonal therapy and alternative treatment of VVA symptoms are often the preferred choice for many patients. These include lifestyle modifications, encouraging sexual activity, use of vaginal lubricants and vaginal moisturizers, vaginal oxytocin gel, vaginal laser therapy, and vitamin D supplementation [17–22].

Vitamin D, a lipid-soluble steroid, enhances the absorption of calcium and phosphate thereby promoting a healthy musculoskeletal system. The Endocrine Society's Practice Guidelines on Vitamin D, published in 2011, describes the range of serum levels of vitamin D seen in patients, Vitamin D deficiency was defined as a serum level of 25-hydroxyvitamin D (25(OH)D) < 20 ng/mL, insufficiency as 21 to 29 ng/mL, and sufficiency level of at least 30 ng/mL [23]. The adequate level of vitamin D attenuates the rising of serum parathyroid hormone (PTH) level, leading to a plateau of bone resorption [24]. Furthermore, vitamin D insufficiency is associated with several health problems including chronic infections, autoimmune disease, and malignancy [25–28]. Recently, connections have been identified between vitamin D insufficiency and female reproductive dysfunction, including polycystic ovarian syndrome (PCOS), uterine leiomyoma, endometriosis, and poor in vitro fertilization (IVF) outcome [29,30]. Vitamin D insufficiency also contributes to the pelvic floor disorder and a thinning of the vaginal epithelium, which are associated with VVA in postmenopausal women [31].

Vitamin D receptors (VDRs) are involved in regulating the development and differentiation of the stratified epithelium of the vagina, as well as, the maturation of vaginal cells. Lee et al. reported that vitamin D positively regulates cell-to-cell junctions through the VDR, Ras homolog gene family (RhoA), and Ezrin pathway. Ezrin protein, extensively expressed in the vaginal wall, regulates actin-binding proteins responsible for plasma membrane interactions and cell-to-cell junctions. These processes help modulate the strength and flexibility of the vaginal membrane. In contrast, RhoA regulates cell motility, epithelial layer adhesion, cytokinesis, and cell polarity [32]. Therefore, vitamin D inadequacy maybe a linked factor to VVA in postmenopausal women.

The primary source of vitamin D is endogenous production following exposure to sunlight. Ultraviolet B radiation from sun exposure causes 7-dehydrocholesterol under the skin to be converted to pre-vitamin D3, and then vitamin D3 (cholecalciferol). Vitamin D3 is metabolized in the liver to 25-hydroxyvitamin D (25(OH)D), the major circulating form of vitamin D and is used to determine an individual's vitamin D status. The circulating 25(OH)D is subsequently metabolized in kidneys to the more biologically more active form, 1,25-dihydroxyvitamin D [33]. The lack of adequate sun exposure is the leading cause of vitamin D deficiency and insufficiency due to modern living conditions [34–36]. Vitamin D from the diet is another important source and oral supplements are typically given as either vitamin D3 (cholecalciferol) or vitamin D2 (ergocalciferol). Vitamin D3 is derived from animal sources such as oily fish; salmon, mackerel and herring; and cod liver oil. In contrast, vitamin D2 is derived from plants and UV irradiated yeast and mushroom.

Vitamin D inadequacy is a global health problem with approximately 50% of adults worldwide estimated to be vitamin D insufficient. Poor vitamin D status is especially prevalent in low- and middle-income countries [37,38]. Among the Asian population, the prevalence of vitamin D insufficiency was reported to be as high as 75% [39]. Based on a nationwide retrospective cohort study in 2019, a prevalence of vitamin D insufficiency among older women of 43.9% was reported. Major factors contributing to insufficient vitamin D in Thai women are sunscreen usage and sun avoidant behavior. In addition, air pollution in urban areas, such as Bangkok, decreases the amount of UVB available for cutaneous vitamin D synthesis. Furthermore, in Thailand, dairy products are not fortified with vitamin D, and very few vitamin D-rich foods are part of the typical Thai diet [40]. Thus, dietary intake of vitamin D in the Thai population is generally low. The Endocrine Society Practice Guideline recommends vitamin D supplementation of 1500–2000 IU per day to maintaining vitamin D adequacy, as judged by a serum level of 25(OH)D $\geq$ 30 ng/mL, in all adults aged more than 50 years. In the case of known vitamin D deficiency, supplementation of vitamin D at 50,000 IU per week is recommended to provide all the potential skeletal and non-skeletal health benefits [23]. Vitamin D2 (ergocalciferol) at a dose of 20,000 IU per capsule is available in Thailand from the Government Pharmaceutical Organization. However, the effects of Vitamin D2 on VVA in postmenopausal women have not been examined. This study aimed to evaluate the effect of oral vitamin D2 supplementation on VVA in postmenopausal women by measuring the vaginal maturation index (VMI), cytological changes in vaginal smear such as a shift from superficial squamous cells towards intermediate epithelial cells, vaginal pH, and the visual analog scale (VAS) of VVA symptoms. This study was initiated based on a hypothesis that adequate oral vitamin D supplementation could improve the vaginal health in Thai menopausal women which have a high prevalence of vitamin D insufficiency.

2. Materials and Methods

A double-blinded, randomized, placebo-controlled trial was conducted to study the effects of oral ergocalciferol on vaginal health including, VMI, vaginal pH, and VAS of VVA symptoms at six and 12 weeks of supplementation. The primary outcome was VMI in the 12 weeks of study compared to vitamin D and the placebo group. The secondary outcomes were vaginal pH, VAS of VVA symptoms, and adverse drug reaction. The study protocol conformed to the principles of the Declaration of Helsinki was approved by the Ethical Clearance Committee on Human Rights Related to Research Involving Human Subjects Faculty of Medicine Ramathibodi Hospital, Mahidol University (MURA2018/90), clinical trial registration number: TCTR20180419001.

2.1. Participants

Postmenopausal women presenting VVA symptoms, who visited the outpatient department of Department of Obstetrics and Gynaecology, Faculty of Medicine, Ramathibodi Hospital, Bangkok, a tertiary care and training hospital between February 2018 and May 2019, were enrolled. Informed consent was provided by all participants. Inclusion criteria were menopausal women, absence of menstruation for at least one year, a previous bilateral oophorectomy or serum FSH level more than 40 IU/L. The exclusion criteria were a history of hormonal treatments or vitamin D supplementation within the previous 12 weeks, abnormal PAP smear, active sexually transmitted disease, active urinary tract infection, abnormal uterine bleeding, or the presence of serious medical conditions, including cardiovascular disease, liver failure, and renal failure. In addition, patients with a history of vitamin D allergy or unwillingness to participate in the study protocol were excluded. The sample size was calculated using the randomized controlled trial for continuous data formula [41], based on previous studies of the results of Rad P. et al. [31]. The ratio of treatment and control groups was 1:1 with α-error and β-error of 0.01 and 0.1, respectively. The calculated sample-size was 33 and the final sample-size was 40 for each group, after add-ons of 20% incomplete or missing data.

2.2. Randomization, Blinding, and Intervention Protocol

All participants, mostly locals who live in the Bangkok Metropolitan area, were randomly distributed into groups using a computerized permutated block with four randomizations. The participants and investigators were blinded to the group allocation. Participants in the study group received oral vitamin D2 (ergocalciferol) at 20,000 IU with two capsules per week for 12 weeks. The placebo group received two identical placebo capsules per week for 12 weeks. Participants in both groups were encouraged to avoid any other drugs and supplements, such as hormonal therapy, herbal remedies, as well as, vaginal lubricants and moisturizers during the study period. Participants were instructed to lead a normal life, without controlling other confounding factors that have an effect on the serum vitamin D level, including sun exposure, sunscreen application, and their diet.

2.3. Data Collection and Measurements

Baseline characteristics were collected at the time of enrollment, including age, menopausal age, body mass index (BMI), parity, current medication, smoking history, drinking history, exercise habits, sexual activity, and VAS of VVA symptoms. In addition, a medical history was taken including hypertension, diabetes mellitus, and dyslipidemia. Participants were categorized as sexually active, having sexual intercourse two times or more per month, and those who exercised regularly, aerobic exercises more than 75 min per week. Pelvic examinations were performed to exclude any genital lesion or infection, the VMI and vaginal pH were subsequently collected. The testing for the serum 25(OH) D level was also performed.

The VMI evaluation was obtained from the bilateral upper one-third of the vaginal wall using Ayre's spatula. Samples were smeared onto a glass slide and immediately fixed in 95% alcohol. VMIs were examined by an experienced laboratory technician. The percentage of superficial (S), intermediate (I), and parabasal (P) cells were used to calculate the VMI as $(1 \times S) + (0.5 \times I) + (0 \times P)$. The vaginal pH was obtained from the posterior fornix and was measured with a SIEMENS Multistix® (Siemens Healthcare GmbH, Erlangen, Germany). VAS of VVA symptoms were recorded during an interview about dryness, pain, itching, and dyspareunia symptoms following a 10 points scale (0 = absent, 5 = moderate, 10 = severe). All parameters were collected at baseline, six, and 12 weeks. Serum vitamin D was collected and measured using the chemiluminescent immunoassay (CLIA) technology with a LIAISON® (DiaSorin, Saluggia, Italy) at baseline and 12 weeks.

At the six and 12 weeks of the study, all participants visited their physician and the allocated supplement bottle was returned to the investigator to count the remaining capsules. Good compliance was defined as those who were taking more than 80% of the medicine. All adverse effects were recorded during interviewing for any abnormal symptoms.

2.4. Statistical Analysis

All statistical analysis was performed using STATA version 15.0 (StataCorp LLC, College Station, TX, USA). The intention-to-treat analysis was used as a method for analyzing the results in this prospective randomized controlled trial study. The baseline characteristics were analyzed and the quantitative variables were tested using the Shapiro-Wilk test for their distribution of data.

The data with normal distribution were presented as mean ± standard deviation (SD). The data with non-normal distribution data were presented as the median, (ranges). The Student *t*-test was used to compare the continuous variables in parametric data. The Mann-Whitney U test was used for comparison of continuous variables in non parametric data. For comparison of the VMI, vaginal pH, and VAS of VVA between time points within the group, the paired *t*-test was used. The statistically significant level was p-value < 0.05.

3. Results

Ninety-two postmenopausal women were invited to participate in the study. Twelve women were excluded: Two had an abnormal PAP smear, four had a history of recent vitamin D supplementation, and six were unable to participate in the study. A total of eight participants were included and sixty-eight participants completed the study at the 12th week. There were a total of 12 losses following up at the 12th week, including four in the treatment groups, and eight in the placebo group, as shown in Figure 1.

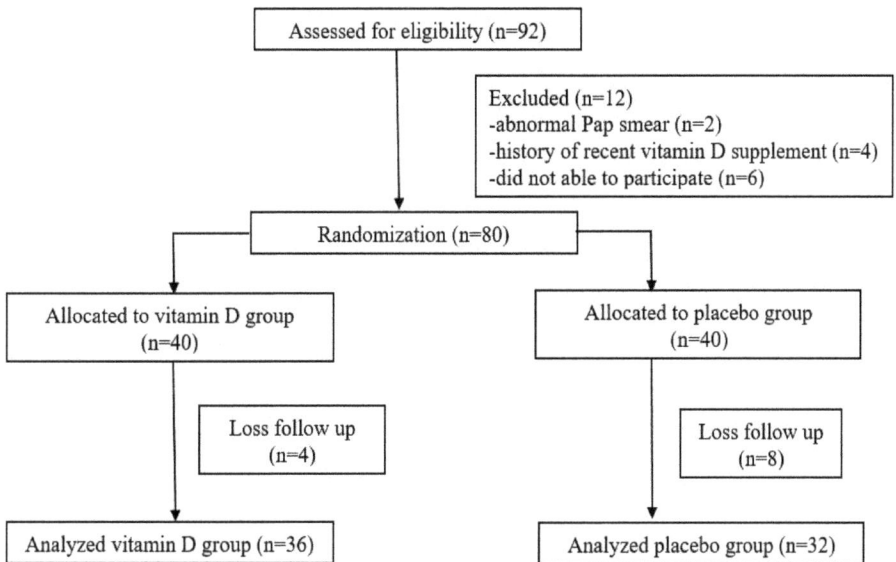

Figure 1. The study flow chart.

All of the sixty-eight participants were of good compliance with taking their assigned tablets. The characteristics of participants in both groups showed a not statistically significant difference including VMI, vaginal pH, and VAS of VVA symptoms, as shown in Table 1. After the 12th week of the study, the mean serum 25(OH) D levels were 39.88 ± 13.48 ng/mL and 22.58 ± 7.03 ng/mL in the vitamin D group and placebo group, respectively. Moreover, there was no report of any adverse outcome in both groups.

Table 1. Baseline characteristics of the participants.

Characteristics	Vitamin D (N = 40)	Placebo (N = 40)
Age (years) [a]	59.95 ± 5.81	58.33 ± 6.25
Age at menopause [a]	48.5 ± 5.35	49.5 ± 4.24
Body mass index (kg/m2) [a]	24.14 ± 3.92	24.63 ± 4.24
Active sexual activity [b]	19 (51.35%)	18 (48.65%)
Nulliparous [b]	7 (17.5%)	9 (22.5%)
Having underlying medical diseases	20 (50%)	26 (65%)
Smoking history [b]	2 (5%)	0 (0%)
Alcohol drinking [b]	2 (5%)	0 (%)
Regular exercise [b]	22 (44%)	28 (56%)
Vaginal maturation index [a]	10.33 ± 19.00	18.56 ± 27.99
Vaginal pH [a]	7.55 ± 1.02	7.51 ± 0.94
VAS of VVA symptoms [a]	7.21 ± 2.20	6.48 ± 2.28
Serum 25(OH)vitamin D level (ng/mL) [a]	24.98 ± 8.25	23.28 ± 7.53

Notes: [a] Data expressed as mean ± standard deviation (SD), [b] data expressed as a percentage. VAS—visual analog scale; VVA—vulvovaginal atrophy.

The comparison of vaginal health outcomes, including VMI, vaginal pH, and VAS of VVA symptoms between vitamin D and control groups at baseline, six, and 12 weeks did not reveal a significant difference, see Table 2 and Figure 2.

Table 2. Comparison of the vaginal health measurement between vitamin D group and placebo group at baseline, six, and 12 weeks.

Vaginal Health Measurement	Vitamin D	Placebo	p-Value
Vaginal Maturation Index			
Baseline	10.33 ± 19.00	18.56 ± 27.99	0.50
Six weeks	15.83 ± 22.81	22.06 ± 28.54	0.44
12 weeks	15.43 ± 24.87	17.36 ± 26.73	0.81
Vaginal pH			
Baseline	7.55 ± 1.02	7.51 ± 0.94	0.86
Six weeks	7.28 ± 0.94	7.31 ± 0.92	0.89
12 weeks	7.39 ± 0.96	7.50 ± 0.8	0.62
VAS of VVA symptoms			
Baseline	7.21 ± 2.20	6.48 ± 2.28	0.15
Six weeks	4.24 ± 2.44	4.06 ± 2.47	0.76
12 weeks	2.94 ± 2.36	2.94 ± 2.47	0.99

Notes: Data expressed as mean ± standard deviation (SD).

However, vitamin D caused a significant difference in the mean difference of VMI between baseline and at six weeks (5.5 ± 16.27, $p < 0.05$). Moreover, vitamin D caused a significant improvement in the mean difference of vaginal pH (−0.24 ± 0.38 and −0.21 ± 0.55, respectively) and for VAS of VVA symptoms (−2.97 ± 2.30 and −4.19 ± 2.66, respectively) both at six and 12 weeks of the study, compared to the baseline, as shown in Table 3.

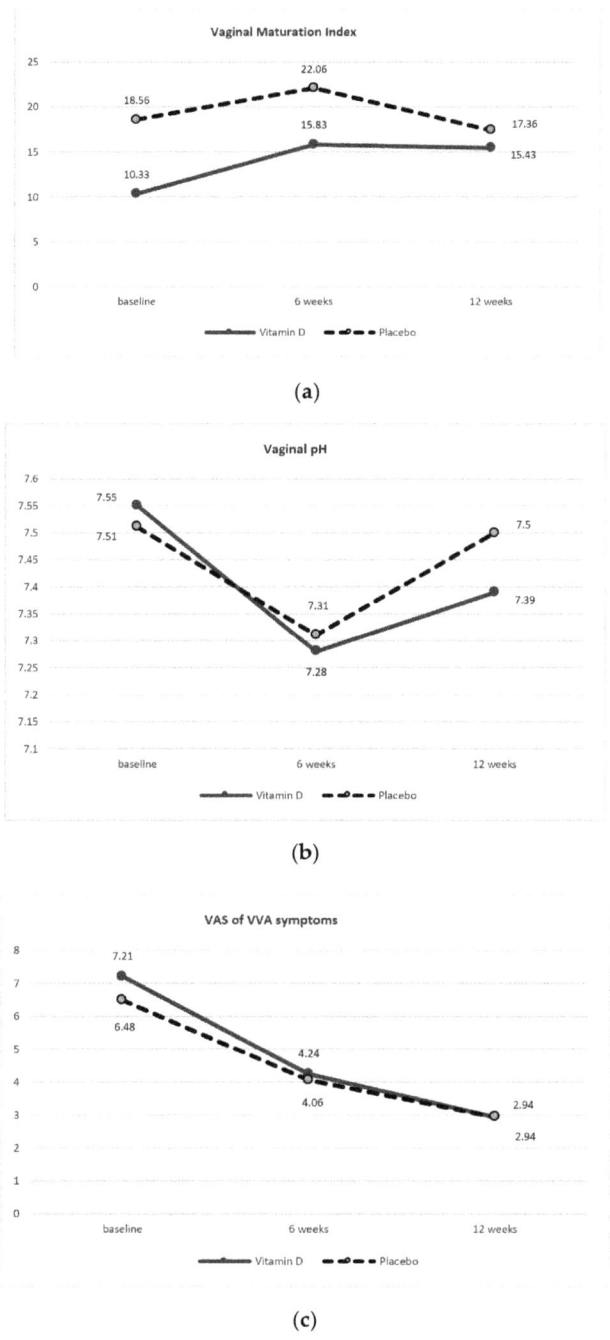

Figure 2. The vaginal health changes between at baseline, six, and 12 weeks with a comparison between the vitamin D group and placebo group: (**a**) Vaginal maturation index (VMI); (**b**) vaginal pH; (**c**) visual analog scale of vulvovaginal atrophy symptoms (VAS of VVA symptoms). VAS—visual analog scale; VVA—vulvovaginal atrophy.

Table 3. Comparison of the mean difference of vaginal health measurement between the vitamin D group and placebo group compared between the baseline and at six weeks and between the baseline and at 12 weeks.

Mean Difference	Vitamin D	p-Value	Placebo	p-Value
Vaginal Maturation Index				
Baseline and at six weeks	5.5 ± 16.27 *	0.04	−3.5 ± 20.42	0.29
Baseline and at 12 weeks	5.1 ± 17.57	0.07	−1.2 ± 16.54	0.65
Vaginal pH				
Baseline and at six weeks	−0.24 ± 0.38 *	<0.05	−0.14 ± 0.54	0.15
Baseline and at 12 weeks	−0.21 ± 0.55 *	0.03	−0.05 ± 0.41	0.52
VAS of VVA symptoms				
Baseline and at six weeks	−2.97 ± 2.30 *	<0.01	−2.47 ± 2.14 *	<0.01
Baseline and at 12 weeks	−4.19 ± 2.66 *	<0.01	−3.59 ± 2.45 *	<0.01

Notes: Data expressed as mean ± standard deviation (SD), * p-value < 0.05.

4. Discussion

Vitamin D supplementation, in the form of ergocalciferol 40,000 IU per week for 12 weeks in postmenopausal women with VVA symptoms did not affect vaginal health in comparison to placebo therapy. However, ergocalciferol supplements potentially improve most of the vaginal health parameters, including VMI, vaginal pH, and VAS of VVA symptoms, represented as a change in the mean difference compared between baseline, six, and 12 weeks. While such changes were rarely seen in the placebo group except for the VAS of the VVA symptoms, which is a personal-based subjective measure. Moreover, our study was not conducted in women with vitamin deficiency, which may limit the effects of supplementation with ergocalciferol. However, the results were relevant to the previous study by Yildirim B. et al. In their analysis, a cross-sectional study of 60 postmenopausal women, in which 30 participants received an oral 1, 25-dihydroxy vitamin D at 0.5 mcg per day, and another 30 postmenopausal women in a controlled group. Following the participants for one-year revealed that subjects in the vitamin D treatment group had a significant increase in the proportion of superficial cells to basal cells and parabasal cells compared to the placebo group [42]. In addition, a study focused on a vitamin D deficient population by Kaur H. et al. reported the effects of oral cholecalciferol. The effect of cholecalciferol supplementation at 60,000 IU weekly for 10 weeks and then 60,000 IU every three months for six months was examined in 100 menopausal female patients aged 65–78 years with vitamin D deficiency and gynecological diseases, including pelvic floor disorders (PFDs) that effected urinary or fecal incontinence, pelvic organ prolapse (POP), and bacterial vaginosis. After the six-month study, the mean score of the vaginal health index (MVHI) for the pelvic floor patients was significantly improved compared to the placebo and healthy groups [43]. Therefore, the effects of oral vitamin D supplementation on improving vaginal health outcomes may depend on the baseline vitamin D status of the patient, the duration of supplementation, dose, and type of vitamin D supplements such as cholecalciferol 60,000 IU per week for 10 weeks or 1, 25-dihydroxy vitamin D 0.5 mcg per day for a year. From our study, ergocalciferol 40,000 IU per week for 12 weeks can improve the mean difference of vaginal health outcomes, but this effect was not statistically significantly different from the placebo. For the modality of treatment, there are a few reports of vaginal vitamin D administration. Local effects of vitamin D on vaginal health as a report by Rad P. et al. from a double-blind study using the vitamin D vaginal suppository at 1000 IU daily for eight weeks on vaginal atrophy in 40 postmenopausal women. A statistically significant improvement was reported in vaginal health, including VMI, vaginal pH, and dryness symptoms in the treatment group compared to the placebo group [31]. A similar analysis by Keshavarzi Z. et al. reported the beneficial effect of an eight week treatment with vaginal suppositories containing 1000 IU of vitamin D plus 1 mg of vitamin E in improving vaginal atrophy among women with breast cancer receiving tamoxifen [44]. Moreover, the latest narrative systematic review of the effect of vitamin D on vaginal health of menopausal women included six trials with a total of 391 participants, in which two studies were individually randomized controlled trials (RCTs) and four were quasi-randomized. The systematic review indicated that vitamin D alone, in the high doses tested or vaginal use format, appeared to have an effect on vaginal epithelial cells especially superficial cells and promoting a decreased in vaginal pH. The duration of vitamin D use of eight to 10 weeks is sufficient for improvement of vaginal health except for vaginal dryness [45].

One limitation of this analysis is that not all study participants are vitamin D deficient. As a result, changes in vaginal health may not be as apparent comparing the placebo and the vitamin D treatment group. Future research to the optimized dosage, route of treatment, form, and duration of vitamin D treatment has the promise to improve the health effects in postmenopausal women with VVA or genitourinary syndrome of menopause, especially in patients with contraindications for hormonal treatment and vitamin D deficiency.

5. Conclusions

Oral vitamin D supplementation, in the form of oral ergocalciferol at 40,000 IU per week for 12 weeks, did not promote a significant difference from the placebo to improve the vaginal health outcomes, including VMI, vaginal pH, and VAS of VVA symptoms in postmenopausal patients with vulvovaginal atrophy. However, vitamin D supplements seemed to improve VMI and vaginal pH both at six and 12 weeks when compared to baseline.

Author Contributions: T.K., J.M., S.A.-O.V. and O.V. conceived the hypothesis. T.K. and O.V. conducted the data collection process and prepared the first draft of the manuscript. S.A.-O.V. and A.S. conducted the statistical analyses and provided insights of its clinical significance. T.K., J.M., S.A.-O.V., A.S., and especially O.V. contributed to the final version of the manuscript. All authors have read and agreed to the published version of the manuscript.

Funding: This research received no external funding.

Conflicts of Interest: The authors declare no conflict of interest.

References

1. Portman, D.J.; Gass, M.L. Vulvovaginal Atrophy Terminology Consensus Conference Panel. Genitourinary syndrome of menopause: New terminology for vulvovaginal atrophy from the International Society for the Study of Women's Sexual Health and the North American Menopause Society. *Menopause* **2014**, *21*, 1063–1068. [CrossRef] [PubMed]
2. Gandhi, J.; Chen, A.; Dagur, G.; Suh, Y.; Smith, N.; Cali, B.; Khan, S.A. Genitourinary syndrome of menopause: An overview of clinical manifestations, pathophysiology, etiology, evaluation, and management. *AJOG* **2016**, *215*, 704–711. [CrossRef] [PubMed]
3. Kim, H.K.; Kang, S.Y.; Chung, Y.J.; Kim, J.H.; Kim, M.R. The Recent Review of the Genitourinary Syndrome of Menopause. *J. Menopausal Med.* **2015**, *21*, 65–71. [CrossRef] [PubMed]
4. Brotman, R.M.; Shardell, M.D.; Gajer, P.; Fadrosh, D.; Chang, K.; Silver, M.I.; Viscidi, R.P.; Burke, A.E.; Ravel, J.; Gravitt, P.E. Association between the vaginal microbiota, menopause status, and signs of vulvovaginal atrophy. *Menopause* **2018**, *25*, 1321–1330. [CrossRef]
5. The North American Menopause Society. Management of symptomatic vulvovaginal atrophy: 2013 position statement of The North American Menopause Society. *Menopause* **2013**, *20*, 888–902. [CrossRef] [PubMed]
6. Panay, N. Genitourinary syndrome of the menopause–dawn of a new era? *Climacteric* **2015**, *18*, 13–17. [CrossRef]
7. Mitchell, C.M.; Waetjen, L.E. Genitourinary Changes with Aging. *Obstet. Gynecol. Clin. N. Am.* **2018**, *45*, 737–750. [CrossRef]
8. Nappi, R.E.; Palacios, S.; Bruyniks, N.; Particco, M.; Panay, N. EVES Study investigators. The burden of vulvovaginal atrophy on women's daily living: Implications on quality of life from a face-to-face real-life survey. *Menopause* **2019**, *26*, 485–491. [CrossRef]
9. Islam, R.M.; Bell, R.J.; Davis, S.R. Prevalence of sexual symptoms in relation to menopause in women in Asia: A systematic review. *Menopause* **2018**, *25*, 231–238. [CrossRef]

10. Moyneur, E.; Dea, K.; Derogatis, L.R.; Vekeman, F.; Dury, A.Y.; Labrie, F. Prevalence of depression and anxiety in women newly diagnosed with vulvovaginal atrophy and dyspareunia. *Menopause* **2020**, *27*, 134–142. [CrossRef]
11. Archer, D.F.; Simon, J.A.; Portman, D.J.; Goldstein, S.R.; Goldstein, I. Ospemifene for the treatment of menopausal vaginal dryness, a symptom of the genitourinary syndrome of menopause. *Exp. Rev. Endocrinol. Metab.* **2019**, *14*, 301–314. [CrossRef] [PubMed]
12. Barton, D.L.; Shuster, L.T.; Dockter, T.; Atherton, P.J.; Thielen, J.; Birrell, S.N.; Sood, R.; Griffin, P.; Terstriep, S.A.; Mattar, B.; et al. Systemic and local effects of vaginal dehydroepiandrosterone (DHEA): NCCTG N10C1 (Alliance). *Support Care Cancer* **2018**, *26*, 1335–1343. [CrossRef]
13. Writing Group for the Women's Health Initiative Investigators. Risks and Benefits of Estrogen Plus Progestin in Healthy Postmenopausal Women: Principal Results From the Women's Health Initiative Randomized Controlled Trial. *JAMA* **2002**, *288*, 321–333. [CrossRef] [PubMed]
14. Clarke, C.A.; Glaser, S.L.; Uratsu, C.S.; Selby, J.V.; Kushi, L.H.; Herrinton, L.J. Recent declines in hormone therapy utilization and breast cancer incidence: Clinical and population-based evidence. *J. Clin. Oncol.* **2006**, *24*, e49–e50. [CrossRef]
15. Lev-Sagie, A. Vulvar and Vaginal Atrophy: Physiology, Clinical Presentation, and Treatment Considerations. *Clin. Obstet. Gynecol.* **2015**, *58*, 476–491. [CrossRef]
16. Jaisamrarn, U.; Triratanachat, S.; Chaikittisilpa, S.; Grob, P.; Prasauskas, V.; Taechakraichana, N. Ultra-low-dose estriol and lactobacilli in the local treatment of postmenopausal vaginal atrophy. *Climacteric* **2013**, *16*, 347–355. [CrossRef]
17. Faubion, S.S.; Larkin, L.C.; Stuenkel, C.A.; Bachmann, G.A.; Chism, L.A.; Kagan, R.; Kaunitz, A.M.; Krychman, M.L.; Parish, S.J.; Partridge, A.H.; et al. Management of genitourinary syndrome of menopause in women with or at high risk for breast cancer: Consensus recommendations from The North American Menopause Society and The International Society for the Study of Women's Sexual Health. *Menopause* **2018**, *25*, 596–608. [CrossRef] [PubMed]
18. Pitsouni, E.; Grigoriadis, T.; Falagas, M.E.; Salvatore, S.; Athanasiou, S. Laser therapy for the genitourinary syndrome of menopause. A systematic review and meta-analysis. *Maturitas* **2017**, *103*, 78–88. [CrossRef]
19. Lima, S.M.; Yamada, S.S.; Reis, B.F.; Postigo, S.; Galvao da Silva, M.A.; Aoki, T. Effective treatment of vaginal atrophy with isoflavone vaginal gel. *Maturitas* **2013**, *74*, 252–258. [CrossRef]
20. Edwards, D.; Panay, N. Treating vulvovaginal atrophy/genitourinary syndrome of menopause: How important is vaginal lubricant and moisturizer composition? *Climacteric* **2016**, *19*, 151–161. [CrossRef]
21. Archer, D.F. Dehydroepiandrosterone intra vaginal administration for the management of postmenopausal vulvovaginal atrophy. *J. Steroid Biochem. Mol. Biol.* **2015**, *145*, 139–143. [CrossRef]
22. Al-Saqi, S.H.; Uvnas-Moberg, K.; Jonasson, A.F. Intravaginally applied oxytocin improves post-menopausal vaginal atrophy. *Post Reprod. Health* **2015**, *21*, 88–97. [CrossRef] [PubMed]
23. Holick, M.F.; Binkley, N.C.; Bischoff-Ferrari, H.A.; Gordon, C.M.; Hanley, D.A.; Heaney, R.P.; Murad, M.H.; Weaver, C.M. Evaluation, treatment, and prevention of vitamin D deficiency: An Endocrine Society clinical practice guideline. *J. Clin. Endocrinol. Metab.* **2011**, *96*, 1911–1930. [CrossRef] [PubMed]
24. Priemel, M.; von Domarus, C.; Klatte, T.O.; Kessler, S.; Schlie, J.; Meier, S.; Proksch, N.; Pastor, F.; Netter, C.; Streichert, T.; et al. Bone mineralization defects and vitamin D deficiency: Histomorphometric analysis of iliac crest bone biopsies and circulating 25-hydroxyvitamin D in 675 patients. *J. Bone Miner. Res.* **2010**, *25*, 305–312. [CrossRef] [PubMed]
25. Staud, R. Vitamin D: More than just affecting calcium and bone. *Curr. Rheumatol. Rep.* **2005**, *7*, 356–364. [CrossRef] [PubMed]
26. Wacker, M.; Holick, M.F. Vitamin D—Effects on skeletal and extraskeletal health and the need for supplementation. *Nutrients* **2013**, *5*, 111–148. [CrossRef]
27. Hossein-nezhad, A.; Holick, M.F. Vitamin D for health: A global perspective. *Mayo Clin. Proc.* **2013**, *88*, 720–755. [CrossRef] [PubMed]
28. Thacher, T.D.; Clarke, B.L. Vitamin D insufficiency. *Mayo Clin. Proc.* **2011**, *86*, 50–60. [CrossRef]
29. Skowrońska, P.; Pastuszek, E.; Kuczyński, W.; Jaszczoł, M.; Kuć, P.; Jakiel, G.; Wocławek-Potocka, I.; Łukaszuk, K. The role of vitamin D in reproductive dysfunction in women—A systematic review. *Ann. Agric. Environ. Med.* **2016**, *23*, 671–676. [CrossRef] [PubMed]

30. Lorenzen, M.; Boisen, I.M.; Mortensen, L.J.; Lanske, B.; Juul, A.; Blomberg Jensen, M. Reproductive endocrinology of vitamin D. *Mol. Cell Endocrinol.* **2017**, *453*, 103–112. [CrossRef]
31. Rad, P.; Tadayon, M.; Abbaspour, M.; Latifi, S.M.; Rashidi, I.; Delaviz, H. The effect of vitamin D on vaginal atrophy in postmenopausal women. *Iran J. Nurs. Midwifery Res.* **2015**, *20*, 211–215. [PubMed]
32. Lee, A.; Lee, M.R.; Lee, H.H.; Kim, Y.S.; Kim, J.M.; Enkhbold, T.; Kim, T.H. Vitamin D Proliferates Vaginal Epithelium through RhoA Expression in Postmenopausal Atrophic Vagina tissue. *Mol. Cells* **2017**, *40*, 677–684. [PubMed]
33. Holick, M.F. Vitamin D deficiency. *N. Engl. J. Med.* **2007**, *357*, 266–281. [CrossRef]
34. Moan, J.; Dahlback, A.; Porojnicu, A.C. At what time should one go out in the sun? *Adv. Exp. Med. Biol.* **2008**, *624*, 86–88.
35. Holick, M.F. The vitamin D deficiency pandemic: Approaches for diagnosis, treatment and prevention. *Rev. Endocr. Metab. Disord.* **2017**, *18*, 153–165. [CrossRef] [PubMed]
36. Wacker, M.; Holick, M.F. Sunlight and vitamin D: A global perspective for health. *Dermato-Endocrinol.* **2013**, *5*, 51–108. [CrossRef]
37. Roth, D.E.; Abrams, S.A.; Aloia, J.; Bergeron, G.; Bourassa, M.W.; Brown, K.H.; Calvo, M.S.; Cashman, K.D.; Combs, G.; De-Regil, L.M.; et al. Global prevalence and disease burden of vitamin D deficiency: A roadmap for action in low- and middle-income countries. *Ann. N. Y. Acad. Sci.* **2018**, *1430*, 44–79. [CrossRef]
38. Daly, R.M.; Gagnon, C.; Lu, Z.X.; Magliano, D.J.; Dunstan, D.W.; Sikaris, K.A.; Zimmet, P.Z.; Ebeling, P.R.; Shaw, J.E. Prevalence of vitamin D deficiency and its determinants in Australian adults age 25 years and older: A national, population-based study. *Clin. Endocrinol.* **2012**, *77*, 26–35. [CrossRef]
39. Man, R.E.; Li, L.J.; Cheng, C.Y.; Wong, T.Y.; Lamoureux, E.; Sabanayagam, C. Prevalence and Determinants of Suboptimal Vitamin D Levels in a Multiethnic Asian Population. *Nutrients* **2017**, *9*, 313. [CrossRef]
40. Siwamogsatham, O.; Ongphiphadhanakul, B.; Tangpricha, V. Vitamin D deficiency in Thailand. *J. Clin. Transl. Endocrinol.* **2014**, *2*, 48–49. [CrossRef]
41. Bernard, R. *Fundamental of Biostatistics*, 5th ed.; Thomson Learning: Duxberry, South Africa, 2000.
42. Yildirim, B.; Kaleli, B.; Duzcan, E.; Topuz, O. The effects of postmenopausal Vitamin D treatment on vaginal atrophy. *Maturitas* **2004**, *49*, 334–337. [CrossRef] [PubMed]
43. Kaur, H.; Bala, R.; Nagpal, M. Role of Vitamin D in urogenital health of geriatric participants. *J. Mid-Life Health* **2017**, *8*, 28–35.
44. Keshavarzi, Z.; Janghorban, R.; Alipour, S.; Tahmasebi, S.; Jokar, A. The effect of vitamin D and E vaginal suppositories on tamoxifen-induced vaginal atrophy in women with breast cancer. *Support Care Cancer* **2019**, *27*, 1325–1334. [CrossRef] [PubMed]
45. Riazi, H.; Ghazanfarpour, M.; Taebi, M.; Abdolahian, S. Effect of Vitamin D on the Vaginal Health of Menopausal Women: A Systematic Review. *J. Menopausal Med.* **2019**, *25*, 109–116. [CrossRef]

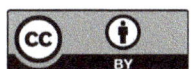

© 2020 by the authors. Licensee MDPI, Basel, Switzerland. This article is an open access article distributed under the terms and conditions of the Creative Commons Attribution (CC BY) license (http://creativecommons.org/licenses/by/4.0/).

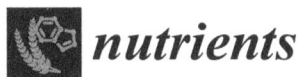

Article

The Association between 25-Hydroxyvitamin D Concentration and Disability Trajectories in Very Old Adults: The Newcastle 85+ Study

Sarah Hakeem [1,2,3], Nuno Mendonca [1,2,4,5], Terry Aspray [6,7], Andrew Kingston [1], Carmen Ruiz-Martin [8], Carol Jagger [1], John C. Mathers [1,2], Rachel Duncan [7] and Tom R. Hill [1,2,*]

1. Population Health Sciences Institute, Faculty of Medical Sciences, Newcastle University, Newcastle upon Tyne NE2 4HH, UK; S.H.M.Hakeem2@ncl.ac.uk (S.H.); nuno.mendonca@nms.unl.pt (N.M.); andrew.kingston@ncl.ac.uk (A.K.); carol.jagger@ncl.ac.uk (C.J.); john.mathers@ncl.ac.uk (J.C.M.)
2. Human Nutrition Research Centre, Faculty of Medical Sciences, Newcastle University, Newcastle upon Tyne NE2 4HH, UK
3. College of Nursing, Umm Al-Quraa University, Makkah 715, Saudi Arabia
4. EpiDoC Unit, NOVA Medical School, Universidade Nova de Lisboa (NMS-UNL), 1150-082 Lisbon, Portugal
5. Comprehensive Health Research Centre (CHRC), NOVA Medical School, Universidade Nova de Lisboa, 1150-082 Lisbon, Portugal
6. Translational and Clinical Research Institute, Faculty of Medical Sciences, Newcastle University, Newcastle upon Tyne NE2 4HH, UK; Terry.Aspray@ncl.ac.uk
7. Freeman Hospital, NHS, Newcastle upon Tyne NE7 7DN, UK; rachel.duncan2@nhs.net
8. Bioscreening Core Facility, Faculty of Medical Sciences, Newcastle University, Newcastle upon Tyne NE4 5 PL, UK; carmen.martin-ruiz@ncl.ac.uk
* Correspondence: tom.hill@ncl.ac.uk

Received: 31 July 2020; Accepted: 7 September 2020; Published: 9 September 2020

Abstract: *Background*: Low vitamin D status is common in very old adults which may have adverse consequences for muscle function, a major predictor of disability. *Aims*: To explore the association between 25-hydroxyvitamin D [25(OH)D] concentrations and disability trajectories in very old adults and to determine whether there is an 'adequate' 25(OH)D concentration which might protect against a faster disability trajectory. *Methodology*: A total of 775 participants from the Newcastle 85+ Study for who 25(OH)D concentration at baseline was available. Serum 25(OH)D concentrations of <25 nmol/L, 25–50 nmol/L and >50 nmol/L were used as cut-offs to define low, moderate and high vitamin D status, respectively. Disability was defined as difficulty in performing 17 activities of daily living, at baseline, after 18, 36 and 60 months. *Results*: A three-trajectory model was derived (low-to-mild, mild-to-moderate and moderate-to-severe). In partially adjusted models, participants with 25(OH)D concentrations <25 nmol/L were more likely to have moderate and severe disability trajectories, even after adjusting for sex, living in an institution, season, cognitive status, BMI and vitamin D supplement use. However, this association disappeared after further adjustment for physical activity. *Conclusions*: Vitamin D status does not appear to influence the trajectories of disability in very old adults.

Keywords: vitamin D status; disability; very old adults

1. Introduction

Life expectancy is increasing worldwide. By 2050, it is predicted that there will be 379 million people aged 80 and above, and almost 10% of the population of developed countries will be aged ≥ 80 (OECD, 2013). Disability is defined as experiencing difficulty in performing activities that are essential for independent living. Such activities comprise the basic activities of daily living (BADL), such as getting up and washing hands, and the instrumental activities of daily living (IADL), such as shopping for groceries and doing housework [1]. The frequency of ADL disability is higher among very old adults (those aged 80 and older) [2]. Difficulty with performing ADL is a predictor of longer hospital stays and of additional general practice (GP) visits [3]. Furthermore, disability increases the risk of mortality 2–3 fold among very old adults [4]. Generally, disability raises the amount of benefits paid for assistance programs and care facilities in developed countries; for example, it increases the cost of care by 22% in the United Kingdom alone [5].

Very old adults are more likely to have lower circulating concentrations of 25-hydroxyvitamin D [25(OH)D]. This is due to many reasons, including decreased production of vitamin D by skin, low exposure to sunlight, and low vitamin D intake as well as catabolism factors such as medication and disease [6]. Following hydroxylation of 25(OH)D in the kidney, 1,25(OH)D binds to its nuclear receptor (VDR) which is expressed in multiple tissues, including muscle. It then influences protein synthesis in the muscle, muscle calcium uptake and type 2 muscle's fibre size and number [7]. Low concentrations of 25(OH)D are associated with poor muscle strength [8]. After controlling for potential confounders, 25(OH)D deficiency prevalence rates were 31 and 43% higher among men and women with muscle weakness than those with normal strength, respectively [9]. Two potential mechanisms have been suggested to explain the association between 25(OH)D and muscle function. First, age-related reduction of 1,25(OH)D reduces the stimulation of VDR expression by muscle. Second, the decline of VDR expression upon aging leads to impaired muscle response to 1,25(OH)D [10].

Maintaining adequate concentrations of 25(OH)D may protect against disability in terms of both musculoskeletal and cognitive function; the few studies that have assessed this association have found inverse associations between 25(OH)D concentration and risk of disability [8,11–13]. However, these studies have several limitations including: use of different definitions of low 25(OH)D concentration; being cross-sectional rather than longitudinal; recruited those aged 65 and over with few studies of the very old; being unrepresentative because they recruited women only [8,13], targeted at a specific ethnic group [12] or involved patients with a specific disease [11]. Consequently there is a need for longitudinal studies of associations between 25(OH)D concentration and disability trajectory and which focus on very-old adults, including those living in institutions.

We have previously reported vitamin D status in participants from the Newcastle 85+ study and found that 33% of the participants had vitamin D concentration < 30 nmol/L [14]. Therefore, this study aims to explore the association between 25(OH)D concentration and disability trajectory over five years in the Newcastle 85+ study participants. It also aims to investigate whether there is a threshold concentration of 25(OH)D above which the disability trajectory among the very old adults is slowed. In line with our previous work on vitamin D status and cognitive decline [15] and all-cause mortality [16] which showed that both lower and higher vitamin D status was associated with adverse biological outcomes, in the current analysis we hypothesized that lower and higher 25(OH)D concentrations are associated with a faster disability trajectory in very old adults.

2. Materials and Methods

2.1. Study Population and Design (The Newcastle 85+ Study)

The participants were from the Newcastle 85+ Study, which is socio-demographically representative study of the general UK population. It included both population-based and institutionalised older adults born in 1921 (age 85 years at recruitment) and living in Newcastle-upon-Tyne and North Tyneside (northeast England). All those who met these inclusion criteria were invited to participate (n = 1459). Only those individuals with end-stage terminal illness (n = 11) were excluded. The recruitment and baseline assessment took place over a 17-month period in 2006–2007. The follow-up phases took place at 18 (Phase 2), 36 (Phase 3) and 60 months (Phase 4) from baseline [17]. A health assessment, comprising questionnaires, measurements, function tests and a fasting blood sample, was carried out in the participants' usual place of residence. In addition, general practice medical records were reviewed to extract data on diagnosed diseases and prescribed medication. Both the health assessment and data extraction were conducted by trained research nurses following a standard protocol. In the UK, patients are registered with a single general practice that acts as a gatekeeper to secondary care and receives details of all hospital admissions and outpatient attendance. The review of the general practice records included hospital correspondence to ensure that all recorded disease diagnoses were extracted, irrespective of where and when the diagnosis was made. Our analysis included all Newcastle 85+ Study participants ($n = 775$) for which data on health assessment, general practice records and serum 25(OH)D concentration were available at baseline (Supplemental Figure S1). From these initial group, data on health assessment and general practice records were available for 631, 484 and 344 participants at phases 2, 3, and 4, respectively.

2.2. Ethical Approval

The research complied with the requirements of the Declaration of Helsinki. Ethical approval was obtained from the Newcastle and North Tyneside 1 Research Ethics Committee (reference number 06/Q0905/2). Written informed consent was obtained from the participants. Where individuals lacked the capacity to give consent, for example because of cognitive impairment, a formal written opinion was sought from a relative or carer. Participants could decline to take part in any element of the study protocol.

2.3. Measurement of Serum 25(OH)D Concentration

Serum 25(OH)D concentration was measured at baseline from blood samples collected between June 2006 and August 2007. After an overnight fast, 40 mL blood was drawn from the antecubital vein between 7:00 and 10:30 a.m. Ninety-five per-cent of the samples were received for processing within 1 h of venepuncture. The total 25(OH)D concentration was determined by the DiaSorin radioimmunoassay (RIA) kit (DiaSorin Corporation, Stillwater, MN, USA) according to the manufacturer's recommendations, using 25(OH)D-specific antibodies and 125I-labelled 25(OH)D (DiaSorin Corporation) as a tracer. The minimum detectable concentration of 25(OH)D was 5 nmol/L, and the inter-assay coefficients of variation ranged from 8.4% to 12.6% [18].

2.4. Disability Measures and Scores

At baseline and at each follow-up assessment, participants were asked about their ability to perform 17 activities comprising the basic and instrumental activities of daily living (BADLs and IADLs) and mobility items (Supplemental Table S1); these activities were taken predominantly from the Groningen Activity Restriction Scale [19]. The ability to perform the ADLs was self-reported by the participants. Each question was framed as 'can you' rather than 'do you', to assess the participants' maximum capability to perform the activities, accounting for situational responses. Each item reported as performed without difficulty scored 0 and each item performed with difficulty scored 1 (for a maximum score of 17). A disability score was calculated based on the total number of ADLs performed with difficulty or requiring an aid/appliance or personal help [17]. Participants were classified as having a disability if they had difficulty with at least one item.

2.5. Other Measures/Confounders

In addition, the following variables, which are known to influence 25(OH)D concentration, were taken into account in the analysis: demographic factors [sex, living arrangements, housing type, years of full-time education], anthropometry [weight, body composition, fat-free mass, BMI] health and morbidity [disease count, cognitive status via SMMSE] and lifestyle factors [smoking, alcohol consumption, physical activity]; details on these have previously been published [20] as well as information on use of supplements containing vitamin D (yes/no) obtained from the interviewer-administered questionnaire and prescribed vitamin D medication from the GP records [14].

However, apart from the vitamin D-containing supplements, no other supplements (including calcium, magnesium or B-vitamins) were included in the analysis owing to the very modest differences to micronutrient intakes when including supplements [21], and the inherent limitations in supplement frequency data. The date on which the blood sample was drawn was recorded and used to derive the season of collection defined as spring (March–May), summer (June–August), autumn (September–November) and winter (December–February).

2.6. Statistical Analysis

Normality was assessed using the Shapiro-Wilk test and confirmed using Q-Q plots and histograms. Summary statistics of normally distributed continuous values are presented as means and standard deviations (SD), and non-Gaussian distributed variables as medians and interquartile ranges (IQR). Categorical data are presented as percentages (with corresponding sample sizes).

Group-based trajectory models (GBTM) were used to derive distinct clusters of participants' disability trajectories from baseline over the subsequent 60 months. Bayesian information criteria (BIC) were used to assess the best number of trajectories within the model. The model was then further assessed by the posterior probability of group membership >75%. Differences between disability trajectory groups were tested using the Kruskal-Wallis test for ordered non-normally distributed continuous variables (weight, BMI, fat-free mass, serum 25(OH)D, chronic disease count) and χ^2 test for categorical variables (sex, physical activity, alcohol drinker, smoker, 25(OH)D, impaired cognitive status, living in an institution).

Multinomial regression was used to determine the association between disability and 25(OH)D concentration in both cross-sectional and longitudinal analysis. The concentration of 25(OH)D was not normally distributed, therefore, non-parametric analysis was used. The following cut-offs were used in the analysis: <25 nmol/L (low), 25 to 50 nmol/L (moderate) and >50 nmol/L (high) [22]. Important confounders were selected based on their clinical and theoretical relevance as well as univariate analysis with the disability trajectory. These confounders were then fitted, removed and refitted until the best possible but parsimonious model was achieved while checking for model fit statistics throughout, using 10% of change-in-estimate. The multi-collinearity between the confounders was assessed using VIF. Model 1 was an unadjusted model. Model 2 was adjusted for sex, living in an institution and season of blood collection. Model 3 was adjusted further for cognitive status, BMI and vitamin D containing medication. Model 4 was adjusted further for physical activity. The models were stratified by sex. Statistical significance was set at $p < 0.05$. All analyses were performed using IBM SPSS Statistics software version 24 (IBM, Armonk, NY, USA) except for the disability trajectory that was derived using STATA v15.0 (package traj).

2.7. Sensitivity Analysis

To investigate the effects of grip strength, FFM (fat-free mass) and disease count, the models were further adjusted for each of these variables. Models were rerun, excluding those participants with evidence of cognitive impairment (SMMSE score < 26). The models were also stratified by season of blood collection using the same categories as [14].

3. Results

3.1. 25(OH)D Concentration and Disability at Baseline

A cross-sectional analysis of the association between 25(OH)D cut-offs and disability baseline data reveals a U-shaped association between 25(OH)D and disability. A significant association was found between 25(OH)D concentration and disability score at baseline, ($p = < 0.001$) and ($p = 0.002$) for low (<25 nmol/L) and high (>50 nmol/L) concentrations, respectively.

3.2. Disability Trajectories

The disability trajectories (DT; one linear (low to mild trajectory) and two quadratic (mild to moderate and moderate to severe trajectories)) from age 85 to 90 years were best presented by a triple-group model. The trajectories are plotted in Figure 1 and the characteristics of the participants with each of these trajectories are described in Table 1. DT1 represents a low-to-mild disability trajectory (group size: n = 249–33.4%), DT2 represents a mild-to-moderate disability trajectory (group size: n = 351–44%) and DT3 represents a moderate-to-severe disability trajectory (group size: n = 175–22.5%). The participants with a low-to-mild disability trajectory had a slightly increased disability trajectory over five years, while the participants with a mild-to-moderate or moderate-to-severe disability trajectory showed serious trajectories with advancing age, with the score (number of activities that the participants were unable to undertake, unaided) increasing from four to 9.5 and from 11 to 15, respectively.

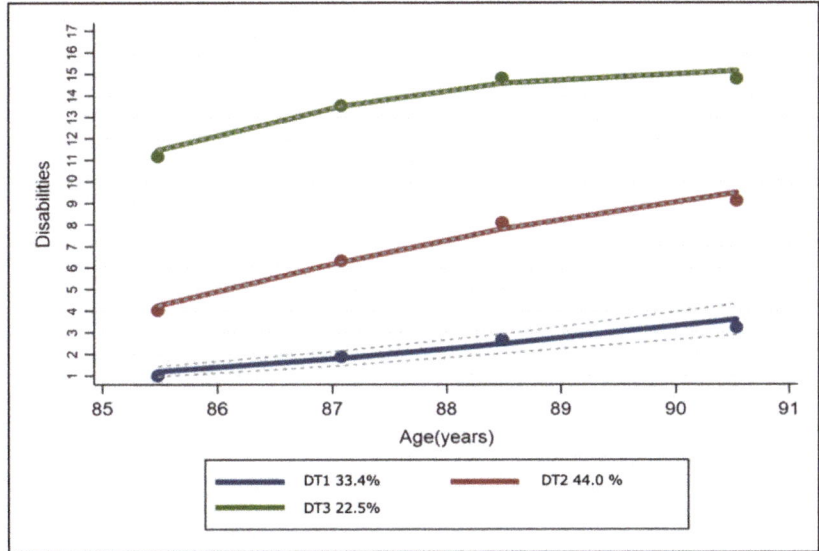

Figure 1. Disability trajectories with 95% confidence intervals in participants who had a serum 25(OH)D measurement available. DT1: Low to mild disability trajectory; DT2: Mild to moderate disability trajectory; DT3: Moderate to severe disability trajectory. Percentages represent group size. Disabilities resulted from calculating ADLs, IADLs and mobility. The grey dotted lines represent the 95% confidence intervals of the disability trajectories. ADL: activities of daily living, IADL: instrumental activities of daily living.

3.3. The Differences in Socioeconomic, Lifestyle and Health Factors between Disability Trajectories

Body weight, total number of years in education, fat-free mass and smoking did not differ significantly between participants in each of the three disability trajectories in. The participants in the three groups showed significant differences regarding their BMI, physical activity level, alcohol intake, vitamin D containing medication use, number of chronic diseases, cognitive status and living in an institution. However, the moderate-to-severe DT group was characterised by a higher percentage of women, a lower proportion of alcohol drinkers, living in an institution, being less physically active, having a higher number of chronic diseases and being cognitively impaired (Table 1). Although there were no significant differences in median serum 25(OH)D concentration between DT groups, the distribution of participants across the three categories of vitamin D adequacy based on 25(OH)D concentration (low, moderate and high) differed significantly across these three trajectories (Table 1).

Table 1. Participant characteristics by the three disability trajectories identified at baseline.

	Low-to-Mild (n = 249)	Mild-to-Moderate (n = 351)	Moderate-to-Severe (n = 175)	p
Women % (n)	48.4 (121)	56.6 (231)	69.3 (122)	<0.001
Weight (kg) mean (SD)	63.9 (11.8)	63.5 (13.4)	63.9 (14.3)	0.732
BMI mean (SD)	23.8 (3.8)	24.7 (4.4)	24.9 (5.2)	0.029
Fat-free mass (kg) mean (SD)	46.5 (9.2)	44.4 (9.1)	45 (8.9)	0.151
Total number of years in education % (n)				
0–9 years	61.9 (153)	62.1 (213)	70.3 (111)	0.241
10–11 years	23.9 (59)	24.2 (83)	22.2 (35)	
12–20 years	14.2 (35)	13.7 (47)	7.6 (12)	
Physical activity % (n)				
Low	2.4 (6)	27.3 (68)	70.3 (175)	<0.001
Moderate	15.8 (55)	58.7 (205)	25.5 (89)	
High	63.2 (110)	33.9 (59)	2.9 (5)	
Alcohol drinkers % (n)	80 (156)	72.4 (168)	55.3 (52)	<0.001
Smoking % (n)	3.6 (9)	8 (28)	4.5 (8)	0.124
Vitamin D containing medication % (n)	10 (25)	13.4 (47)	31.8 (56)	<0.001
Supplement users % (n)	23.3 (58)	20.8 (73)	12 (21)	0.012
Serum 25(OH)D nmol/L median (IQR)	42 (29–59)	36 (23–58)	39 (21–70)	0.178
25(OH)D				
<25 nmol/L (low) % (n)	26.4 (66)	36 (90)	37.6 (94)	0.02
25–50 nmol/L (moderate) % (n)	34.7 (122)	31.8 (112)	33.5 (118)	
>50 nmol/L (high) % (n)	38.1 (67)	19.9 (35)	42 (74)	
Chronic disease count mean (SD)	4.1 (1.5)	4.93 (1.75)	5.6 (1.9)	<0.001
Impaired cognitive status % (n)	12 (30)	23.3 (82)	57.5 (100)	<0.001
Living in institution % (n)	0.4 (1)	3.4 (12)	30.7 (54)	<0.001

BMI: body mass index. SD: standard deviations. IQR: medians and interquartile ranges. p, p-value: Kruskal-Wallis test for continuous non-normally distributed variables or χ2 test for categorical variables 25(OH)D: <25 nmol/L (low), 25–50 nmol/L (moderate), >50 nmol/L (high).

3.4. 25(OH)D Concentration and Disability Trajectory

The results of the analysis show that participants with low concentrations of 25(OH)D (<25 nmol/L) were more likely to have a mild-to-moderate disability trajectory (OR = 2.01, 95% CI = 1.29–3.14, p = 0.002) or a moderate-to-severe disability trajectory (OR = 3.39, 95% CI = 1.99–5.76, p = 0.001) than a low-to-mild disability trajectory compared to those with higher 25(OH)D concentrations in the unadjusted model, after adjusting for sex, living in an institution and season (OR = 2.01, 95% CI = 1.27–3.19, p = 0.003) and (OR = 3.02, 95% CI = 1.70–5.38, p = 0.001) and after further adjustment for cognitive status, BMI and vitamin D containing medication (OR = 1.97, 95% CI = 1.22–3.17, p = 0.005) and (OR = 3.12, 95% CI = 1.67–5.85, p = 0.001), respectively. However, this association disappeared after adjustment for physical activity (Table 2). The results also show that participants with high 25(OH)D concentrations were more likely to have a moderate-to-severe disability trajectory compared to those with moderate concentrations over five years but only in the unadjusted model (OR = 1.94, 95% CI = 1.23–3.06, p = 0.004). However, in the adjusted models, no association was found between high concentration of 25(OH)D and disability trajectory.

Table 2. Association between 25(OH)D concentration and disability trajectories.

Trajectories	25(OH)D	Model 1 OR	Model 1 95% CI	p	Model 2 OR	Model 2 95% CI	p	Model 3 OR	Model 3 95% CI	p	Model 4 OR	Model 4 95% CI	p
DT1: Low-to-mild	<25 nmol/L		(ref)			(ref)			(ref)			(ref)	
	25–50 nmol/L	2.01	1.29–3.14	0.002	2.01	1.27–3.19	0.003	1.97	1.22–3.17	0.005	1.61	0.95–2.74	0.074
DT2: Mild-to-moderate	>50 nmol/L		(ref)			(ref)			(ref)			(ref)	
	<25 nmol/L	1.05	0.73–1.52	0.774	0.94	0.64–1.38	0.771	0.92	0.61–1.38	0.707	1.07	0.69–1.67	0.749
	25–50 nmol/L	3.39	1.99–5.76	0.001	3.02	1.70–5.38	0.001	3.12	1.67–5.85	0.001	1.95	0.94–4.06	0.071
DT3: Moderate-to-severe	>50 nmol/L		(ref)			(ref)			(ref)			(ref)	
		1.94	1.23–3.06	0.004	1.34	0.80–2.22	0.254	0.83	0.45–1.55	0.577	1.02	0.49–2.12	0.945

CI: confidence interval. BMI: body mass index. OR: odd ratio. ref: reference. 25(OH)D cut-offs: <25 nmol/L (low), 25–50 nmol/L (moderate) and >50 nmol/L (high); Number of participants with low, moderate and high 25(OH)D for DT1 is 66, 122, 67; DT2 is 89, 111, 34; DT3 is 94, 118, 74; Model 1 is the unadjusted model. Model 2 is further adjusted for sex, living in an institution and season. Model 3 is further adjusted for cognitive status, BMI and vitamin D containing medication. Model 4 is further adjusted for physical activity.

3.5. 25(OH)D Concentration and Disability Trajectory by Sex

Men with low concentrations of 25(OH)D were more likely to have a moderate-to-severe disability trajectory (OR = 3.55, 95% CI = 1.56–8.09, $p = 0.003$) than a low-to-mild disability trajectory compared to those with moderate concentrations in the unadjusted model, even after adjusting for living in an institution and season (OR = 4.42, 95% CI = 1.79–10.90, $p = 0.001$) and after further adjustment for cognitive status, BMI and vitamin D containing medication (OR = 3.83, 95% CI = 1.44–10.17, $p = 0.007$). However, this association disappeared after future adjustment for physical activity (Supplemental Table S2).

Women with low concentrations were more likely to have mild-to-moderate and moderate-to-severe disability trajectories than a low-to-mild disability trajectory compared to those with moderate concentrations in the unadjusted model (OR = 1.87, 95% CI = 1.03–3.39, $p = 0.039$) and (OR = 3.03, 95% CI = 1.50–6.13, $p = 0.002$), respectively. This association was maintained even after adjusting for sex, living in an institution and season (OR = 2.06, 95% CI = 1.12–3.83, $p = 0.020$) and (OR = 2.58, 95% CI = 1.21–5.50, $p = 0.014$), respectively. It also continued after further adjustment for cognitive status, BMI and vitamin D containing medication (OR = 1.95, 95%CI = 1.02–3.72, $p = 0.041$) and (OR = 2.70, 95% CI = 1.16–6.27, $p = 0.020$), respectively, but it disappeared after future adjustment for physical activity. Women showed a U-shaped association between 25(OH)D and a moderate-to-severe disability trajectory but only in the unadjusted model (OR = 2.29, 95% CI = 1.25–4.17, $p = 0.007$).

3.6. Sensitivity Analysis

Using the same models with further adjustment for grip strength, fat-free mass and disease count separately, no association was found between 25(OH)D concentration and disability trajectory. However, when physical activity was removed from the model, after adjusting for grip strength, fat-free mass and disease count, participants with a low concentration were more likely to have mild-to-moderate and moderate-to-severe disability trajectories.

The models were also rerun excluding individuals with cognitive impairment (SMMSE < 26). Participants with normal cognitive status ($n = 561$) who had a low concentration were more likely to have a moderate-to-severe disability trajectory (OR = 2.30, 95% CI = 1.15–4.58, $p = 0.017$) than a low-to-mild disability trajectory in the unadjusted model. This was also maintained in the adjusted models for the same confounders: sex, living in an institution and season (OR = 2.14, 95% CI = 1.04–4.39, $p = 0.038$) and even after adjustment for BMI and vitamin D containing medication (OR = 2.44, 95% CI = 1.13–5.27, $p = 0.022$) (Supplemental Table S3). This association disappeared after further adjustment for physical activity.

Participants' characteristics by season have been described previously. Stratifying the analysis by season, no association was found between 25(OH)D and disability trajectory in Spring ($n = 121$). Participants with low concentrations were more likely to have a moderate-to-severe disability trajectory compared to those with moderate concentrations in the unadjusted model for Summer ($n = 309$) and Autumn ($n = 180$) (OR = 2.96, 95% CI = 1.17–7.48, $p = 0.021$) and (OR = 6.03, 95% CI = 1.47–24.77, $p = 0.013$), respectively. However, the association disappeared in the adjusted models. For Winter ($n = 168$), participants with low concentrations were more likely to have a moderate-to-severe disability trajectory (OR = 5.83, 95% CI = 1.81–18.74, $p = 0.003$) compared to normal concentrations in the unadjusted model and after adjustment for sex and living in an institution (OR = 6.44, 95% CI = 1.79–23.12, $p = 0.004$) and after further adjustment for cognitive status, BMI and vitamin D containing medication (OR = 5.10, 95% CI = 1.28–20.37, $p = 0.021$). This association disappeared after adjustment for physical activity. On the other hand, participants with high concentrations were more likely to have a moderate-to-severe disability trajectory (OR = 6.92, 95% CI = 2.23–21.43, $p = 0.001$) compared to normal concentrations in the unadjusted model and after adjustment for sex, living in an institution and season (OR = 4.51, 95% CI = 1.24–16.37, $p = 0.022$). After adjustment for cognitive status, BMI and vitamin D containing medication, the association was attenuated although it became stronger after adjustment for physical activity (OR = 6.11, 95% CI = 1.01–36.75, p = 0.048) (Supplemental Table S4).

Serum 25(OH)D was used as a continuous variable in the analysis, but no association was found between 25(OH)D and disability (baseline data) or disability trajectory (follow up phase data) in the unadjusted or adjusted models.

4. Discussion

4.1. Main Findings

For the current analysis, the disability trajectories model was best presented by the triple-group model. These trajectories differed from two previously derived disability trajectories in different samples of the Newcastle 85+ Study [23,24]. We showed that, in partially adjusted models, people aged 85+ years with a 25(OH)D concentration (25–50 nmol/L) were more likely to have less disability at baseline and a slower disability trajectory over the following five years. However, in fully adjusted models, our results did not show a protective effect of any 25(OH)D concentration on trajectories of disability over five years.

4.2. Evidence from Other Studies

The lack of an association between 25(OH)D concentration and disability trajectories in our study is inconsistent with the findings of prospective cohort studies that investigate the association between vitamin D status and disability in those age 65 years and over. For example, two studies found that a 25(OH)D < 50 nmol/L increased the risk of disability in arthritis and multiple sclerosis patients, respectively [11,12]. Likewise, Semba, et al. [13] found that a 25(OH)D < 50 nmol/L was associated with a higher possibility of disability in women aged over 65 years and living in the community. The higher risk of a disability trajectory amongst participants with a concentration higher than 50 nmol/L in the cross-sectional analysis and in unadjusted models in the prospective analyses could be driven largely by those with cognitive impairment or those taking vitamin D containing medication or prescribed medication. First, our overall analysis showed that the association between a high concentration and disability trajectory disappeared after adjusting for these variables. Moreover, excluding participants with low SMMSE scores supports this finding. On the other hand, participants with a normal cognitive status did not show an association between high concentration and disability trajectories. In addition, there is no general agreement amongst researchers regarding the optimal concentration of 25(OH)D in relation to disability trajectory. The Institute of Medicine (IoM) defines vitamin D deficiency as a concentration of 25(OH)D < 30 nmol/L, and vitamin D adequacy as a concentration of >50 nmol/L for all age groups based on integrating data from several health outcomes and PTH [25]. In contrast, the UK Scientific Advisory Committee on Nutrition (SACN) defines vitamin D deficiency at a 25(OH)D concentration < 25 nmol/L [26]. However, our previous findings from the Newcastle 85+ study have documented a U-shaped association between 25(OH)D and muscle strength and performance [27].

Generally, the main role of vitamin D is to support musculoskeletal health. Therefore, maintaining an moderate 25(OH)D concentration is essential in order to slow the effect of ageing on the bones and muscles. Ageing is accompanied by a redistribution of the cortical and trabecular bone [28]. Moreover, a low 25(OH)D concentration increases osteoblastic activity and bone turnover [29,30]. A significant positive association has also been documented between 25(OH)D concentration, BMD [31] and type II muscle fibre [32] in older people. In addition, the VDR expression is reduced in the muscles as part of ageing [33]. A positive association between 25(OH)D concentration and muscle strength has been reported [32]. Therefore, a lack of VDR, which is expected in very-old adults, leads to reduced muscle mass and strength, as explained previously. Furthermore, studies in rats have demonstrated that a high PTH, due to a low concentration of 25(OH)D, induces muscle catabolism and reduces calcium transport in the skeletal muscle [32], thereby leading to low muscle strength. Combined, this can explain the effect of a low concentration of 25(OH)D on the onset and progression of disability.

In addition, the association between moderate 25(OH)D concentration and physical performance and strength has been confirmed previously [10]. Kotlarczyk, et al. [34] found that slower gait speed and lower IADL scores were associated with low 25(OH)D concentration. Moreover, a positive association between the 8-foot walk test and the sit-to-stand test, with a concentration of 25(OH)D, was also found [35]. These results indicate that a low concentration of 25(OH)D was associated with low muscle strength, which is a predictor of disability. Consistent with our results, Granic, et al. [27] demonstrated that a 25(OH)D concentration of > 30 nmol/L maintains muscle strength, but a concentration of > 50 nmol/L did not have further muscular or musculoskeletal benefits in the very old adults. However, whilst we appreciate that muscle function and disability per se are different parameters, a comparison nonetheless is relevant because of the role of muscle function in contributing to disability.

Physical activity is clearly a predictor of disability [11], although the association between PA and 25(OH)D was conflicted between the studies. First, a high concentration of 25(OH)D can positively influence the intensity of PA [36]. However, a converse association is also suggested [37]. In the same vein, a study analysing the data from NHANES reported that PA is generally associated with a high concentration of 25(OH)D, whether this activity occurs indoors or outdoors [38]. Therefore, restricted PA, which is associated with disability, can have an adverse effect on 25(OH)D concentration, possibly due either to a defect in metabolism or limited exposure to sunlight. Besides, PA is accompanied by improved health, stronger muscles and a lower BMI, which are all associated with 25(OH)D concentration [13,39,40]. Furthermore, the progression of disability is accompanied by a greater risk of feeding disability onset [41]; this contributes to the risk of nutrient deficiency, including vitamin D. Our results show that the association between 25(OH)D and the disability trajectory disappeared after adjusting for PA. This suggests that the association between 25(OH)D concentration and disability could be due the effect of PA rather than 25(OH)D concentration. This means those with a higher PA have a better vitamin D status and, obviously, those with a high PA have less disability.

Age-related changes also result in body composition changes. For that reason, a lean body mass is significantly lower in older adults compared to younger ones—a change that accelerates after the age of 60 [42]. The univariate analysis of our data showed an association between fat-free mass and disability trajectories. However, the evidence demonstrated that the amount of fat mass but not fat-free mass was associated with muscle function and disability. For instance, Sternfeld, et al. [43] and Visser, et al. [44] agreed that there was no association between physical disability and total body skeletal muscle mass, while a high percentage of fat mass was associated with physical disability.

Even though a higher lean-to-fat ratio was associated with a faster walking speed, this suggests that the impact of a lean mass is important in relation to the amount of body fat. Indeed, fat-free mass was not a significant predictor of mobility-related disability in the regression model [45]. The association between 25(OH)D concentration and fat and lean mass could be explained by the escalation in fat mass, which may enhance the storage of vitamin D and, consequently, lower the circulating 25(OH)D [40]. However, the adjustment for BMI in the model, and for FFM in the sensitivity analysis, did not affect the association between 25(OH)D concentration and disability trajectory in the current study.

Our results also suggest that in partially adjusted models, men with a low concentration of 25(OH)D were more likely to develop only a severe disability trajectory, while women with a low concentration were more likely to develop either a moderate or a severe disability trajectory. This could be explained by the findings of Granic, et al. [46], who demonstrated that men had better muscle strength and physical performance (measured by grip strength and timed-up-and-go), but a steeper decline in both grip strength and timed-up-to-go over five years. Similarly, Millán-Calenti et al. [3]. reported that older men and women (80+ years) have a higher risk of being dependent (OR = 1.10) using ADL and IADL compared to younger adults (65+), but the risk among women is even higher (OR = 2.48). Conversely, our results are inconsistent with the findings of Semba, et al. [13], who demonstrated that only women with a low 25(OH)D concentration were at risk of having a disability. This difference could be due to the smaller number of men included in the studies compared to women.

The association between 25(OH)D concentration and disability trajectories in the current study varies by season. In the spring, no association was found, whereas a significant adverse association was found between a 25(OH)D concentration lower than 25 nmol/L and disability trajectory, but only in the unadjusted model. However, in Winter, a U-shaped association was found between 25(OH)D concentration and disability trajectory. This conflicting results between the seasons could be explained by the differences between the participants' cognitive status, PA and vitamin D containing medication usage. The total number of participants in the Spring was the lowest ($n = 121$); consequently, Spring was associated with the lowest percentage of participants who had normal cognitive status (14.5%), were physically active (14.5%) and who took vitamin D containing medication (15.5%) when compared to the other seasons. This may explain the failure to detect the association. On the contrary, the data showed that, in the Winter, of the 165 participants, 14 were cognitively impaired and took vitamin D containing medication; nine of the cognitively impaired participants were physically active compared to the 52 participants who had a normal cognitive status and were physically active. Therefore, a potential negative effect of the highest 25(OH)D tertile on disability trajectory could be partly driven by those who have an impaired cognitive status, that influences their PA, and by those who have reached a higher concentration through taking vitamin D containing medication shortly before the baseline assessments.

4.3. Strengths and Limitations

Our study has several strengths, including its prospective design, its broad representativeness of the population in England and Wales, large number of participants, the five-year follow up to measure disability, the robustness of the clustering technique (GBTM) used to derive disability trajectory, and the adjustment for several potential confounders associated with disability and 25(OH)D concentration. Physical activity and season, which could reflect UV exposure, were also considered in the models. Determining the disability by using 17 ADLs that compromise BADL, IADL and mobility items is also a strength of this study. Moreover, our study used prevalent cut-offs of serum 25(OH)D to determine the concentration required to predict the onset and progress of disability trajectory.

However, the findings reported here should be interpreted with caution due to the following limitations. First, the concentration of 25(OH)D was only measured at baseline, so it might change during the subsequent five years depending on sun exposure, season, supplement intake, physical activity and disease. However, the changes in these variables are unlikely across the follow-up phases, if only disease/disability may increase but not the others. Another limitation was that the frequency or dose of supplements used as well as UV exposure were not measured. Finally, it is possible that some disability transitions were not fully captured during the follow up phases, as these were 18 or 24 months apart.

5. Conclusions

We found a U-shaped association between 25(OH)D and disability at baseline with both low (<25 nmol/L) and high (>50 nmol/L) 25(OH)D concentrations associated with faster disability. However these findings should be interpreted with caution as residual confounding is very likely driving these associations. In fully adjusted models, we failed to find a significant association between any 25(OH)D concentration and disability trajectories over 5 years. However, it should be noted that sample size limitations may have precluded the detection of statistically significant findings and that larger studies are needed for this research question.

Supplementary Materials: The following are available online at http://www.mdpi.com/2072-6643/12/9/2742/s1, Supplementary Figure S1: The Newcastle 85+ Study recruitment. Supplementary Table S1. Self-reported activities of daily living. Supplementary Table S2. Association between different 25(OH)D cut-offs and disability trajectories by sex. Supplementary Table S3. Association between 25(OH)D concentration and disability trajectories of people with normal cognitive status. Supplementary Table S4. Association between different 25(OH)D cut-offs and disability trajectories by season.

Author Contributions: S.H., T.R.H., T.A. and N.M. were responsible for conception and designed the manuscript; S.H. was responsible for statistical analyses; S.H. wrote the paper, and had primary responsibility for the final content of the manuscript; T.R.H., T.A., N.M., J.C.M., A.K., C.R.-M., C.J. and R.D. critically reviewed and revised the manuscript for scientific content, and approved the final version. All authors have read and agreed to the published version of the manuscript.

Funding: This particular research received no external funding.

Acknowledgments: The Newcastle 85+ study was jointly funded by the Medical Research Council and Biotechnology and Biomedical Science Research Council (G0500997), now part of UK Research and Innovation (UKRI) in addition to the Newcastle Healthcare Charity. The following waves were funded by the Dunhill Medical Trust (R124/0509), Newcastle University, UK Medical Research Council and the British Heart Foundation Nutrients 2020, 12, 2068 16 of 22 (606013333). Overall, the project was supported by National Institute for Health Research Newcastle Biomedical Research Centre based at Newcastle upon Tyne Hospitals NHS Foundation Trust and Newcastle University (A.G.). We thank the operational support from the North of England Commissioning Support Unit and the local general practitioners and staff in addition to the research, management and administrative teams and of course the study participants and their family for providing the data.

Conflicts of Interest: Competing interests S.H., N.M., T.A., A.K., C.R.-M., C.J., J.C.M., R.D. and T.R.H. have no conflicts of interest. The opinions expressed in this paper are those of the authors and do not necessarily reflect the views of the organizations they work with.

References

1. Gobbens, R.J.; van Assen, M.A. The prediction of ADL and IADL disability using six physical indicators of frailty: A longitudinal study in the Netherlands. *Curr. Gerontol. Geriatr. Res.* **2014**, *2014*. [CrossRef] [PubMed]
2. Yu, R.; Wong, M.; Chang, B.; Lai, X.; Lum, C.M.; Auyeung, T.W.; Lee, J.; Tsoi, K.; Lee, R.; Woo, J. Trends in activities of daily living disability in a large sample of community-dwelling Chinese older adults in Hong Kong: An age-period-cohort analysis. *BMJ Open* **2016**, *6*. [CrossRef]
3. Millán-Calenti, J.C.; Tubío, J.; Pita-Fernández, S.; González-Abraldes, I.; Lorenzo, T.; Fernández-Arruty, T.; Maseda, A. Prevalence of functional disability in activities of daily living (ADL), instrumental activities of daily living (IADL) and associated factors, as predictors of morbidity and mortality. *Arch. Gerontol. Geriatr.* **2010**, *50*, 306–310. [CrossRef] [PubMed]
4. Majer, I.M.; Nusselder, W.J.; Mackenbach, J.P.; Klijs, B.; van Baal, P.H.M. Mortality risk associated with disability: A population-based record linkage study. *Am. J. Public Health* **2011**, *101*, e9–e15. [CrossRef] [PubMed]
5. Ali, Z. *Economics of Disability in Bangladesh*; The National Archives: Richmond, UK, 2014.
6. Gallagher, J.C. Vitamin D and Aging. *Endocrinol. Metabol. Clin. N. Am.* **2013**, *42*, 319–332. [CrossRef]
7. Ceglia, L. Vitamin D and its role in skeletal muscle. *Curr. Opin. Clin. Nutr. Metab. Care* **2009**, *12*, 628–633. [CrossRef]
8. Zamboni, M.; Zoico, E.; Tosoni, P.; Zivelonghi, A.; Bortolani, A.; Maggi, S.; Di Francesco, V.; Bosello, O. Relation between vitamin D, physical performance, and disability in elderly persons. *J. Gerontol. Ser. A Biol. Sci. Med. Sci.* **2002**, *57*, M7–M11. [CrossRef]
9. Orces, C.H. Prevalence of clinically relevant muscle weakness and its association with vitamin D status among older adults in Ecuador. *Aging Clin. Exp. Res.* **2017**, *29*, 943–949. [CrossRef]
10. Bischoff-Ferrari, H.A.; Borchers, M.; Gudat, F.; Durmuller, U.; Stahelin, H.B.; Dick, W. Vitamin D receptor expression in human muscle tissue decreases with age. *J. Bone Miner. Res.* **2004**, *19*, 265–269. [CrossRef]
11. Oliveira, S.R.; Simão, A.N.C.; Alfieri, D.F.; Flauzino, T.; Kallaur, A.P.; Mezzaroba, L.; Lozovoy, M.A.B.; Sabino, B.S.; Ferreira, K.P.Z.; Pereira, W.L.C.J.; et al. Vitamin D deficiency is associated with disability and disease progression in multiple sclerosis patients independently of oxidative and nitrosative stress. *J. Neurol. Sci.* **2017**, *381*, 213–219. [CrossRef]
12. Valderrama-Hinds, L.M.; Al Snih, S.; Rodriguez, M.A.; Wong, R. Association of arthritis and vitamin D insufficiency with physical disability in Mexican older adults: Findings from the Mexican Health and Aging Study. *Rheumatol. Int.* **2017**, *37*, 607–616. [CrossRef] [PubMed]
13. Semba, R.D.; Garrett, E.; Johnson, B.A.; Guralnik, J.M.; Fried, L.P. Vitamin D deficiency among older women with and without disability. *Am. J. Clin. Nutr.* **2000**, *72*, 1529–1534. [CrossRef] [PubMed]

14. Hill, T.R.; Granic, A.; Davies, K.; Collerton, J.; Martin-Ruiz, C.; Siervo, M.; Mathers, J.C.; Adamson, A.J.; Francis, R.M.; Pearce, S.H.; et al. Serum 25-hydroxyvitamin D concentration and its determinants in the very old: The Newcastle 85+ Study. *Osteoporos. Int.* **2016**, *27*, 1199–1208. [CrossRef] [PubMed]
15. Granic, A.; Hill, T.R.; Kirkwood, T.B.L.; Davies, K.; Collerton, J.; Martin-Ruiz, C.; von Zglinicki, T.; Saxby, B.K.; Wesnes, K.A.; Collerton, D.; et al. Serum 25-hydroxyvitamin D and cognitive decline in the very old: The Newcastle 85+ study. *Eur. J. Neurol.* **2015**, *22*, e6–e7. [CrossRef]
16. Granic, A.; Aspray, T.; Hill, T.; Davies, K.; Collerton, J.; Martin-Ruiz, C.; von Zglinicki, T.; Kirkwood, T.B.; Mathers, J.C.; Jagger, C. 25-hydroxyvitamin D and increased all-cause mortality in very old women: The Newcastle 85+ study. *J. Int. Med.* **2015**, *277*, 456–467. [CrossRef]
17. Collerton, J.; Davies, K.; Jagger, C.; Kingston, A.; Bond, J.; Eccles, M.P.; Robinson, L.A.; Martin-Ruiz, C.; von Zglinicki, T.; James, O.F.W.; et al. Health and disease in 85 year olds: Baseline findings from the Newcastle 85+ cohort study. *BMJ* **2009**, *339*. [CrossRef]
18. Martin-Ruiz, C.; Jagger, C.; Kingston, A.; Collerton, J.; Catt, M.; Davies, K.; Dunn, M.; Hilkens, C.; Keavney, B.; Pearce, S.H.S.; et al. Assessment of a large panel of candidate biomarkers of ageing in the Newcastle 85+ study. *Mech. Ageing Dev.* **2011**, *132*, 496–502. [CrossRef]
19. Kempen, G.I.J.M.; Miedema, I.; Ormel, J.; Molenaar, W. The assessment of disability with the Groningen Activity Restriction Scale. Conceptual framework and psychometric properties. *Soc. Sci. Med.* **1996**, *43*, 1601–1610. [CrossRef]
20. Collerton, J.; Barrass, K.; Bond, J.; Eccles, M.; Jagger, C.; James, O.; Martin-Ruiz, C.; Robinson, L.; von Zglinicki, T.; Kirkwood, T. The Newcastle 85+ study: Biological, clinical and psychosocial factors associated with healthy ageing: Study protocol. *BMC Geriatr.* **2007**, *7*, 14. [CrossRef]
21. Mendonça, N.; Hill, T.; Granic, A.; Mathers, J.; Wrieden, W.; Siervo, M.; Seal, C.; Jagger, C.; Adamson, A. Micronutrient intake and food sources in the very old. *Br. J. Nutr.* **2016**, *16*, 751–761.
22. Vieth, R.; Holick, M.F. Chapter 57B—The IOM—Endocrine Society Controversy on Recommended Vitamin D Targets: In Support of the Endocrine Society Position. In *Vitamin D*, 4th ed.; Feldman, D., Ed.; Academic Press: Cambridge, MA, USA, 2018; pp. 1091–1107. [CrossRef]
23. Mendonça, N.; Granic, A.; Hill, T.R.; Siervo, M.; Mathers, J.C.; Kingston, A.; Jagger, C. Protein Intake and Disability Trajectories in Very Old Adults: The Newcastle 85+ Study. *J. Am. Geriatr. Soc.* **2018**, *67*, 50–56. [CrossRef]
24. Kingston, A.; Davies, K.; Collerton, J.; Robinson, L.; Duncan, R.; Kirkwood, T.B.; Jagger, C. The enduring effect of education-socioeconomic differences in disability trajectories from age 85 years in the Newcastle 85+ Study. *Arch. Gerontol. Geriatr.* **2015**, *60*, 405–411. [CrossRef] [PubMed]
25. Ross, A.C.; Manson, J.E.; Abrams, S.A.; Aloia, J.F.; Brannon, P.M.; Clinton, S.K.; Durazo-Arvizu, R.A.; Gallagher, J.C.; Gallo, R.L.; Jones, G.; et al. The 2011 Report on Dietary Reference Intakes for Calcium and Vitamin D from the Institute of Medicine: What Clinicians Need to Know. *J. Clin. Endocrinol. Metab.* **2011**, *96*, 53–58. [CrossRef] [PubMed]
26. Scientific Advisory Committee on Nutrition. Vitamin D and Health. 2016. Available online: https://assets.publishing.service.gov.uk/government/uploads/system/uploads/attachment_data/file/537616/SACN_Vitamin_D_and_Health_report.pdf (accessed on 7 September 2020).
27. Granic, A.; Hill, T.R.; Davies, K.; Jagger, C.; Adamson, A.; Siervo, M.; Kirkwood, T.B.; Mathers, J.C.; Sayer, A.A. Vitamin D Status, Muscle Strength and Physical Performance Decline in Very Old Adults: A Prospective Study. *Nutrients* **2017**, *9*, 379. [CrossRef] [PubMed]
28. Bouxsein, M.L.; Karasik, D. Bone geometry and skeletal fragility. *Curr. Osteoporos. Rep.* **2006**, *4*, 49–56. [CrossRef]
29. Van de Peppel, J.; Franceschi, R.T.; Li, Y.; van der Eerden, B.C.J. Chapter 17—Vitamin D Regulation of Osteoblast Function A2—Feldman, David. In *Vitamin D*, 4th ed.; Academic Press: Cambridge, MA, USA, 2018; pp. 295–308. [CrossRef]
30. Lips, P.; van Schoor, N.M. The effect of vitamin D on bone and osteoporosis. *Best Pract. Res. Clin. Endocrinol. Metab.* **2011**, *25*, 585–591. [CrossRef]
31. Bischoff-Ferrari, H.A.; Dietrich, T.; Orav, E.J.; Dawson-Hughes, B. Positive association between 25-hydroxy vitamin D levels and bone mineral density: A population-based study of younger and older adults. *Am. J. Med.* **2004**, *116*, 634–639. [CrossRef]
32. Ceglia, L. Vitamin D and skeletal muscle tissue and function. *Mol. Aspects Med.* **2008**, *29*, 407–414. [CrossRef]

33. Visser, M.; Deeg, D.J.H.; Lips, P. Low Vitamin D and High Parathyroid Hormone Levels as Determinants of Loss of Muscle Strength and Muscle Mass (Sarcopenia): The Longitudinal Aging Study Amsterdam. *J. Clin. Endocrinol. Metab.* **2003**, *88*, 5766–5772. [CrossRef]
34. Kotlarczyk, M.P.; Perera, S.; Ferchak, M.A.; Nace, D.A.; Resnick, N.M.; Greenspan, S.L. Vitamin D deficiency is associated with functional decline and falls in frail elderly women despite supplementation. *Osteoporos. Int.* **2017**, *28*, 1347–1353. [CrossRef]
35. Bischoff-Ferrari, H.A.; Dietrich, T.; Orav, E.J.; Hu, F.B.; Zhang, Y.; Karlson, E.W.; Dawson-Hughes, B. Higher 25-hydroxyvitamin D concentrations are associated with better lower-extremity function in both active and inactive persons aged ≥ 60 y. *Am. J. Clin. Nutr.* **2004**, *80*, 752–758. [CrossRef] [PubMed]
36. Al-Eisa, E.S.; Alghadir, A.H.; Gabr, S.A. Correlation between vitamin D levels and muscle fatigue risk factors based on physical activity in healthy older adults. *Clin. Interv. Aging* **2016**, *11*, 513. [PubMed]
37. Van den Heuvel, E.; Van Schoor, N.; De Jongh, R.T.; Visser, M.; Lips, P. Cross-sectional study on different characteristics of physical activity as determinants of vitamin D status; inadequate in half of the population. *Eur. J. Clin. Nutr.* **2013**, *67*, 360–365. [CrossRef] [PubMed]
38. Fernandes, M.R.; Barreto, W.D. Association between physical activity and vitamin D: A narrative literature review. *Rev. Assoc. Med. Bras.* **2017**, *63*, 550–556. [CrossRef] [PubMed]
39. Stewart, J.W.; Alekel, D.L.; Ritland, L.M.; Van Loan, M.; Gertz, E.; Genschel, U. Serum 25-hydroxyvitamin D is related to indicators of overall physical fitness in healthy postmenopausal women. *Menopause* **2009**, *16*, 1093. [CrossRef] [PubMed]
40. Toffanello, E.D.; Perissinotto, E.; Sergi, G.; Zambon, S.; Musacchio, E.; Maggi, S.; Coin, A.; Sartori, L.; Corti, M.-C.; Baggio, G. Vitamin D and physical performance in elderly subjects: The Pro. VA study. *PLoS ONE* **2012**, *7*, e34950. [CrossRef]
41. Dunlop, D.D.; Hughes, S.L.; Manheim, L.M. Disability in activities of daily living: Patterns of change and a hierarchy of disability. *Am. J. Public Health* **1997**, *87*, 378–383. [CrossRef]
42. Kyle, U.; Genton, L.; Hans, D.; Karsegard, L.; Slosman, D.; Pichard, C. Age-related differences in fat-free mass, skeletal muscle, body cell mass and fat mass between 18 and 94 years. *Eur. J. Clin. Nutr.* **2001**, *55*, 663. [CrossRef]
43. Sternfeld, B.; Ngo, L.; Satariano, W.A.; Tager, I.B. Associations of body composition with physical performance and self-reported functional limitation in elderly men and women. *Am. J. Epidemiol.* **2002**, *156*, 110–121. [CrossRef]
44. Visser, M.; Harris, T.; Langlois, J.; Hannan, M.; Roubenoff, R.; Felson, D.; Wilson, P.; Kiel, D. Body fat and skeletal muscle mass in relation to physical disability in very old men and women of the Framingham Heart Study. *J. Gerontol. Ser. A Biol. Sci. Med. Sci.* **1998**, *53*, M214–M221. [CrossRef]
45. Visser, M.; Langlois, J.; Guralnik, J.M.; Cauley, J.A.; Kronmal, R.A.; Robbins, J.; Williamson, J.D.; Harris, T.B. High body fatness, but not low fat-free mass, predicts disability in older men and women: The Cardiovascular Health Study. *Am. J. Clin. Nutr.* **1998**, *68*, 584–590. [CrossRef] [PubMed]
46. Granic, A.; Davies, K.; Jagger, C.; Kirkwood, T.B.; Syddall, H.E.; Sayer, A.A. Grip strength decline and its determinants in the very old: Longitudinal findings from the Newcastle 85+ Study. *PLoS ONE* **2016**, *11*, e0163183.

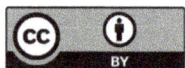

© 2020 by the authors. Licensee MDPI, Basel, Switzerland. This article is an open access article distributed under the terms and conditions of the Creative Commons Attribution (CC BY) license (http://creativecommons.org/licenses/by/4.0/).

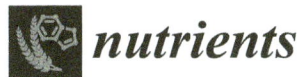

Article

Disparities in Head and Neck Cancer: A Case for Chemoprevention with Vitamin D

Mirela Ibrahimovic [1,2], Elizabeth Franzmann [3,4], Alison M. Mondul [1,2], Katherine M. Weh [1,5], Connor Howard [1,5], Jennifer J. Hu [3,6], W. Jarrard Goodwin [3,6] and Laura A. Kresty [1,5,*]

1. The Rogel Cancer Center, University of Michigan, Ann Arbor, MI 48109, USA; imirela@umich.edu (M.I.); amondul@umich.edu (A.M.M.); kweh@med.umich.edu (K.M.W.); conhow@med.umich.edu (C.H.)
2. Department of Epidemiology, School of Public Health, University of Michigan, Ann Arbor, MI 48109, USA
3. Sylvester Comprehensive Cancer Center, University of Miami School of Medicine, Miami, FL 33136, USA; efranzman@med.miami.edu (E.F.); jhu@med.miami.edu (J.J.H.); wgoodwin@med.miami.edu (W.J.G.)
4. Department of Otolaryngology, University of Miami School of Medicine, Miami, FL 33136, USA
5. Department of Surgery, Thoracic Surgery Section, University of Michigan, Ann Arbor, MI 48109, USA
6. Department of Public Health Sciences, University of Miami School of Medicine, Miami, FL 33136, USA
* Correspondence: lkresty@med.umich.edu; Tel.: +1-734-647-0723

Received: 31 July 2020; Accepted: 26 August 2020; Published: 29 August 2020

Abstract: Blacks experience disproportionate head and neck cancer (HNC) recurrence and mortality compared to Whites. Overall, vitamin D status is inversely associated to HNC pointing to a potential protective linkage. Although hypovitaminosis D in Blacks is well documented it has not been investigated in Black HNC patients. Thus, we conducted a prospective pilot study accessing vitamin D status in newly diagnosed HNC patients stratified by race and conducted in vitro studies to investigate mechanisms associated with potential cancer inhibitory effects of vitamin D. Outcome measures included circulating levels of vitamin D, related nutrients, and risk factor characterization as well as dietary and supplemental estimates. Vitamin D-based in vitro assays utilized proteome and microRNA (miR) profiling. Nineteen patients were enrolled, mean circulating vitamin D levels were significantly reduced in Black compared to White HNC patients, 27.3 and 20.0 ng/mL, respectively. Whites also supplemented vitamin D more frequently than Blacks who had non-significantly higher vitamin D from dietary sources. Vitamin D treatment of HNC cell lines revealed five significantly altered miRs regulating genes targeting multiple pathways in cancer based on enrichment analysis (i.e., negative regulation of cell proliferation, angiogenesis, chemokine, MAPK, and WNT signaling). Vitamin D further altered proteins involved in cancer progression, metastasis and survival supporting a potential role for vitamin D in targeted cancer prevention.

Keywords: head and neck cancer; racial disparities; vitamin D; chemoprevention; UVB; microRNA; proteomic profiling

1. Introduction

Head and neck cancer (HNC) is the ninth most commonly diagnosed cancer in the United States and is associated with significant morbidity, mortality, and economic loss [1,2]. Important racial disparities persist for HNC [3]. Historically, HNC was more common in Black Americans than Whites, however, the incidence rate in the latter has increased since the 1990s in parallel with human papillomavirus (HPV)—positive HNC, which is diagnosed more among White males [4]. Black Americans tend to have lower rates of HPV-associated HNC which generally present as oropharyngeal cancers and are associated with better response to treatment and improved five-year survival rates compared to HPV-negative HNC [5,6]. Overall, HNC in Black patients is associated with a much lower five-year survival rate, about 30% compared to 57% in White patients [5,6]. Disparate survival rates have been investigated in recent years, yet consensus regarding the causative factors remains to be fully elucidated. Published reports document that Black HNC patients present with more advanced disease at initial diagnosis, experience greater delays in treatment initiation, and experience more gaps in health insurance coverage compared to Whites [7–9]. Still, our understanding of racial disparities in HNC remains incomplete. Research assessing potential biological mechanisms underlying HNC in racially diverse populations is lacking, as is information on the contribution of modifiable dietary factors to HNC incidence and progression. An inverse association between vitamin D status and cancer incidence, prognosis, and mortality has been reported in several cancer types, HNC included [10–14]. Moreover, it is well documented that Black Americans are at a higher risk for low vitamin D status, yet the link between HNC and vitamin D status has not been evaluated among Black patients [15,16].

Studies investigating vitamin D have identified a multitude of health benefits including improved calcium absorption, improved immune function, and an increase in bone density [17,18]. It has been speculated that vitamin D has potential anticarcinogenic effects through multiple biologic functions; however, clinical interventions and observational studies evaluating vitamin D have yielded mixed results across different cancers [10]. Nonetheless, a recent prospective cohort study targeting HNC in a population without race reported shows that higher vitamin D intake levels are associated with decreased risk of HNC recurrence [13]. Conversely, vitamin D deficiency has been linked to lymphatic metastasis among HNC patients [19].

The goal of this prospective pilot study was to assess vitamin D status in newly diagnosed Black and White HNC patients and to conduct in vitro studies to improve our understanding of mechanisms associated with the potential cancer inhibitory effects of vitamin D in the context of HNC. To our knowledge, there have been no studies evaluating the association between vitamin D levels and HNC in Black patients despite their increased risk of vitamin D deficiency and increased risk of HNC recurrence as well as reduced five-year survival rates compared to White patients. In the present analysis, we examine vitamin D levels and other characteristics in Black and White HNC patients treated for HNC in Miami, Florida. Further, to explore anti-cancer mechanisms of vitamin D microRNA (miR) and proteomic profiling was conducted on human HNC cancer cell lines following vitamin D treatment.

Our research findings support that Black HNC patients present at an earlier age and with reduced levels of circulating vitamin D levels compared to Whites even in sunny South Florida. In addition, none of our Black HNC patients had vitamin D levels greater than or equal to 30 ng/mL, the level associated with optimal regulation of parathyroid hormone (PTH), calcium absorption, and bone health. Parallel in vitro studies revealed that vitamin D treatment of HNC cell lines significantly altered miRs regulating genes involved in many cancer pathways (i.e., steroid biosynthesis, cell proliferation, angiogenesis, chemokine, stem cell pluripotency, MAPK, and WNT signaling). Similarly, proteomic profiling following vitamin D treatment revealed modulation of proteins with roles in HNC cancer progression, metastasis, chemoresistance, and cancer recurrence and further supporting a potential role vitamin D in targeted cancer prevention [20–23].

2. Materials and Methods

2.1. Characteristics of the Head and Neck Cancer Patient Population

Nineteen HNC patients (10 non-Hispanic Whites and 9 Blacks) were recruited from the Sylvester Cancer Center or Jackson Memorial Hospital in Miami, Florida. Patients 18 years of age or older were included if they had a new diagnosis of HNC cancer (including primary lesions of the oral cavity, excluding HPV-linked cancers of the oropharynx); primary lesions of stage I–IV were included. All subjects gave their informed consent for inclusion before they participated in the study. The study was conducted in accordance with the Declaration of Helsinki, and the protocol was approved by the Institutional Review Board and Ethics Committee of the University of Miami (Project ID: 81110). Both male and female patients were enrolled in the study on a rolling basis. If the participant was pregnant, suffered from other illnesses or used chronic medication known to impact vitamin D metabolism they were excluded from the study. Human subject inclusion codes were G1A, M1A, and C3A. Additional information collected included basic demographic and socioeconomic factors (i.e., age, sex, height, weight, residency, annual income, highest education level completed, risk factors, and occupational history).

2.2. Dietary Intake Information and Risk Factor Characterization

Block Dietary Data Systems screeners were used to collect data on the patients' dietary intake including fruit and vegetable consumption as well as calcium and vitamin D intake. In addition to this, physical activity and sun exposure data were collected. Smoking status and alcohol consumption data were acquired by utilizing Tobacco Product Assessment Consortium (TobPRAC) tools.

2.3. Blood Measures

Blood levels of both the circulating metabolite (25-hydroxyvitamin D) and active metabolite (1,25-dihydroxyvitamin D) of vitamin D were measured from serum. Plasma was utilized to determine calcium and PTH levels. Levels of 25-hydroxyvitamin D and 1,25-dihydroxyvitamin D were determined using a two-step process involving rapid extraction and purification and (radioimmunoassay) RIA with specific antibodies (DiaSorin, Stillwater, MN, USA). PTH levels were determined utilizing the Immulite Immunometric assay (Diagnostic Products Corp., Los Angeles, CA, USA). Quest Diagnostics (San Juan Capistrano, CA, USA and Miramar, FL, USA) analyzed the samples utilizing well validated methods as previously reported [24]. Patients were categorized on the basis of four serum concentrations informed by the literature. 25-hydroxyvitamin D: <10.0 ng/mL, 10.0–19.9 ng/mL, 20.0–29.9 ng/mL, and >30.0 ng/mL. The first cut point is the classic definition of vitamin D deficiency and the second the level at which blood PTH homeostasis is achieved, the third a level proposed to classify an insufficient state and the fourth a level postulated for optimal regulation of PTH, calcium absorption and bone density [25]. The other two blood-based markers were assessed on a continuous scale. Students T-test were used to determine if there were statistically significant differences in blood or nutrient levels between Black and White patients. Chi-Square test was utilized to determine differences between racial groups by level and a p-value of 0.05 was considered statistically significant.

2.4. Head and Neck Cancer Cell Lines

SCC-25 (CR-1628™) and CAL-27 (CRL-2095™) cell lines were both obtained from American Type Culture Collection (ATCC). SCC-25 cells were isolated from a 70 year old White male who had squamous cell carcinoma of the tongue at T2N1 [26]. Likewise, CAL-27 cells were isolated from squamous cell carcinoma of the tongue in a White male who was 56 years old [27]. The two cell lines were plated at 3.5E06 and 1E06, respectively, and allowed to adhere for 30 h in T-75 flasks with DMEM:F12 complete medium, 10% FBS. Cells were then treated with either 2 µM of vitamin D in the form of cholecalciferol (vitamin D3, Sigma, St Louis, MO, USA) or vehicle (dilute EtOH) and harvested 24 h post-treatment utilizing a cell scraper. Cells were placed in D-PBS (without calcium or magnesium) and centrifuged at low speed (500× g) to pellet. The pellets were snap frozen in liquid nitrogen and stored at −80 °C until they were processed for RNA isolation, proteomic profiling, or evaluation of individual vitamin D linked proteins. The concentration of Vitamin D3 utilized for the HNSCC cell line studies were based on our preliminary viability investigations as shown (Figure S1) which show the LD50 in the range or 0.5 to 2uM as well as consideration of the published literature, both in preclinical and clinical studies [28–33]. As discussed above, circulating levels of vitamin D in humans have been targeted at >30 ng/mL (75 nmol/L or 0.075uM) [33] for optimal health. However, precise dose extrapolation from cell lines to physiological relevant human concentrations of vitamin D is complicated by the fact that levels may not accurately reflect tissue or intracellular concentrations [34]. Furthermore, human intervention studies or supplementation in free-living populations frequently involve daily vitamin D intake or in some intervention studies multiple times a day, whereas the in vitro studies herein are based on a single dose of vitamin D. Considering these factors a concentration of 2 µM was chosen for all cell-based assays.

2.5. RNA Isolation and microRNA Assay

RNA was isolated utilizing standard phenol-chloroform extraction procedures as previously described [35]. RNA quality was determined by Nanodrop using the 8000 Spectrophotometer (Thermo Scientific, Wilmington, NC, USA) and RNA integrity and presence of the small RNA fraction was determined using the Bioanalyzer 2100 capillary electrophoresis system (Agilent, Santa Clara, CA, USA). Sixty nanograms of total RNA was reverse transcribed using the human Megaplex Primer Pools A and B and the TaqMan miR reverse transcription kit (Applied Biosystems, Foster City, CA, USA) [35]. Each sample was pre-amplified for 12 cycles using human pool A and B Taqman® Megaplex™ PreAmp Primers and PreAmp Master Mix (Applied Biosystems) and the preamplification reactions diluted, combined with TaqMan ® Gene-Expression Master Mix (Applied Biosystems) divided into eight aliquots and each aliquot was added to one of the eight sample ports of the TaqMan® Array A or B (v2.0), respectively. The TaqMan® Array Human miR Card Set v2.0 (Thermo Fisher Scientific, Waltham, MA, USA) enables detection of 667 human miRs, 3 miR endogenous reference controls, and 1 miR assay not related to human as a negative control. Table S1 includes relevant miR platform and sequence information. The real-time PCR reactions were run according to the manufacturer's instructions. RealTime Statminer Software (Integromics, Philadelphia, PA, USA) was used to analyze the data. The global geometric mean of all expressed miR assays was used to normalize the data. Significantly altered miRs were determined based on the most stringent criteria with a *p*-value cutoff of 1E-05 was used to determine statistically significant miRs.

2.6. MiR Gene Targets and Enrichment Analysis

Validated gene targets from miRs significantly altered by vitamin D treatment were determined using miRTarBase (The Chinese University of Hongkong, Shenzhen, China) [36]. The miRTarBase software and database enables users to search for validated gene targets based on the miR ID. This database was chosen as it is relatively stable and miRTarBase has been shown to be broader and more comprehensive when compared to other miR target validation databases [37]. Database for Annotation, Visualization, and Integrated Discovery (DAVID, v6.8, Frederick National Laboratory for Cancer Research, Frederick, MD, USA) was utilized to analyze the validated gene targets regulated by up or down-regulated miRs. Additionally, MetaCore software (Clarviate Analytics, Philadelphia, PA, USA) was used to further explore functional analysis of common gene targets for CAL-27 and SCC-25. *p*-values are calculated for the terms in each ontology after enrichment; the terms are then tested as separate hypotheses. The resultant *q*-value illustrates the corrected-values accounting for the total terms in the ontology including the rank of each term. This provides an estimate of the Benjamini False Discovery Rate (FDR).

2.7. Proteomic Profiling

Protein resuspension was achieved in 2-D cell lysis buffer (30 mM Tris-HCl, pH 8.8, containing 7 M urea, 2 M thiourea, and 4% CHAPS). This mixture was then sonicated at 4 °C followed by shaking for 30 min at room temperature, centrifugation at 4 °C (14,000 rpm) for 30 min and supernatant collection. Bio-Rads protein assay was used to measure protein concentration. The protein lysate was further processed for global proteome profiling including CyDye labeling, running of SDS gels, gel imaging, resolving protein spots, spot digestion, and MALDI-TOF MS and TOF/TOF tandem MS/MS methods were conducted in collaboration with Applied Biomics (Hayward, CA, USA).

2.8. Lysate Collection and Western Blot Analysis of HNC Cancer Cells Following Vitamin D

CAL-27 (7E5) and SCC-25 (7E5) cells were seeded in T-25 flasks (Corning, Thermofisher Scientific, Waltham, MA, USA) and adhered overnight prior to treatment with 2 µM vitamin D (Sigma Aldrich,

Saint Louis, MO, USA) or vehicle (dilute ethanol) dissolved in phenol red free complete RPMI medium (Thermo Fisher Scientific, Scientific, Waltham, MA, USA). Cell lysates were harvested at 24 and 48 h post-treatment using RPPA lysis buffer (1% Triton X-100, 50 mM HEPES, pH 7.4, 150 mM NaCl, 1.5 mM $MgCl_2$, 1 mM EGTA, 100 mM NaF, 10 mM sodium pyrophosphate, 1 mM sodium orthovanadate, and 10% glycerol) with complete EDTA-free protease and PhosSTOP phosphatase inhibitors (Sigma Aldrich, Saint Louis, MO, USA). Protein was quantified using the DC protein assay (Bio-Rad, Hercules, CA, USA). Approximately 15 µg of protein was loaded in precast 4–20% Criterion TGX gels (Bio-Rad, Hercules, CA, USA), ran for 1 h, transferred to a PVDF membrane with the Trans-Blot® Turbo™ system (Bio-Rad, Hercules, CA, USA) for 30 min, blocked for 1 h at room temperature, incubated overnight with primary antibodies and incubated with the secondary antibody for 1 h. Images were captured via the ChemiDoc Molecular Imager and band quantification with ImageLab analysis software (both Bio-Rad, Hercules, CA, USA). Expression values were determined by chemiluminescent immunodetection and normalized to appropriate loading controls. Immunoblotting was performed using commercially available antibodies from Abcam (Cambridge, MA USA): DAB2 (#ab33441; 1:500), Cell Signaling Technology (Danvers, MA USA): GAPDH (#2118; 1:25,000), LsBio (Seattle, WA USA): LRP2 (#LS-c667890; 1:250), Santa Cruz Biotechnology (Dallas, TX USA): Vitamin D receptor (#sc-13133; 1:100), GAPDH (#sc-32233; 1:40,000), and Thermo Fisher Scientific, Scientific, Waltham, MA, USA): Vitamin D binding protein (#PA5-29082; 1:500).

3. Results

3.1. Patient Characteristics

Patient demographics, tobacco and alcohol use, and nutrient levels are summarized in Table 1. A total of nineteen HNC patients enrolled, 9 Black and 10 White. Black patients were significantly younger (53.6 years ± 9.4) upon HNC diagnosis compared to White patients (64.3 years ± 14.4) (*p*-value = 0.036). One hundred percent of the participants reported alcohol use. Compared to White patients, Black patients were both more likely to have a history of smoking and reported higher current smoking status. Ever smoking was reported by 66.7% of Black patients versus 30% of Whites. Among patients who smoked the average years of smoking was 24.6 years among Blacks and 34.7 years among White patients, in alignment with Whites being diagnosed at a later age. Black patients had non-significantly elevated mean body mass index (BMI) compared to Whites. All patients reported low fruit and vegetable consumption, two servings per day. Whites reported significantly higher rates of sun protection via sunscreen or protective clothing when sun exposure was ≥2 h/daily (*p*-value = 0.003, Chi-square). All Blacks reporting protecting from the sun did so by clothing or hats, not sunscreen use, whereas Whites protected with both sunscreen and apparel. Both groups reported similar sun exposure in terms of intense sun exposure, weekly sun exposure, and exposure during summer and winter months. Blacks and Whites did not differ significantly based on months living in Florida. Blacks averaged 11.0 months and Whites 10.4 months in Florida, with one Black and 3 White patients reporting living outside of Florida for at least three months. Black and White HNC patients differed significantly in terms of education, with Whites reporting significantly higher rates of college graduation as well as completing graduate or professional degrees. In contrast the highest level of education for Blacks was high school graduation, 55.6% vs. 10% among White patients. Reported annual income levels were significantly lower among Black compared to White HNC patients. Physical activity levels were low for both Black and White patients with over 70% reporting rarely or never exercising.

Table 1. Characteristics of newly diagnosed head and neck cancer patients.

Characteristics	Race	
	Black	White
Average Age (years, ±SD)	53.6 (±9.4)	64.3 (±14.4) #
Ratio of Men:Women (n)	5:4	8:2
Alcohol Use	100%	100%
Current Smoker	33.3%	20%
Ever Smoker	66.7%	30%
Body Mass Index (mean kg/m^2)	27.1	24.2
Fruit & Vegetable Servings/Daily	2.0	2.1
Sun Protection, Never or Seldom	89.9%	20.0%
Sun Protection, Always or Mostly	11.1%	80.0% #
Middle School or Some High School (n)	22.2% (2)	0%
High School Graduate (n)	55.6% (5)	10% (1)
Some College (n)	11.1% (1)	30.0% (3)
College Graduate or Professional Degree (n)	11.1% (1)	60.0% (6) #

Education is reported as highest level achieved; Sun protection use refers to using clothing or sunscreen for periods of sun exposer ≥2 h a day; and # Statistically significantly different based on Students T-Test or the Chi-Square test statistic for population differences across categories (p-value < 0.05).

3.2. Blood Levels of Vitamin D, Parathyroid, and Calcium Among Head and Neck Cancer Patients

Table 2 reports serum and plasma measurements by patient racial group. Generally, the circulating metabolite, 25-Hydroxyvitamin D (25-OH) vitamin D is considered the most valid indicator of vitamin D status as it reflects the last 15 days; compared to the active metabolite which reflects approximately the last 15 h. The mean level of 25-Hydroxyvitamin D among Blacks diagnosed with HNC (20 ng/mL) was significantly lower than the mean among Whites (27.30 ng/mL, p-value = 0.04). In addition, to mean 25-Hydroxyvitamin D levels being lower in Blacks, no Black HNC patients had vitamin D levels greater than or equal to 30 ng/mL, the level associated with optimal regulation of PTH, calcium absorption and bone density. In contrast, 30% of White patients had 25-Hydroxyvitamin D levels over 30 ng/mL. About 50% of Blacks presented with 25-Hydroxyvitamin D levels in the 10–19.9 ng/mL range compared to only 10% of Whites further supporting that even in sunny South Florida vitamin D levels are lower in Blacks HNC patients compared to White HNC patients. There were no differences noted in 1,25-Dihydroxyvitamin D, which has relatively short half-life and is not considered an indicator of true vitamin D status, but rather a marker modulated only in cases of severe deficiency. Similarly, there were no differences in circulating PTH or calcium levels between the two patient populations.

Table 2. Blood levels of vitamin D, parathyroid, and calcium among head and neck cancer patients.

Measurement	Race		p-Value
	Black	White	
25-Hydroxyvitamin D (ng/mL)	20.00 (±5.98)	27.30 (±9.86)	0.04
1,25-Dihydroxyvitamin D (pg/mL)	43.86 (±20.80)	36.80 (±14.33)	0.21
Patients with Low Vitamin D (<19.9 ng/mL)	50%	10%	
Patients with Intermediate Vitamin D (20.0–29.9 ng/mL)	50%	60%	
Patients with Sufficient Vitamin D (≥30 ng/mL)	0%	30%	0.06
Parathyroid (pg/mL)	35.50 (±23.95)	35.89 (±14.93)	0.48
Calcium (pg/mL)	9.34 (0.58)	9.09 (±0.68)	0.21

p-value based on Students T-test for nutrient levels and Chi-square test statistic for vitamin D differences by concentrations in the populations (<0.05 considered statistically significant).

3.3. Nutrient Levels of Vitamin D and Calcium Based on Dietary Screeners

Block Vitamin D and Calcium Screeners were utilized to gain insight into how dietary and supplement sources of vitamin D may impact circulating levels with the results summarized in Table 3.

Black HNC patients reported (non-significantly) lower total vitamin D intake compared to Whites. Interestingly, compared to Whites, Black patients reported marginally higher intake of vitamin D from dietary sources (p-value = 0.07), whereas White patients reported non-significantly higher supplemental intake of both vitamin D and also calcium; 50% of Whites reported use of supplemental vitamin D compared to 22.2% of Black HNC patients.

Table 3. Nutrient levels of vitamin D and calcium based on dietary screeners.

Measurement	Race		p-Value
	Black	White	
Total Vitamin D (IU)	174.70 (±154.37)	276.93 (±206.03)	0.23
Dietary Vitamin D (IU)	121.24 (±113.77)	62.92 (±40.10)	0.07
Supplemental Vitamin D (IU)	88.89 (±176.38)	200.00 (±210.82)	0.12
Patients Supplementing Vitamin D	22.2%	50.0%	0.21
Total Calcium (mg)	678.40 (±450.42)	542.93 (±280.74)	0.22
Dietary Calcium (mg)	535.16 (±317.30)	447.87 (±286.89)	0.27
Supplemental Calcium (mean, mg)	25.28 (±56.10)	83.69 (±82.94)	0.31
Patients Supplementing Calcium	44.4%	60.0%	0.34

p-Value based on Students T-test or Chi-square test for population measures (<0.05 considered statistically significant).

3.4. Top miRs Dysregulated in HNC Cell Lines by Vitamin D

A total of 5 miRs were highly significantly dysregulated ($p < 5.00E-04$) in either CAL-27 or SCC-25 cell lines following vitamin D treatment as shown in Figure 1. In CAL-27 cells, hsa-miR-7-1-3p and hsa-miR-632 were significantly dysregulated by vitamin D as compared to a vehicle treated cells (p-value = 2.36E-05, −26.459 Fold-change and p-value = 9.56E-05 and 47.487 Fold-change, respectively) (Figure 1A). Vitamin D treatment of the SCC-25 cells resulted in significantly altered hsa-miR-331-5p (p-value = 3.82E-05, −45.008 Fold Change), hsa-miR-335 (p-value = 3.83E-05, −63.611 Fold Change), and hsa-miR-616 (p-value = 6.73E-05, 66.355 Fold Change), respectively (Figure 1A).

Figure 1C,D illustrate the total gene targets for all significantly down and up-regulated miRs, respectively, and overlapping gene targets of miRs altered in the same direction by vitamin D treatment (detailed in Table S4). The total 157 validated genes stem from the three up-regulated miRs which contrasts to 3082 genes regulated by the two down-regulated miRs. In Figure 1C, down-regulated miR-335 contributes the majority of presumably up-regulated gene targets compared to miR-7-1-3p. The two down-regulated miRs share 32 validated gene targets (Table S4) with diverse cancer-associated functions. Figure 1D illustrates the lack of overlapping genes among up-regulated miRs. There is only one common gene target, POLD3, that is shared between miR-632 and miR-331-5p, but not miR-616-3p. Overall, there is a considerably reduced number of validated gene targets for the up-regulated miRs compared to the down-regulated; still, a number of resultant genes have documented roles in cell proliferation, DNA damage response, cancer stemness, extracellular matrix organization, and genome stability (Table S5). In contrast with the down-regulated miRs, all three of the up-regulated miRs have similar numbers of validated gene targets.

Next, validated gene targets regulated by the vitamin D altered miRNAs were determined using miRTarBase. The number of validated gene targets associated with significantly altered miRs in each cell line are depicted in Figure 1B. In SCC-25 and CAL-27 cells a total of 3014 and 225 validated gene targets were identified, respectively (Figure 1B). Specifically, 63 validated gene targets were identified for hsa-miR-331-5p, 2898 for hsa-miR-335, and 53 for hsa-miR-616 in SCC-25 cells, respectively. In CAL-27 cells, 184 validated gene targets were stemmed from hsa-miR-7-1 and 41 from hsa-miR-632. Figure 1B shows the total number of validated gene targets regulated by vitamin D altered miRs stratified by cell line, including 45 common or overlapping genes. A comprehensive list of validated gene targets and their respective miRs is available in Table S2, with Table S3 ($n = 45$) and Table S4 ($n = 32$), showing the identity of overlapping genes depicted in Figure 1B–D, respectively.

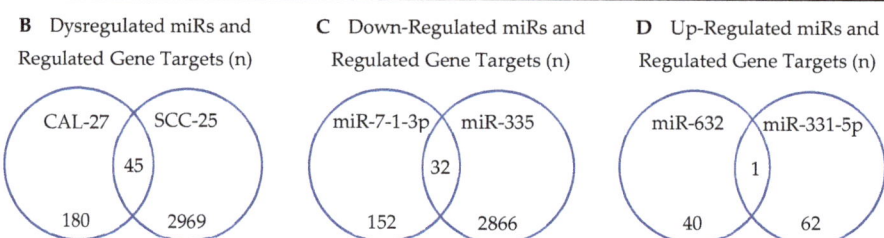

Figure 1. Summary of Significantly Dysregulated miRs following Vitamin D Treatment of Head and Neck Cancer Cell Lines. (**A**) Vitamin D altered miRs in CAL-27 and SCC-25 cells, the direction of change, and the number of validated gene targets regulated by each miR with 45 overlapping genes. (**B**) Validated gene targets regulated by Vitamin D modulated miRs in CAL-27 and SCC-25 cells and overlapping gene targets. (**C**) Specific miRs down regulated by Vitamin D in CAL-27 and SCC-25 cells, with overlapping genes identified (n = 32). (**D**) Up-regulated miRs showing individual results and overlapping gene targets (n = 1).

3.5. DAVID Enrichment Analysis

Two approaches of enrichment analysis were applied. The first based on the direction of miR change and resultant genes (157 and 3082) regulated by those miRs altered by vitamin D and the second based on all miRs and resultant common genes altered in both cell lines by vitamin D treatment (n = 45). The genes regulated by vitamin D driven miR dysregulation were analyzed for their respective Kyoto Encyclopedia of Genes and Genomes (KEGG) pathways, biological processes, molecular function, and disease linkages. Table 4 summarizes the top most significantly altered functional terms based on all up or down-regulated miRs and subsequent validated gene targets (n = 157 and 3082). The top KEGG pathway for the up-regulated miRs, presumably down-regulated gene targets, is Pathways in cancer (p-value = 0.01, FDR = 0.90) with nine genes contributing (*CKD4, DVL3, ETS1, MSH6, XIAP, RHOA, SMAD4, CCDC6,* and *LPAR2*). Expanded results, beyond the top changes, are detailed in Table S5. Stemming from vitamin D down-regulated miRs, the most significant identified KEGG pathway (Table 4) is Steroid biosynthesis (p-value = 7.72E-06, FDR = 2.2E-03, 13 genes), followed by MAPK signaling pathway (p-value = 3.89E-05, FDR = 5.52E-03, 65 genes), and Signaling pathways regulating pluripotency of stem cells (p-value = 6.80E-05, FDR = 6.43E-03, 41 genes). Additional significantly altered pathways linked to down-regulated miRs include Estrogen, PI3K-AKT, RAS, and Chemokine signaling (Table S5).

Table 4. Top pathways, biological processes, and molecular functions and diseases for altered MiR. Target Genes following vitamin D Treatment of CAL-27 and SCC-25 head and neck cell lines.

Functional Parameter	MiR Alteration	Term (n)	p-Value	Benjamini-Hochberg FDR
KEGG Pathway	Up-regulated	Pathways in Cancer (9)	0.01	0.90
	Down-regulated	Steroid Biosynthesis (13)	7.72E-06	2.2E-03
Biological Process	Up-regulated	Positive regulation of transcription from RNA polymerase II promoter (18)	3.31E-03	0.97
	Down-regulated	Negative regulation of cell proliferation (95)	5.27E-06	0.03
Molecular Function	Up-regulated	Protein binding (96)	1.50E-04	0.04
	Down-regulated	Transcription factor activity, sequence-specific DNA binding (194)	1.47E-05	0.03
Diseases	Up-regulated	Cancer (95)	4.30 E-04	7.71E-03
	Down-regulated	Chemodependency (736)	2.91E-12	5.53E-11

FDR: False Discovery Rate.

Nine biological processes were significantly altered by vitamin D based on genes linked to down-regulated miRs including Negative regulation of cell proliferation (p-value = 5.27E-06, FDR = 0.03, 95 genes), Angiogenesis (p-value = 1.03E-05, FDR = 0.03, 60 genes), and Canonical WNT signaling (p-value = 2.26E-05, FDR = 0.03, 29 genes) as well as Extracellular matrix and Cell adhesion. Genes stemming from up-regulated miRs resulted in Positive regulation of transcription from RNA polymerase II promoter as the top process, but it was not significant once FDR corrected.

In terms of molecular function, vitamin D linked up-regulated miRs and subsequent genes identified only Protein binding (p-value = 1.50E-04, FDR = 0.04, 96 genes) as a significant function.

Down-regulated miRs and related genes revealed only Transcription factor activity, sequence-specific DNA binding (p-value = 1.47E-05, FDR = 0.03, 194 genes). Finally, top diseases identified based on miRs up and down-regulated by vitamin D include Cancer and Chemodependency, respectively.

In addition, enrichment analysis was conducted based on the 45 validated gene targets shared in both vitamin D treated HNC cell lines (as illustrated in Figure 1A and detailed in Table S3) revealing Focal adhesion as the only significant pathway (p-value = 3.20E-04, FDR = 2.90E-02, 6 genes) following vitamin D treatment. Genes included *COL4A1, EGFR, IGF1R, ITGA1, PAK3*, and *VEGFA*, many with relevance to HNC. Similar to the results stemming from up or down-regulated miR driven genes (Figure 1C,D), Protein binding was the top molecular function identified based on the 45 shared genes in CAL-27 and SCC-25 cells.

3.6. Protein Level Changes in HNC Cells Following Vitamin D Treatment

Western blot results implicate response differences to vitamin D treatment between CAL-27 cells and SCC-25 cells (Figure 2). Western results show that levels of LRP2 and DAB2 proteins are constitutively lower in CAL-27 cells as compared to SCC-25 cells. The vitamin D receptor is expressed more strongly in SCC-25 as well. However, vitamin D binding protein is expressed more strongly in CAL-27 cells. Vitamin D treatment increased levels of the vitamin D receptor in both HNC cell lines, with strongest effects noted in SCC-25 cells. Vitamin D treatment modestly increased DAB2 levels only in CAL-27 cells. Vitamin D driven LRP2 increases were only observed in SCC-25 cells supporting differential responses between the cell lines. Findings may reflect that HNC cells increase their ability to endocytose vitamin D and bind vitamin D at the nuclear receptor in response to vitamin D treatment. The observed differences between cell lines may be due to molecular differences between them, raising the possibility that there may also be different molecular profiles in patient populations; expression of these proteins should be examined in patient samples. These findings may have relevance to the relative importance of free versus bound vitamin D in HNC and to the metabolism and processing of vitamin D in vivo [38,39].

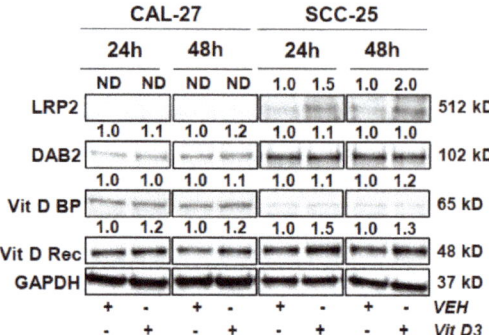

Figure 2. Modulation of vitamin D related proteins. Western blot results for CAL-27 and SCC-25 HNC cell lines following 2 μM vitamin D treatment. ND indicates no detection. Quantitation was normalized to GAPDH as a loading control and fold-change from vehicle reported.

Proteomic profiling was also employed as an untargeted approach to determine additional proteins modified by vitamin D utilizing of SCC-25 and CAL-27 human HNC cell lines with results summarized in Table 5. A total of six proteins were identified as highly dysregulated by vitamin D. Nucleophosmin, Lactoylglutathione lyase, Heat shock protein beta-1, and Ras-related protein Rap-2b were markedly downregulated in SCC-25 cells. In CAL-27 cells, Peroxiredoxin-1 and Histone H2A type 1-J were down and up-regulated, respectively (Table 5).

Table 5. Proteins modified by vitamin D treatment of head and neck cancer cell lines.

Cells	Spot	Protein	Symbol	Fold-Change	Uniprot No.
SCC-25	15/16 *	Nucleophosmin	NPM_HUMAN	−2.36	P06748
	28	Lactoylglutathione lyase	LGUL_HUMAN	−2.73	Q04760
	31	Heat shock protein beta-1	HSPB1_HUMAN	−2.57	P04792
	51	Ras-related protein Rap-2b	RAP2B_HUMAN	−3.39	P61225
CAL-27	30	Peroxiredoxin-1	PRDX1_HUMAN	−2.60	Q06830
	31	Histone H2A type 1-J	H2A1J_HUMAN	+2.48	Q99878

* The fold-change for Nucleophosmin is an average of the two detected spots 15 and 16 following treatment with vitamin D.

4. Discussion

Many studies have investigated the underlying factors that contribute to racial disparities in HNC patients pointing to a complex and multifactorial etiology. Black HNC patients have a 20–30% reduction in five-year relative survival compared to Whites [40,41]. In turn, Black Americans have higher age-adjusted HNC mortality rates compared to Whites [42]. The literature supports that Black patients are more likely to be diagnosed with higher stage disease and distant metastases, and experience increased mortality following a diagnosis of HNC [9,43,44]. Black HNC patients are also significantly less likely to undergo surgical treatment, even among patients with similar health insurance status [9,45,46]. Sociodemographic factors are frequently cited as dominate causes to cancer disparities, including HNC [47–50]. However, a recent meta-analysis including ten studies with greater than 100,000 patients reported poorer survival among Black HNC patients after controlling for socioeconomic factors as well as tumor stage and treatment variables supporting that additional factors contribute to the observed racial differences [51]. Thus, the objective of this prospective pilot study was to assess vitamin D status in newly diagnosed HNC patients stratified by race and to gain potential mechanistic insight by performing in vitro studies utilizing human HNC cell lines. Among Whites vitamin D status is inversely associated with HNC, low vitamin D levels in White HNC patients is also linked to cancer progression, increased recurrence, and metastatic disease [13,14,19]. Despite well documented hypovitaminosis D in Blacks, vitamin D status has not been assessed in HNC patients stratified by race.

Our pilot study results showed significantly lower levels of circulating vitamin D (25-hydroxyvitamin D) in newly diagnosed Black HNC patients (20.0 ng/mL) compared to the White patients (27.3 ng/mL). Although this is the first such report in Blacks with HNC, it does align with earlier research in Blacks without cancer which also reported reduced vitamin D levels in the range of 18.0–25.1 ng/mL [15,16,52–55]. Higher levels of melanin pigmentation in darker skin is known to be a contributory cause of lower levels of vitamin D among Blacks. In addition, an inverse association between BMI and vitamin D level has been noted previously, including during interventional studies [56–58]. Although the mean BMI was higher among Black HNC patients and more Blacks were overweight based on BMI, the differences were not statistically significant. Sun exposure is also known to impact vitamin D levels and to interact with obesity [59]. All HNC patients reported similar levels of sun exposure, but Whites reported more frequent use of sunscreen compared to Blacks. Overall, both groups of HNC patients had low levels of vitamin D, with none of the Black patients and only 30% of the White patients having levels ≥30 ng/mL, which is required for optimal PTH regulation, calcium absorption, and bone density [25]. Moreover, 50% of Black HNC patients had deficient vitamin D levels, below 20 ng/mL. Interestingly, dietary and supplement intake measures also indicated that Black HNC patients had lower total vitamin D, but they received more from dietary sources, whereas White patients supplemented more frequently. Two previous studies have also reported lower supplemental vitamin D intake in Blacks compared to Whites [60,61]. Although randomized clinical trials and interventional studies with vitamin D have had mixed results, targeting deficient populations may prove beneficial, especially in the context of racial disparities [10,62,63].

Similar to previous larger studies and published metanalysis focused on racial disparities in HNC [8,9,64,65], our pilot study results support that Black and White HNC patients differ significantly in terms of highest educational obtainment and annual income level. Exposure to other known HNC risk factors appeared similar between Whites and Blacks, including alcohol use and current smoking status. Blacks HNC patients did have non-significantly increased rates of ever smoking compared to Whites, and they were diagnosed about ten years earlier than Whites with HNC for reasons that remain unclear. In addition, Blacks who smoked, did so on average for 10 fewer years compared to Whites when diagnosed with HNC, raising the possibility that other, less well characterized factors may indeed be contributing to HNC progression and disparate survival among Blacks.

Tobacco, alcohol, and HPV are considered among the major modifiable risk factors for HNC [5]. Tobacco use has declined in the United States reducing tobacco linked HNC and in turn reducing age adjusted HNC incidence rates among Blacks [8,66]; yet, Blacks still have elevated age adjusted mortality rates for HNC compared to Whites [3,8,42,67]. In addition, HPV-positive HNC has markedly increased in recent years, but is generally more common among White males and has more favorable treatment outcomes [68–71]; thus, neither tobacco use or HPV prevalence patterns appear to fully explain the racial disparity in HNC outcomes. Although this is a small pilot study, we report differences in vitamin D levels among newly diagnosed Black and White HNC patients which may contribute to disparities in HNC outcomes. The topic merits further investigation in a larger cohort study incorporating additional relevant clinical variables such as cancer stage, grade, subsite analysis, treatment choice and survival outcomes.

In vitro studies were undertaken to explore potential mechanisms of vitamin D activity in two human HNC cell lines, CAL-27 and SCC-25, both of squamous cell origin. Vitamin D treatment significantly altered five miRs, each regulating between 41 to 2898 genes. Of the miRs modulated by vitamin D, Hsa-miR-7-1 and hsa-miR-335 were significantly down-regulated; whereas, hsa-miR-331-5p, hsa-miR-616, and hsa-miR-632 were significantly up-regulated. Enrichment analysis via DAVID was conducted based on the genes regulated by each miR within a cell line, and also separately based on genes regulated by vitamin D induced up or down-regulated miRs revealing effects on multiple cancer relevant pathways and processes. There is evidence that both down-regulated miRs have oncogenic activity in HNC or precursors lesions [72–85]. Analysis of genes regulated by down-regulated miRs revealed modulation of multiple pathways relevant to HNC including MAPK, PI3K, RAS, and Chemokine signaling. Additionally, the top biological processes altered based on genes regulated by down-regulated miRs was Negative regulation of cellular proliferation followed by Angiogenesis; Canonical WNT signaling and Cell adhesion were also among the significant processes. Two previous studies investigating the role of miR-7 in lung cancer, which shares risk factors with HNC, reported that miR-7 is induced by EGFR/Ras/ERK/Myc signaling leading to aberrant cell proliferation and migration [75,86]. Together these results support a cancer inhibitory role for vitamin D through impacting key drivers identified in HNC [87]. Considering that HPV-positive HNC are documented to have double the PI3-kinase activating mutations (50% as compared to HPV-negative ones, which have about 25%) future studies should expand evaluations to include HPV-positive models or tissues [88].

Vitamin D treatment of HNC cell lines up-regulated hsa- miR-331-5p, hsa-miR-616-3p, and hsa-miR-632. Combined, these miRs presumably down-regulate 157 gene targets, many with well documented roles in cell proliferation, signal transduction, DNA damage response, cancer stemness, adhesion, extracellular matrix (EMT) organization, and genome stability (i.e., *MDM4, CDK4, MSH6, XIAP, ETS1, RHOA, SMAD4, POLD3, COL3A1, FGF2, FOXF2,* and *SOX5*). Notably, *MDM4* plays a role in regulating p53 and has been linked to cancer recurrence and poor outcomes in HNC patients [89–91]. As another example, the transcription of *CDK4* is linked to tobacco mediated oral carcinogenesis and acts as a potent cyclin dependent Kinase 4 Regulatory Factor (KRF) and a potential cancer target [92]. In terms of specific miRs, vitamin D treatment increased miR-331-5p. Reports support that miR-331-5p, as well as the 3p strand, differ in patients with laryngeal squamous cell carcinoma [80,82,93]. Moreover, overexpression of miR-331-3p inhibits cell proliferation and invasion while promoting apoptosis via reduced expression of elF4B and subsequent inhibition of the phosphorylation of PI3K/AKT signaling molecules [94]. Similarly, in lung cancer, increased expression of miR-331 has cancer inhibitory effects through down-regulation of MAPK, suppression of EMT as well as inhibition of metastatic ability of cancer cells in vitro and in vivo [95,96]. Results for miR-632 in the context of HNC appear mixed. One study reported that under-expression of miR-632 in saliva from oral squamous cell carcinoma patients compared to healthy controls suggesting increasing levels by vitamin D may prove favorable [97]. Similarly, Lu et al. suggested miR-632 to be a tumor suppressor in laryngeal cancers where it is down-regulated potentially via CCR6 and p38 dependent mechanisms [98]. Conversely, another study reported that increased expression of miR-632 in laryngeal tissues and cell lines accelerates cell proliferation, migration, and invasion supporting a more oncogenic function [99]. Contradictory finding may be due to heterogeneity of cell lines and even patient samples. It is well documented that miRs can act in a cancer specific manner, but there is less research documenting site specific effects within a target or evaluating additional sources of heterogeneity. To our knowledge miR-616-3p has not been reported as dysregulated in HNC. Our data supports that vitamin D modulates a select panel of miRs in HNC cell lines, which ultimately interferes with many cancer hallmarks. Additional research has evaluated vitamin D modulation of miRs in lung, cervical, and breast cancers [66]. However, the miRs identified in previously published studies do not overlap with those identified as significantly modulated by vitamin D in HNC cell lines.

Proteomic profiling was conducted to assess whether vitamin D held potential to impact or correct known defects in protein machinery associated with HNC. In total, vitamin D markedly increased one protein and down-regulated five proteins, all with documented roles in cancer [22,100–104]. Nucleophosmin (NPM), is associated with evasion of apoptosis, increased cancer cell viability, growth, and cell proliferation [105], and was down-regulated following vitamin D treatment of SCC-25 cells.

In a recent study increased expression of NPM was reported in 82% of laryngeal cancer tissues and NPM knockdown inhibited laryngeal cancer cell survival [23]. The full results revealed an oncogenic role for NPM in laryngeal cancer through its effects on apoptosis and cellular growth. Overexpression of NPM has been documented in oral squamous cell carcinoma (OSCC); immunohistochemistry and immunofluorescent staining showed significantly elevated expression levels in OSCC patient samples compared to control [106]. Another OSCC focused study reported NPM silencing induced genes involved in apoptosis and downregulated of procarcinogenesis genes [107]. The down-regulation of NPM following vitamin D treatment is consistent with our enrichment analysis results given NPM has a role in the Myc-ARF-p53 pathway and the molecule functions as a histone chaperone [108,109]. The latter may also explain the reduction noted in Histone H2A type 1-j (H2A1J) following vitamin D. Similarly, lactoylglutathione lyase (GLO1), was down-regulated in HNC cell lines after vitamin D treatment and is documented to be significantly overexpressed in OSCC tissues [110]. Importantly, there is recent evidence that GLO1 plays a critical role in invasion and metastasis of oropharyngeal tumors, in addition to initiation and maintenance of tumor growth. It has been reported that patients with high GLO1 expression have significantly shorter disease-specific survival [110]. GLO1 has only been characterized in a small number of HNC studies as cited; however, it is shown to have multiple roles in promoting cancer cell survival, proliferation, and is a likely target for chemotherapy based on the broader literature [111].

Vitamin D down-regulated Heat shock protein beta-1 (HSP27), a multi-functional protein with well documented roles in HNC inflammation, proliferation, cancer progression, stemness, EMT, and more recently radio-sensitization and therapeutic resistance [21,112–117]. Moreover, in SCC of the tongue HSP27 inhibition represses apoptosis and enhances sensitivity to chemotherapies [21] supporting a role for agents that reduce or impair HSP27. HSP27 is also a downstream target of the PI3K/AKT signaling pathway [112] which links our proteomic results to our enrichment analysis based on vitamin D induced miR alterations. Finally, expression levels of a number of RAB family members segregate metastatic versus non-metastatic oral cancers, including *RAB2B* [118]. In addition, the latter study reported knock-down of *RAB5, RAB7*, and *RAB11* in SCC-25 cells inhibits cancer cell migration and invasion supporting that agents downregulating RAB family members may impart cancer inhibitory potential.

Two additional proteins were altered by vitamin D treatment specifically in CAL-27 HNC cells. H2A1-J was up-regulated by vitamin D but has not been reported on in HNC. However, H2A1 depletion is linked to induction of cancer cell stemness in hepatocellular carcinoma [119] which aligns with gene enrichment analysis conducted based on miRs dysregulated by vitamin D in our study. Additionally, modulated by vitamin D in CAL-27 cells was Peroxiredoxin-1 (PRX-1). It was down-regulated, further supporting a role for vitamin D in suppressing HNC associated pathways. An evaluation of Prx-1 in human OSCC tissues showed elevated expression in OSCC samples compared to controls; interestingly investigators also saw a dose-dependent elevation in Prx-1 such that expression was highest in smokers with OSCC and lowest in control tissues [120]. Additional research has shown silencing of Prx-1 in CAL-27 and SCC-15 blocks promotion of proliferation and migration and Prx-1 has the ability to promote EMT processes via NFκB linked activity, as has been reported for NPM and HSP27 [120,121]. Thus, vitamin D treatment of HNC cell lines results in potent down-regulation of proteins implicated in multiple aspects of cancer, from inflammation, to aberrant proliferation, to migration, altered EMT, adhesion, and therapeutic resistance. Interestingly, a number of the vitamin D inhibited proteins are known to converge on a common transcription factor, NFkB which has also been proposed as a potential target for increased therapeutic efficacy in HNC [122].

5. Conclusions

Limitations of our research include a relatively small sample size, but this was intended to be a first assessment for determining whether a larger study was warranted. In addition, our small sample size of 19 HNC patients precludes making any linkages to sex, stage, grade, site-specific effects, or survival. Finally, to our knowledge there are no HNC cell lines available for research which are derived from Black patients; thus, our in vitro work was limited to HNC cell lines derived from White HNC patients.

Still, our data shows for the first time that circulating vitamin D levels are significantly depressed in newly diagnosed Black HNC patients compared to Whites. Furthermore, in vitro studies targeting mechanisms by which vitamin D may inhibit HNC revealed activity targeting early to late cancer related events; spanning from inflammation and chemokine changes to alterations in EMT, drivers of recurrence, and therapeutic resistance. Despite mixed results from vitamin D trials in other targets, our results support that vitamin D modulates a number of cancer pathways, biological processes, genes, and proteins with well documented roles in HNC development, response to therapy and disease recurrence which remains a significant issue. Study results support conducting future research to evaluate vitamin D in larger cohorts stratified by race and with sufficient power to interpret key clinical correlates and survival outcomes. Our results also revealed new vitamin D induced miR alterations which paralleled changes in many HNC relevant proteins paving the way for future genetic studies to interrogate miR dysregulation relative protein function. Ultimately, our results may inform and guide future in vitro, in vivo, and clinical chemoprevention studies assessing the efficacy of vitamin D as an intervention strategy for vulnerable or high risk populations, whether it be based on race or other variables imparting increased risk for HNC.

Supplementary Materials: The following are available online at http://www.mdpi.com/2072-6643/12/9/2638/s1, Figure S1: Vitamin D3 inhibits HNC cell viability, Table S1: MicroRNA platform and sequence information, Table S2: Comprehensive list of vitamin D altered miRs stratified by direction of change and individual validated gene targets, Table S3: Validated gene targets altered in both CAL-27 and SCC-25 HNC cell lines by vitamin D (n = 45), Table S4: Overlapping target genes of miRs altered in the same direction by vitamin D (n = 32), Table S5: Top pathways, biological processes, molecular functions and diseases for vitamin D altered miRs and validated gene targets in HNC cell Lines.

Author Contributions: Conceptualization, L.A.K., W.J.G., J.J.H., and E.F.; methodology, L.A.K., E.F., J.J.H., W.J.G., and A.M.M.; validation, K.M.W., M.I., and C.H.; formal analysis, M.I., C.H., and L.A.K.; investigation, W.J.G., E.F., K.M.W., and L.A.K.; resources, L.A.K. and W.J.G.; data curation, L.A.K., M.I., C.H., and K.M.W.; writing—original draft preparation, L.A.K. and M.I.; writing—review and editing, M.I., A.M.M., K.M.W., J.J.H., C.H., and L.A.K.; visualization, L.A.K., and M.I.; supervision, W.J.G. and L.A.K.; project administration, L.A.K.; and funding acquisition, W.J.G. and L.A.K. All authors have read and agreed to the published version of the manuscript.

Funding: This research was mainly funded by the UM Sylvester Cancer Center at the University of Miami with additional support from the Rogel Cancer Center and The Section of Thoracic Surgery, Department of Surgery at the University of Michigan.

Acknowledgments: We thank the patients who participated in the research and clinical and technical support staff.

Conflicts of Interest: The authors declare no conflict of interest.

References

1. Rettig, E.M.; D'Souza, G. Epidemiology of Head and Neck Cancer. *Surg. Oncol. Clin. N. Am.* **2015**, *24*, 379–396. [CrossRef] [PubMed]
2. Wissinger, E.; Griebsch, I.; Lungershausen, J.; Foster, T.; Pashos, C.L. The Economic Burden of Head and Neck Cancer: A Systematic Literature Review. *Pharmacoeconomics* **2014**, *32*, 865–882. [CrossRef] [PubMed]
3. Daraei, P.; Moore, C.E. Racial Disparity among the Head and Neck Cancer Population. *J. Cancer Educ.* **2015**, *30*, 546–551. [CrossRef] [PubMed]
4. Chaturvedi, A.K.; Engels, E.A.; Pfeiffer, R.M.; Hernandez, B.Y.; Xiao, W.; Kim, E.; Jiang, B.; Goodman, M.T.; Sibug-Saber, M.; Cozen, W.; et al. Human Papillomavirus and Rising Oropharyngeal Cancer Incidence in the United States. *J. Clin. Oncol.* **2011**, *29*, 4294–4301. [CrossRef] [PubMed]
5. Benson, E.; Li, R.; Eisele, D.; Fakhry, C. The Clinical Impact of HPV Tumor Status upon Head and Neck Squamous Cell Carcinomas. *Oral Oncol.* **2014**, *50*, 565–574. [CrossRef]
6. O'Rorke, M.A.; Ellison, M.V.; Murray, L.J.; Moran, M.; James, J.; Anderson, L.A. Human Papillomavirus Related Head and Neck Cancer Survival: A Systematic Review and Meta-Analysis. *Oral Oncol.* **2012**, *48*, 1191–1201. [CrossRef]

7. Al-Othman, M.O.F.; Morris, C.G.; Logan, H.L.; Hinerman, R.W.; Amdur, R.J.; Mendenhall, W.M. Impact of Race on Outcome after Definitive Radiotherapy for Squamous Cell Carcinoma of the Head and Neck. *Cancer* **2003**, *98*, 2467–2472. [CrossRef]
8. Goodwin, W.J.; Thomas, G.R.; Parker, D.F.; Joseph, D.; Levis, S.; Franzmann, E.; Anello, C.; Hu, J.J. Unequal Burden of Head and Neck Cancer in the United States. *Head Neck* **2008**, *30*, 358–371. [CrossRef]
9. Kompelli, A.; Cartmell, K.B.; Sterba, K.R.; Alberg, A.J.; Xiao, C.C.; Sood, A.J.; Garrett-Mayer, E.; White-Gilbertson, S.J.; Rosenzweig, S.A.; Day, T.A. An Assessment of Racial Differences in Epidemiological, Clinical and Psychosocial Factors among Head and Neck Cancer Patients at the Time of Surgery. *World J. Otorhinolaryngol. Head Neck Surg.* **2020**, *6*, 41–48. [CrossRef]
10. Mondul, A.M.; Weinstein, S.J.; Layne, T.M.; Albanes, D. Vitamin D and Cancer Risk and Mortality: State of the Science, Gaps, and Challenges. *Epidemiol. Rev.* **2017**, *39*, 28–48. [CrossRef]
11. Zhao, Y.; Chen, C.; Pan, W.; Gao, M.; He, W.; Mao, R.; Lin, T.; Huang, J. Comparative Efficacy of Vitamin D Status in Reducing the Risk of Bladder Cancer: A Systematic Review and Network Meta-Analysis. *Nutrition* **2016**, *32*, 515–523. [CrossRef] [PubMed]
12. Xu, Y.; Shao, X.; Yao, Y.; Xu, L.; Chang, L.; Jiang, Z.; Lin, Z. Positive Association between Circulating 25-Hydroxyvitamin D Levels and Prostate Cancer Risk: New Findings from an Updated Meta-Analysis. *J. Cancer Res. Clin. Oncol.* **2014**, *140*, 1465–1477. [CrossRef] [PubMed]
13. Yokosawa, E.B.; Arthur, A.E.; Rentschler, K.M.; Wolf, G.T.; Rozek, L.S.; Mondul, A.M. Vitamin D Intake and Survival and Recurrence in Head and Neck Cancer Patients. *Laryngoscope* **2018**, *128*, E371–E376. [CrossRef] [PubMed]
14. Vaughan-Shaw, P.G.; O'Sullivan, F.; Farrington, S.M.; Theodoratou, E.; Campbell, H.; Dunlop, M.G.; Zgaga, L. The Impact of Vitamin D Pathway Genetic Variation and Circulating 25-HydroxyVitamin D on Cancer Outcome: Systematic Review and Meta-Analysis. *Br. J. Cancer* **2017**, *116*, 1092–1110. [CrossRef]
15. Chan, J.; Jaceldo-Siegl, K.; Fraser, G.E. Determinants of Serum 25 Hydroxyvitamin D Levels in a Nationwide Cohort of Blacks and Non-Hispanic Whites. *Cancer Causes Control* **2010**, *21*, 501–511. [CrossRef]
16. Freedman, D.M.; Cahoon, E.K.; Rajaraman, P.; Major, J.M.; Doody, M.M.; Alexander, B.H.; Hoffbeck, R.W.; Kimlin, M.G.; Graubard, B.I.; Linet, M.S. Sunlight and Other Determinants of Circulating 25-Hydroxyvitamin D Levels in Black and White Participants in a Nationwide US Study. *Am. J. Epidemiol.* **2013**, *177*, 180–192. [CrossRef]
17. Aranow, C. Vitamin D and the Immune System. *J. Investig. Med.* **2011**, *59*, 881–886. [CrossRef]
18. Dawson-Hughes, B.; Harris, S.S.; Krall, E.A.; Dallal, G.E. Effect of Calcium and Vitamin D Supplementation on Bone Density in Men and Women 65 Years of Age or Older. *N. Engl. J. Med.* **1997**, *337*, 670–676. [CrossRef]
19. Bochen, F.; Balensiefer, B.; Körner, S.; Bittenbring, J.T.; Neumann, F.; Koch, A.; Bumm, K.; Marx, A.; Wemmert, S.; Papaspyrou, G.; et al. Vitamin D Deficiency in Head and Neck Cancer Patients–Prevalence, Prognostic Value and Impact on Immune Function. *Oncoimmunology* **2018**, *7*. [CrossRef]
20. Coutinho-Camillo, C.M.; Lourenço, S.V.; Nishimoto, I.N.; Kowalski, L.P.; Soares, F.A. Nucleophosmin, P53, and Ki-67 Expression Patterns on an Oral Squamous Cell Carcinoma Tissue Microarray. *Hum. Pathol.* **2010**, *41*, 1079–1086. [CrossRef]
21. Zheng, G.; Zhang, Z.; Liu, H.; Xiong, Y.; Luo, L.; Jia, X.; Peng, C.; Zhang, Q.; Li, N.; Gu, Y.; et al. Hsp27-Mediated Extracellular and Intracellular Signaling Pathways Synergistically Confer Chemoresistance in Squamous Cell Carcinoma of Tongue. *Clin. Cancer Res.* **2018**, *24*, 1163–1175. [CrossRef] [PubMed]
22. Yanagawa, T.; Omura, K.; Harada, H.; Ishii, T.; Uwayama, J.; Nakaso, K.; Iwasa, S.; Koyama, Y.; Onizawa, K.; Yusa, H.; et al. Peroxiredoxin I Expression in Tongue Squamous Cell Carcinomas as Involved in Tumor Recurrence. *Int. J. Oral Maxillofac. Surg.* **2005**, *34*, 915–920. [CrossRef]
23. Wang, H.T.; Tong, X.; Zhang, Z.X.; Sun, Y.Y.; Yan, W.; Xu, Z.M.; Fu, W.N. MYCT1 Represses Apoptosis of Laryngeal Cancerous Cells through the MAX/MiR-181a/NPM1 Pathway. *FEBS J.* **2019**, *286*, 3892–3908. [CrossRef] [PubMed]
24. QuestAssureD ™ 25-Hydroxy and 1,25-Dihydroxyvitamin D. Test Detail. Quest Diagnostics. Available online: https://testdirectory.questdiagnostics.com/test/test-detail/16761/questassured-25-hydroxy-and-125-dihydroxyvitamin-d?p=r&q=25-hydroxyvitaminD&cc=MASTER (accessed on 23 April 2020).
25. Holick, M.F.; Binkley, N.C.; Bischoff-Ferrari, H.A.; Gordon, C.M.; Hanley, D.A.; Heaney, R.P.; Murad, M.H.; Weaver, C.M. Evaluation, Treatment, and Prevention of Vitamin D Deficiency: An Endocrine Society Clinical Practice Guideline. *J. Clin. Endocrinol. Metab.* **2011**, *96*, 1911–1930. [CrossRef] [PubMed]

26. Rheinwald, J.G.; Beckett, M.A. Tumorigenic Keratinocyte Lines Requiring Anchorage and Fibroblast Support Cultured from Human Squamous Cell Carcinomas1. *Cancer Res.* **1981**, *41*, 1657–1663.
27. Gioanni, J.; Samson, M.; Zanghellini, E.; Mazeau, C.; Ettore, F.; Demard, F.; Chauvel, P.; Duplay, H.; Schneider, M.; Laurent, J.-C.; et al. Characterization of a New Surface Epitope Specific for Human Epithelial Cells Defined by a Monoclonal Antibody and Application to Tumor Diagnosis. *Cancer Res.* **1987**, *47*, 4417–4424.
28. Bhoora, S.; Pather, Y.; Marais, S.; Punchoo, R. Cholecalciferol Inhibits Cell Growth and Induces Apoptosis in the CaSki Cell Line. *Med. Sci. (Basel)* **2020**, *8*. [CrossRef]
29. Shruthi, N.; Prashanthkumar, M.; Venugopalreddy, B.; Suma, M.; Subba Rao, V. Analysis of the Cytotoxic Effects of Vitamin D3 on Colorectal, Breast and Cervical Carcinoma Cell Lines. *Biochem. Anal. Biochem.* **2017**, *6*. [CrossRef]
30. Baek, S.; Lee, Y.S.; Shim, H.E.; Yoon, S.; Baek, S.Y.; Kim, B.S.; Oh, S.O. Vitamin D3 regulates cell viability in gastric cancer and cholangiocarcinoma. *Anat. Cell Biol.* **2011**, *44*, 204–209. [CrossRef]
31. Bennett, R.G.; Wakeley, S.E.; Hamel, F.G.; High, R.R.; Korch, C.; Goldner, W.S. Gene expression of vitamin D metabolic enzymes at baseline and in response to vitamin D treatment in thyroid cancer cell lines. *Oncology* **2012**, *83*, 264–272. [CrossRef]
32. Santos, J.M.; Khan, Z.S.; Munir, M.T.; Tarafdar, K.; Rahman, S.M.; Hussain, F. Vitamin D3 decreases glycolysis and invasiveness, and increases cellular stiffness in breast cancer cells. *J. Nutr. Biochem.* **2018**, *53*, 111–120. [CrossRef] [PubMed]
33. Charoenngam, N.; Holick, M.F. Immunologic Effects of Vitamin D on Human Health and Disease. *Nutrients* **2020**, *12*. [CrossRef] [PubMed]
34. Berlin, J.L.; Shantha, G.P.; Yeager, H.; Thomas-Hemak, L. Serum vitamin D levels may not reflect tissue-level vitamin D in sarcoidosis. *BMJ Case Rep.* **2014**, *2014*. [CrossRef] [PubMed]
35. Kresty, L.; Clarke, J.; Ezell, K.; Exum, A.; Howell, A.; Guettouche, T. MicroRNA Alterations in Barrett's Esophagus, Esophageal Adenocarcinoma, and Esophageal Adenocarcinoma Cell Lines Following Cranberry Extract Treatment: Insights for Chemoprevention. *J. Carcinog.* **2011**, *10*. [CrossRef]
36. Chou, C.H.; Shrestha, S.; Yang, C.D.; Chang, N.W.; Lin, Y.L.; Liao, K.W.; Huang, W.C.; Sun, T.H.; Tu, S.J.; Lee, W.H.; et al. MiRTarBase Update 2018: A Resource for Experimentally Validated MicroRNA-Target Interactions. *Nucleic Acids Res.* **2018**, *46*, D296–D302. [CrossRef]
37. Lee, Y.J.; Kim, V.; Muth, D.C.; Witwer, K.W. Validated MicroRNA Target Databases: An Evaluation. *Drug Dev. Res.* **2015**, *76*, 389–396. [CrossRef]
38. Tsuprykov, O.; Chen, X.; Hocher, C.F.; Skoblo, R.; Yin, L.; Hocher, B. Why Should We Measure Free 25(OH) Vitamin D? *J. Steroid Biochem. Mol. Biol.* **2018**, *180*, 87–104. [CrossRef]
39. Nagai, J.; Christensen, E.I.; Morris, S.M.; Willnow, T.E.; Cooper, J.A.; Nielsen, R. Mutually Dependent Localization of Megalin and Dab2 in the Renal Proximal Tubule. *Am. J. Physiol. Ren. Physiol.* **2005**, *289*. [CrossRef]
40. Rose, B.S.; Jeong, J.H.; Nath, S.K.; Lu, S.M.; Mell, L.K. Population-Based Study of Competing Mortality in Head and Neck Cancer. *J. Clin. Oncol.* **2011**, *29*, 3503–3509. [CrossRef]
41. American Cancer Society. *Cancer Facts & Figures 2020*; American Cancer Society: Atlanta, GA, USA, 2020.
42. American Cancer Society. *Cancer Facts and Figures for African Americans 2019–2021*; American Cancer Society: Atlanta, GA, USA, 2019.
43. Mahal, B.A.; Inverso, G.; Aizer, A.A.; Bruce Donoff, R.; Chuang, S.K. Impact of African-American Race on Presentation, Treatment, and Survival of Head and Neck Cancer. *Oral Oncol.* **2014**, *50*, 1177–1181. [CrossRef]
44. Zakeri, K.; Macewan, I.; Vazirnia, A.; Cohen, E.E.W.; Spiotto, M.T.; Haraf, D.J.; Vokes, E.E.; Weichselbaum, R.R.; Mell, L.K. Race and Competing Mortality in Advanced Head and Neck Cancer. *Oral Oncol.* **2014**, *50*, 40–44. [CrossRef] [PubMed]
45. Subramanian, S.; Chen, A. Treatment Patterns and Survival among Low-Income Medicaid Patients with Head and Neck Cancer. *JAMA Otolaryngol. Head Neck Surg.* **2013**, *139*, 489–495. [CrossRef] [PubMed]
46. Du, X.L.; Liu, C.C. Racial/Ethnic Disparities in Socioeconomic Status, Diagnosis, Treatment and Survival among Medicare-Insured Men and Women with Head and Neck Cancer. *J. Health Care Poor Underserved* **2010**, *21*, 913–930. [CrossRef] [PubMed]

47. Molina, M.A.; Cheung, M.C.; Perez, E.A.; Byrne, M.M.; Franceschi, D.; Moffat, F.L.; Livingstone, A.S.; Goodwin, W.J.; Gutierrez, J.C.; Koniaris, L.G. African American and Poor Patients Have a Dramatically Worse Prognosis for Head and Neck Cancer: An Examination of 20,915 Patients. *Cancer* **2008**, *113*, 2797–2806. [CrossRef]
48. Arbes, S.J. Factors Contributing to the Poorer Survival of Black Americans Diagnosed with Oral Cancer (United States). *Cancer Causes Control* **1999**, *10*, 513–523. [CrossRef]
49. Ellis, L.; Canchola, A.J.; Spiegel, D.; Ladabaum, U.; Haile, R.; Gomez, S.L. Racial and Ethnic Disparities in Cancer Survival: The Contribution of Tumor, Sociodemographic, Institutional, and Neighborhood Characteristics. *J. Clin. Oncol.* **2018**, *36*, 25–33. [CrossRef]
50. Saini, A.T.; Genden, E.M.; Megwalu, U.C. Sociodemographic Disparities in Choice of Therapy and Survival in Advanced Laryngeal Cancer. *Am. J. Otolaryngol. Head Neck Med. Surg.* **2016**, *37*, 65–69. [CrossRef]
51. Russo, D.P.; Tham, T.; Bardash, Y.; Kraus, D. The Effect of Race in Head and Neck Cancer: A Meta-Analysis Controlling for Socioeconomic Status. *Am. J. Otolaryngol.* **2020**, *41*, 102624. [CrossRef]
52. Yetley, E.A. Assessing the Vitamin D Status of the US Population. *Am. J. Clin. Nutr.* **2008**, *88*, 558–564. [CrossRef]
53. Harris, S.S.; Soteriades, E.; Coolidge, J.A.S.; Mudgal, S.; Dawson-Hughes, B. Vitamin D Insufficiency and Hyperparathyroidism in a Low Income, Multiracial, Elderly Population. *J. Clin. Endocrinol. Metab.* **2000**, *85*, 4125–4130. [CrossRef]
54. Jacobs, E.T.; Alberts, D.S.; Foote, J.A.; Green, S.B.; Hollis, B.W.; Yu, Z.; Martínez, M.E. Vitamin D Insufficiency in Southern Arizona. *Am. J. Clin. Nutr.* **2008**, *87*, 608–613. [CrossRef] [PubMed]
55. Shea, M.K.; Houston, D.K.; Tooze, J.A.; Davis, C.C.; Johnson, M.A.; Hausman, D.B.; Cauley, J.A.; Bauer, D.C.; Tylavsky, F.; Harris, T.B.; et al. Correlates and Prevalence of Insufficient 25-Hydroxyvitamin D Status in Black and White Older Adults: The Health, Aging and Body Composition Study. *J. Am. Geriatr. Soc.* **2011**, *59*, 1165–1174. [CrossRef] [PubMed]
56. Camozzi, V.; Frigo, A.C.; Zaninotto, M.; Sanguin, F.; Plebani, M.; Boscaro, M.; Schiavon, L.; Luisetto, G. 25-Hydroxycholecalciferol Response to Single Oral Cholecalciferol Loading in the Normal Weight, Overweight, and Obese. *Osteoporos. Int.* **2016**, *27*, 2593–2602. [CrossRef]
57. Gallagher, J.C.; Yalamanchili, V.; Smith, L.M. The Effect of Vitamin D Supplementation on Serum 25OHD in Thin and Obese Women. *J. Steroid Biochem. Mol. Biol.* **2013**, 195–200. [CrossRef]
58. Blum, M.; Dawson-Hughes, B.; Dallal, G.E. Body Size and Serum 25 Hydroxy Vitamin D Response to Oral Supplements in Healthy Older Adults. *J. Am. Coll. Nutr.* **2008**, *27*, 274–279. [CrossRef] [PubMed]
59. Savastano, S.; Barrea, L.; Savanelli, M.C.; Nappi, F.; Di Somma, C.; Orio, F.; Colao, A. Low Vitamin D Status and Obesity: Role of Nutritionist. *Rev. Endocr. Metab. Disord.* **2017**, *18*, 215–225. [CrossRef] [PubMed]
60. Rock, C.L. Multivitamin-Multimineral Supplements: Who Uses Them? *Am. J. Clin. Nutr.* **2007**, *85*, 277–279. [CrossRef]
61. Radimer, K.; Bindewald, B.; Hughes, J.; Ervin, B.; Swanson, C.; Picciano, M.F. Dietary Supplement Use by US Adults: Data from the National Health and Nutrition Examination Survey, 1999–2000. *Am. J. Epidemiol.* **2004**, *160*, 339–349. [CrossRef]
62. Giammanco, M.; Di Majo, D.; La Guardia, M.; Aiello, S.; Crescimannno, M.; Flandina, C.; Tumminello, F.M.; Leto, G. Vitamin D in Cancer Chemoprevention. *Pharm. Biol.* **2015**, *53*, 1399–1434. [CrossRef]
63. Kennel, K.A.; Drake, M.T. Vitamin D in the Cancer Patient. *Curr. Opin. Support. Palliat. Care* **2013**, *7*, 272–277. [CrossRef]
64. Lenze, N.R.; Farquhar, D.R.; Mazul, A.L.; Masood, M.M.; Zevallos, J.P. Racial Disparities and Human Papillomavirus Status in Oropharyngeal Cancer: A Systematic Review and Meta-Analysis. *Head Neck* **2019**, *41*, 256–261. [CrossRef] [PubMed]
65. Peterson, C.E.; Khosla, S.; Chen, L.F.; Joslin, C.E.; Davis, F.G.; Fitzgibbon, M.L.; Freels, S.; Hoskins, K. Racial Differences in Head and Neck Squamous Cell Carcinomas among Non-Hispanic Black and White Males Identified through the National Cancer Database (1998–2012). *J. Cancer Res. Clin. Oncol.* **2016**, *142*, 1715–1726. [CrossRef] [PubMed]
66. Sturgis, E.M.; Cinciripini, P.M. Trends in Head and Neck Cancer Incidence in Relation to Smoking Prevalence: An Emerging Epidemic of Human Papillomavirus-Associated Cancers? *Cancer* **2007**, *110*, 1429–1435. [CrossRef] [PubMed]

67. Morse, D.E.; Kerr, A.R. Disparities in Oral and Pharyngeal Cancer Incidence, Mortality and Survival among Black and White Americans. *J. Am. Dent. Assoc.* **2006**, *137*, 203–212. [CrossRef]
68. Gillison, M.L.; D'Souza, G.; Westra, W.; Sugar, E.; Xiao, W.; Begum, S.; Viscidi, R. Distinct Risk Factor Profiles for Human Papillomavirus Type 16-Positive and Human Papillomavirus Type 16-Negative Head and Neck Cancers. *J. Natl. Cancer Inst.* **2008**, *100*, 407–420. [CrossRef]
69. Schwartz, S.R.; Yueh, B.; McDougall, J.K.; Daling, J.R.; Schwartz, S.M. Human Papillomavirus Infection and Survival in Oral Squamous Cell Cancer: A Population-Based Study. *Otolaryngol. Head Neck Surg.* **2001**, *125*, 1–9. [CrossRef]
70. Dayyani, F.; Etzel, C.J.; Liu, M.; Ho, C.H.; Lippman, S.M.; Tsao, A.S. Meta-Analysis of the Impact of Human Papillomavirus (HPV) on Cancer Risk and Overall Survival in Head and Neck Squamous Cell Carcinomas (HNSCC). *Head Neck Oncol.* **2010**, *2*. [CrossRef]
71. Fakhry, C.; Westra, W.H.; Li, S.; Cmelak, A.; Ridge, J.A.; Pinto, H.; Forastiere, A.; Gillison, M.L. Improved Survival of Patients with Human Papillomavirus-Positive Head and Neck Squamous Cell Carcinoma in a Prospective Clinical Trial. *J. Natl. Cancer Inst.* **2008**, *100*, 261–269. [CrossRef]
72. Huang, Q.; Yang, J.; Zheng, J.; Hsueh, C.; Guo, Y.; Zhou, L. Characterization of Selective Exosomal MicroRNA Expression Profile Derived from Laryngeal Squamous Cell Carcinoma Detected by next Generation Sequencing. *Oncol. Rep.* **2018**, *40*, 2584–2594. [CrossRef]
73. Zeljic, K.; Supic, G.; Magic, Z. New Insights into Vitamin D Anticancer Properties: Focus on MiRNA Modulation. *Mol. Genet. Genom.* **2017**, *292*, 511–524. [CrossRef]
74. Kalinowski, F.C.; Giles, K.M.; Candy, P.A.; Ali, A.; Ganda, C.; Epis, M.R.; Webster, R.J.; Leedman, P.J. Regulation of Epidermal Growth Factor Receptor Signaling and Erlotinib Sensitivity in Head and Neck Cancer Cells by MiR-7. *PLoS ONE* **2012**, *7*. [CrossRef] [PubMed]
75. Horsham, J.; Kalinowski, F.; Epis, M.; Ganda, C.; Brown, R.; Leedman, P. Clinical Potential of MicroRNA-7 in Cancer. *J. Clin. Med.* **2015**, *4*, 1668–1687. [CrossRef]
76. Yang, J.H.; Lin, L.K.; Zhang, S. Epigenetic Silencing of MicroRNA-335 Contributes to Nasopharyngeal Carcinoma Metastasis. *Am. J. Otolaryngol. Head Neck Med. Surg.* **2020**, *41*. [CrossRef] [PubMed]
77. Ou, D.; Wu, Y.; Liu, J.; Lao, X.; Zhang, S.; Liao, G. MiRNA-335 and MiRNA-182 Affect the Occurrence of Tongue Squamous Cell Carcinoma by Targeting Survivin. *Oncol. Lett.* **2016**, *12*, 2531–2537. [CrossRef] [PubMed]
78. Cheng, A.M.; Byrom, M.W.; Shelton, J.; Ford, L.P. Antisense Inhibition of Human MiRNAs and Indications for an Involvement of MiRNA in Cell Growth and Apoptosis. *Nucleic Acids Res.* **2005**, *33*, 1290–1297. [CrossRef] [PubMed]
79. Sethi, N.; Wright, A.; Wood, H.; Rabbitts, P. MicroRNAs and Head and Neck Cancer: Reviewing the First Decade of Research. *Eur. J. Cancer* **2014**, 2619–2635. [CrossRef] [PubMed]
80. Ayaz, L.; Görür, A.; Yaroğlu, H.Y.; Özcan, C.; Tamer, L. Differential Expression of MicroRNAs in Plasma of Patients with Laryngeal Squamous Cell Carcinoma: Potential Early-Detection Markers for Laryngeal Squamous Cell Carcinoma. *J. Cancer Res. Clin. Oncol.* **2013**, *139*, 1499–1506. [CrossRef]
81. MacLellan, S.A.; Lawson, J.; Baik, J.; Guillaud, M.; Poh, C.F.Y.; Garnis, C. Differential Expression of MiRNAs in the Serum of Patients with High-Risk Oral Lesions. *Cancer Med.* **2012**, *1*, 268–274. [CrossRef]
82. Yang, Y.; Li, Y.X.; Yang, X.; Jiang, L.; Zhou, Z.J.; Zhu, Y.Q. Progress Risk Assessment of Oral Premalignant Lesions with Saliva MiRNA Analysis. *BMC Cancer* **2013**, *13*. [CrossRef]
83. Hsu, C.M.; Lin, P.M.; Wang, Y.M.; Chen, Z.J.; Lin, S.F.; Yang, M.Y. Circulating MiRNA Is a Novel Marker for Head and Neck Squamous Cell Carcinoma. *Tumour Biol.* **2012**, *33*, 1933–1942. [CrossRef]
84. Ramdas, L.; Giri, U.; Ashorn, C.L.; Coombes, K.R.; El-Naggar, A.; Ang, K.K.; Story, M.D. MiRNA Expression Profiles in Head and Neck Squamous Cell Carcinoma and Adjacent Normal Tissue. *Head Neck* **2009**, *31*, 642–654. [CrossRef] [PubMed]
85. Rentoft, M.; Fahlén, J.; Coates, P.J.; Laurell, G.; Sjöström, B.; Rydén, P.; Nylander, K. MiRNA Analysis of Formalin-Fixed Squamous Cell Carcinomas of the Tongue Is Affected by Age of the Samples. *Int. J. Oncol.* **2011**, *38*, 61–69. [CrossRef]
86. Chou, Y.T.; Lin, H.H.; Lien, Y.C.; Wang, Y.H.; Hong, C.F.; Kao, Y.R.; Lin, S.C.; Chang, Y.C.; Lin, S.Y.; Chen, S.J.; et al. EGFR Promotes Lung Tumorigenesis by Activating MiR-7 through a Ras/ERK/Myc Pathway That Targets the Ets2 Transcriptional Repressor ERF. *Cancer Res.* **2010**, *70*, 8822–8831. [CrossRef] [PubMed]

87. Alsahafi, E.; Begg, K.; Amelio, I.; Raulf, N.; Lucarelli, P.; Sauter, T.; Tavassoli, M. Clinical Update on Head and Neck Cancer: Molecular Biology and Ongoing Challenges. *Cell Death Dis.* **2019**. [CrossRef]
88. Lechner, M.; Frampton, G.M.; Fenton, T.; Feber, A.; Palmer, G.; Jay, A.; Pillay, N.; Forster, M.; Cronin, M.T.; Lipson, D.; et al. Targeted Next-Generation Sequencing of Head and Neck Squamous Cell Carcinoma Identifies Novel Genetic Alterations in HPV+ and HPV- Tumors. *Genome Med.* **2013**, *5*, 49. [CrossRef]
89. Jackson-Weaver, O.; Ungvijanpunya, N.; Yuan, Y.; Qian, J.; Gou, Y.; Wu, J.; Shen, H.; Chen, Y.; Li, M.; Richard, S.; et al. PRMT1-P53 Pathway Controls Epicardial EMT and Invasion. *Cell Rep.* **2020**, *31*. [CrossRef] [PubMed]
90. Lu, Z.; Sturgis, E.M.; Zhu, L.; Zhang, H.; Tao, Y.; Wei, P.; Wei, Q.; Li, G. Mouse Double Minute 4 Variants Modify Susceptibility to Risk of Recurrence in Patients with Squamous Cell Carcinoma of the Oropharynx. *Mol. Carcinog.* **2018**, *57*, 361–369. [CrossRef]
91. Ach, T.; Schwarz-Furlan, S.; Ach, S.; Agaimy, A.; Gerken, M.; Rohrmeier, C.; Zenk, J.; Iro, H.; Brockhoff, G.; Ettl, T. Genomic Aberrations of MDM2, MDM4, FGFR1 and FGFR3 Are Associated with Poor Outcome in Patients with Salivary Gland Cancer. *J. Oral Pathol. Med.* **2016**, *45*, 500–509. [CrossRef]
92. Mishra, R.; Ranjan Das, B. Early Overexpression of Cdk4 and Possible Role of KRF and C-Myc in Chewing Tobacco Mediated Oral Cancer Development. *Mol. Biol. Rep.* **2003**, *30*, 207–213. [CrossRef]
93. Yu, C.; Xing, F.; Zhang, J.; Xu, J.; Li, Y. A Combination of MRNA Expression Profile and MiRNA Expression Profile Identifies Detection Biomarkers in Different Tumor Stages of Laryngeal Squamous Cell Carcinoma. *Eur. Rev. Med. Pharmacol. Sci.* **2018**, *22*, 7296–7304.
94. Xuefang, Z.; Ruinian, Z.; Liji, J.; Chun, Z.; Qiaolan, Z.; Jun, J.; Yuming, C.; Junrong, H. MiR-331-3p Inhibits Proliferation and Promotes Apoptosis of Nasopharyngeal Carcinoma Cells by Targeting Elf4B-PI3K-AKT Pathway. *Technol. Cancer Res. Treat.* **2020**, *19*, 153303381989225. [CrossRef]
95. Li, X.; Zhu, J.; Liu, Y.; Duan, C.; Chang, R.; Zhang, C. MicroRNA-331-3p Inhibits Epithelial-mesenchymal Transition by Targeting ErbB2 and VAV2 through the Rac1/PAK1/B-catenin Axis in Non-small-cell Lung Cancer. *Cancer Sci.* **2019**, *110*, cas.14014. [CrossRef]
96. Zhan, J.; Jiao, D.; Wang, Y.; Song, J.; Wu, J.; Wu, L.; Chen, Q.; Ma, S. Integrated MicroRNA and Gene Expression Profiling Reveals the Crucial MiRNAs in Curcumin Anti-Lung Cancer Cell Invasion. *Thorac. Cancer* **2017**, *8*, 461–470. [CrossRef] [PubMed]
97. Momen-Heravi, F.; Trachtenberg, A.J.; Kuo, W.P.; Cheng, Y.S. Genomewide Study of Salivary MicroRNAs for Detection of Oral Cancer. *J. Dent. Res.* **2014**, *93*, 86S–93S. [CrossRef]
98. Lu, E.; Su, J.; Zhou, Y.; Zhang, C.; Wang, Y. CCL20/CCR6 Promotes Cell Proliferation and Metastasis in Laryngeal Cancer by Activating P38 Pathway. *Biomed. Pharmacother.* **2017**, *85*, 486–492. [CrossRef]
99. Zhou, Z.X.; Zhang, Z.P.; Tao, Z.Z.; Tan, T.Z. MiR-632 Promotes Laryngeal Carcinoma Cell Proliferation, Migration, and Invasion through Negative Regulation of GSK3β. *Oncol. Res.* **2020**, *28*, 21–31. [CrossRef]
100. Grisendi, S.; Mecucci, C.; Falini, B.; Pandolfi, P.P. Nucleophosmin and Cancer. *Nat. Rev. Cancer* **2006**, 493–505. [CrossRef] [PubMed]
101. Saini, J.; Sharma, P.K. Clinical, Prognostic and Therapeutic Significance of Heat Shock Proteins in Cancer. *Curr. Drug Targets* **2018**, *19*, 1478–1490. [CrossRef] [PubMed]
102. Rabbani, N.; Xue, M.; Weickert, M.O.; Thornalley, P.J. Multiple Roles of Glyoxalase 1-Mediated Suppression of Methylglyoxal Glycation in Cancer Biology—Involvement in Tumour Suppression, Tumour Growth, Multidrug Resistance and Target for Chemotherapy. *Semin. Cancer Biol.* **2018**, 83–93. [CrossRef]
103. Kumar, N.; Prasad, P.; Jash, E.; Saini, M.; Husain, A.; Goldman, A.; Sehrawat, S. Insights into Exchange Factor Directly Activated by CAMP (EPAC) as Potential Target for Cancer Treatment. *Mol. Cell. Biochem.* **2018**, *447*, 77–92. [CrossRef]
104. Monteiro, F.L.; Baptista, T.; Amado, F.; Vitorino, R.; Jerónimo, C.; Helguero, L.A. Expression and Functionality of Histone H2A Variants in Cancer. *Oncotarget* **2014**, *5*, 3428–3443. [CrossRef]
105. Dhar, S.K.; St. Clair, D.K. Nucleophosmin Blocks Mitochondrial Localization of P53 and Apoptosis. *J. Biol. Chem.* **2009**, *284*, 16409–16418. [CrossRef]
106. Jeon, Y.J.; Cho, J.H.; Lee, S.Y.; Choi, Y.H.; Park, H.; Jung, S.; Shim, J.H.; Chae, J.I. Esculetin Induces Apoptosis Through EGFR/PI3K/Akt Signaling Pathway and Nucleophosmin Relocation. *J. Cell. Biochem.* **2016**, *117*, 1210–1221. [CrossRef] [PubMed]
107. Shandilya, J.; Swaminathan, V.; Gadad, S.S.; Choudhari, R.; Kodaganur, G.S.; Kundu, T.K. Acetylated NPM1 Localizes in the Nucleoplasm and Regulates Transcriptional Activation of Genes Implicated in Oral Cancer Manifestation. *Mol. Cell. Biol.* **2009**, *29*, 5115–5127. [CrossRef] [PubMed]

108. Onikubo, T.; Nicklay, J.J.; Xing, L.; Warren, C.; Anson, B.; Wang, W.L.; Burgos, E.S.; Ruff, S.E.; Shabanowitz, J.; Cheng, R.H.; et al. Developmentally Regulated Post-Translational Modification of Nucleoplasmin Controls Histone Sequestration and Deposition. *Cell Rep.* **2015**, *10*, 1735–1748. [CrossRef]
109. Lindström, M.S. NPM1/B23: A Multifunctional Chaperone in Ribosome Biogenesis and Chromatin Remodeling. *Biochem. Res. Int.* **2011**, *2011*. [CrossRef] [PubMed]
110. Kreycy, N.; Gotzian, C.; Fleming, T.; Flechtenmacher, C.; Grabe, N.; Plinkert, P.; Hess, J.; Zaoui, K. Glyoxalase 1 Expression Is Associated with an Unfavorable Prognosis of Oropharyngeal Squamous Cell Carcinoma. *BMC Cancer* **2017**, *17*. [CrossRef] [PubMed]
111. Geng, X.; Ma, J.; Zhang, F.; Xu, C. Glyoxalase i in Tumor Cell Proliferation and Survival and as a Potential Target for Anticancer Therapy. *Oncol. Res. Treat.* **2014**, *37*, 570–574. [CrossRef] [PubMed]
112. Ernst, B.P.; Wiesmann, N.; Gieringer, R.; Eckrich, J.; Brieger, J. HSP27 Regulates Viability and Migration of Cancer Cell Lines Following Irradiation. *J. Proteom.* **2020**, *226*, 103886. [CrossRef]
113. Guttmann, D.M.; Hart, L.; Du, K.; Seletsky, A.; Koumenis, C. Inhibition of Hsp27 Radiosensitizes Head-and-Neck Cancer by Modulating Deoxyribonucleic Acid Repair. *Int. J. Radiat. Oncol. Biol. Phys.* **2013**, *87*, 168–175. [CrossRef]
114. Zhu, Z.K.; Wang, Y.S.; Xu, X. Biology Behavior of Head and Neck Squamous Cell Cancer Cells Changes after Knocking down Heat Shock Protein 27. *Hua Xi Kou Qiang Yi Xue Za Zhi* **2020**, *38*, 139–144. [CrossRef] [PubMed]
115. Berggren, K.L.; Restrepo Cruz, S.; Hixon, M.D.; Cowan, A.T.; Keysar, S.B.; Craig, S.; James, J.; Barry, M.; Ozbun, M.A.; Jimeno, A.; et al. MAPKAPK2 (MK2) Inhibition Mediates Radiation-Induced Inflammatory Cytokine Production and Tumor Growth in Head and Neck Squamous Cell Carcinoma. *Oncogene* **2019**, *38*, 7329–7341. [CrossRef] [PubMed]
116. Chen, W.; Ren, X.; Wu, J.; Gao, X.; Cen, X.; Wang, S.; Sheng, S.; Chen, Q.; Tang, Y.J.; Liang, X.H.; et al. HSP27 Associates with Epithelial–Mesenchymal Transition, Stemness and Radioresistance of Salivary Adenoid Cystic Carcinoma. *J. Cell. Mol. Med.* **2018**, *22*, 2283–2298. [CrossRef] [PubMed]
117. Kim, J.; Lim, H.; Kim, S.; Cho, H.; Kim, Y.; Li, X.; Choi, H.; Kim, O. Effects of HSP27 Downregulation on PDT Resistance through PDT-Induced Autophagy in Head and Neck Cancer Cells. *Oncol. Rep.* **2016**, *35*, 2237–2245. [CrossRef]
118. da Silva, S.D.; Marchi, F.A.; Xu, B.; Bijian, K.; Alobaid, F.; Mlynarek, A.; Rogatto, S.R.; Hier, M.; Kowalski, L.P.; Alaoui-Jamali, M.A. Predominant Rab-GTPase Amplicons Contributing to Oral Squamous Cell Carcinoma Progression to Metastasis. *Oncotarget* **2015**, *6*, 21950–21963. [CrossRef]
119. Lo Re, O.; Fusilli, C.; Rappa, F.; Van Haele, M.; Douet, J.; Pindjakova, J.; Rocha, S.W.; Pata, I.; Valčíková, B.; Uldrijan, S.; et al. Induction of Cancer Cell Stemness by Depletion of Macrohistone H2A1 in Hepatocellular Carcinoma. *Hepatology* **2018**, *67*, 636–650. [CrossRef]
120. Niu, W.; Zhang, M.; Chen, H.; Wang, C.; Shi, N.; Jing, X.; Ge, L.; Chen, T.; Tang, X. Peroxiredoxin 1 Promotes Invasion and Migration by Regulating Epithelial-to-Mesenchymal Transition during Oral Carcinogenesis. *Oncotarget* **2016**, *7*, 47042–47051. [CrossRef]
121. Jiang, Y.; Cao, W.; Wu, K.; Qin, X.; Wang, X.; Li, Y.; Yu, B.; Zhang, Z.; Wang, X.; Yan, M.; et al. LncRNA LINC00460 Promotes EMT in Head and Neck Squamous Cell Carcinoma by Facilitating Peroxiredoxin-1 into the Nucleus. *J. Exp. Clin. Cancer Res.* **2019**, *38*, 1–19. [CrossRef]
122. Monisha, J.; Kishor Roy, N.; Bordoloi, D.; Kumar, A.; Golla, R.; Kotoky, J.; Padmavathi, G.; B. Kunnumakkara, A. Nuclear Factor Kappa B: A Potential Target to Persecute Head and Neck Cancer. *Curr. Drug Targets* **2016**, *18*, 232–253. [CrossRef]

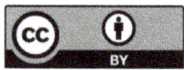

© 2020 by the authors. Licensee MDPI, Basel, Switzerland. This article is an open access article distributed under the terms and conditions of the Creative Commons Attribution (CC BY) license (http://creativecommons.org/licenses/by/4.0/).

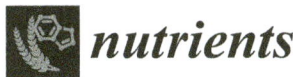

Article

Effect of Vitamin D Treatment on Dynamics of Stones Formation in the Urinary Tract and Bone Density in Children with Idiopathic Hypercalciuria

Joanna Milart [1], Aneta Lewicka [2,*], Katarzyna Jobs [1], Agata Wawrzyniak [1], Małgorzata Majder-Łopatka [3] and Bolesław Kalicki [1]

1. Clinic of Paediatrics, Nephrology and Paediatric Allergology, Military Institute of Medicine, 128, 04-141 Warsaw Szaserów, Poland; jfurgal@wim.mil.pl (J.M.); kjobs@wim.mil.pl (K.J.); awawrzyniak@wim.mil.pl (A.W.); kalicki@wim.mil.pl (B.K.)
2. Laboratory of Food and Nutrition Hygiene, Military Institute of Hygiene and Epidemiology, Kozielska, 4, 01-163 Warsaw, Poland
3. The Main School of Fire Service, Slowackiego 52/54, 01-629 Warsaw, Poland; mmajder@sgsp.edu.pl
* Correspondence: aneta.lewicka@wihe.pl; Tel.: +48-261-853-101

Received: 30 July 2020; Accepted: 17 August 2020; Published: 20 August 2020

Abstract: Vitamin D supplementation in patients with urolithiasis and hypercalciuria is considered to be unsafe. We analyzed the impact of vitamin D supplementation on selected health status parameters in children with idiopathic hypercalciuria. The study included 36 children with urolithiasis resulting from excessive calcium excretion. The level of calcium and 25(OH)D (hydroxylated vitamin D - calcidiol) in serum, urinary calcium excretion and the presence of stones in urinary tract were assessed prospectively. Blood and urine samples were collected at the time when the patient was qualified for the study and every three months up to 24 month of vitamin D intake at a dose of 400 or 800 IU/day. At time zero and at 12, and 24 months of vitamin D supplementation, densitometry was performed. Supplementation with vitamin D caused a statistically significant increase in the concentration of 25(OH)D in serum. There were no significant changes in calcium concentration in serum, excretion of calcium in urine but also in bone density. There was no significant increase in the risk of formation or development of stones in the urinary tract. Supplementation with vitamin D (400–800 IU/day) in children with idiopathic hypercalciuria significantly increases 25(OH)D concentration, does not affect calciuria, but also does not improve bone density.

Keywords: vitamin D treatment; idiopathic hypercalciuria; urolithiasis; children; bone density

1. Introduction

Vitamin D is a fat-soluble steroid hormone, which regulates calcium and phosphate metabolism. The skin exposed to UVB radiation produces pre-vitamin D, which binds to the DBP protein (vitamin D binding protein), and is transported to the liver cells, where is hydroxylated to 25(OH)D (calcidiol). Subsequently, in the proximal tubules of the kidney, the 1α-hydroxylase 25(OH)D converts it to 1.25(OH)D (calcitriol). The production of 25(OH)D unlike 1.25(OH)D is not strictly regulated. Due to the relatively long half-life (about 3 weeks) and chemical stability, this metabolite is an indicator of the level of vitamin D resources in the organism [1,2]. Patients with idiopathic hypercalciuria and urolithiasis were until recently included in the group of people whose supplementation with vitamin D is considered unsafe due to the possibility of increased calciuria and the formation of new stones in the urinary tract [3].

Idiopathic hypercalciuria (IH) is one of the most common metabolic causes of urolithiasis, both in children and adults (30–60% adults and 40–80% children). Urinary calcium excretion in children is considered increased when above 4 mg/kg body weight/24 h. [4]. The calcium-creatinine (Ca/Cr) ratio, calculated from the second morning urine sample, can also be used to estimate the level of hypercalciuria. The reference values of this indicator depend on age and range from 0.8 in infants to 0.2 in adults [4]. Symptoms of hypercalciuria are non-characteristic, including abdominal pain, haematuria, erythrocyturia [5–7]. The hypercalciuria may be the cause of formation of stones in urinary tract.

Urolithiasis (UL) is a condition in which in the urinary tract deposits are formed from chemicals that are normal or pathological constituents of urine [8–11]. In Europe, the incidence of this disease is estimated at about 4% in the adult population and 1–2% in children [8,12].

Both urolithiasis and hypercalciuria predispose to skeletal mineralization disorders, leading to a decreased bone density [8,9]. The human skeletal system is constantly changing. The most significant period is childhood and adolescence. Then, there is a rapid increase in the structure of the bone skeleton, which continues until the bone epiphysis is closed, i.e., until the age of 20. By this time, approximately 90% of bone mass is formed. The peak of bone mass is reached around 30 years of age. If insufficient, it is associated with an increased risk of osteoporosis in later life [9,13].

The gold standard in diagnosing bone density disorders is densitometry. In children, the bone density of the whole body is measured. The test result is expressed by means of indicators comparing the bone density of the tested person with the bone density of healthy people (Z-score). Z-score between (−2) and (−1) is considered as osteopenia in children, while osteoporosis is diagnosed at Z score > (−2), and accompanying clinical symptoms [1,9].

The identification of patients who are at risk of osteopenia and osteoporosis among patients with urolithiasis and idiopathic hypercalciuria allows the implementation of a preventive strategy that includes appropriate supplementation with vitamin D [1,14].

In this study, we evaluated the effect of vitamin D supplementation in children with idiopathic hypercalciuria on 25(OH)D blood level, caciuria, development of new stones in urinary tract and bone mineral density.

2. Materials and Methods

2.1. Patients

The research project was approved by Bioethics Committee at the Military Institute of Medicine (Resolution No. 26/WIM/2013 of 22 May 2013). The study included 36 children (18 boys, 18 girls) with urolithiasis in the course of idiopathic hypercalciuria and low levels of vitamin D, hospitalized in Pediatrics, Nephrology, and Paediatric Allergology Department of Military Institute of Medicine. Inclusion criteria were age 5–16, urolithiasis in the course of idiopathic hypercalciuria, good cooperation with medical staff. Exclusion criteria were chronic kidney disease, urinary tract infections, urinary tract defects, systemic diseases, bone diseases (except osteopenia), endocrine disorders, and patients treated with glucocorticosteroids.

The written consent of legal guardians was obtained and, in the case of children over 15 years of age, also the consent of the child.

2.2. Experimental Study

The medical interview included information about the onset of the problem with urolithiasis, accompanying diseases, and medications. All studied children were subjected to physical examination. The study was performed in four stages (Figure 1). Seven patients were followed up for 1 year, and 29 children for 2 years. The 1 year observation period was associated with reaching adulthood during the study period or resigning from the study after a year of observation.

Studied patients were supplemented with cholecalciferol tablets. We recommended to take the pill with a meal. During the study, vitamin D doses were adjusted to the season of the year and serum 25(OH)D concentrations (400 IU or 800 IU vitamin D dose) (Figure 1). Urolithiasis activity was assessed by ultrasound examination of the urinary system (no stones vs. new ones). In all cases in which calciuria would increase significantly during the treatment, intention was returning the patient to previous treatment and discontinuation of vitamin D.

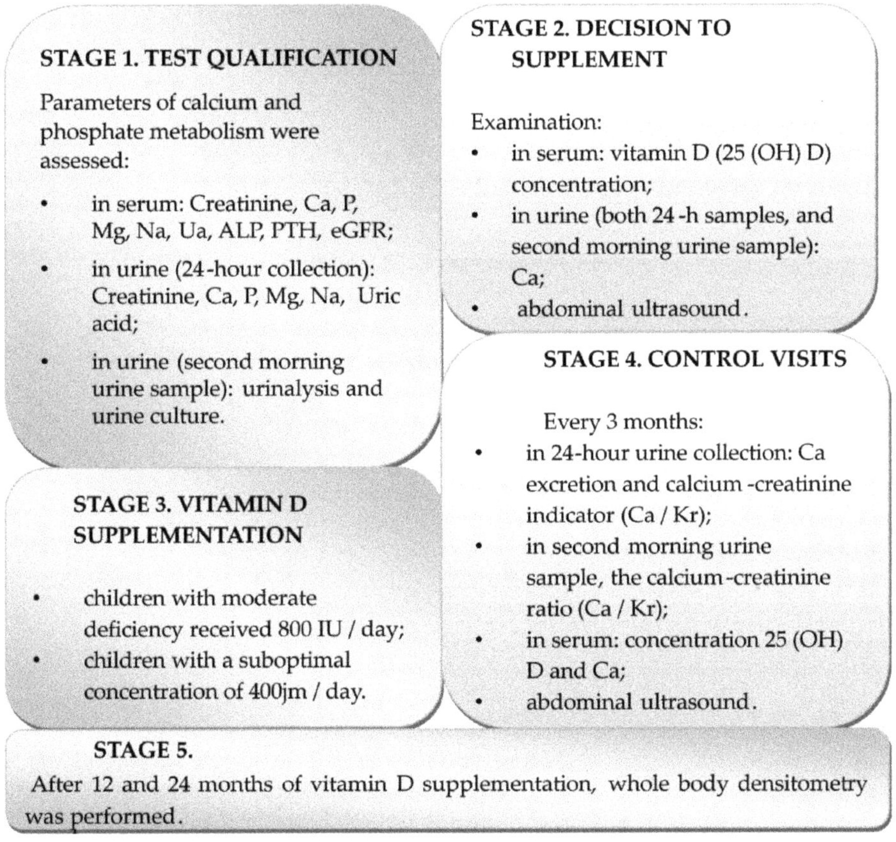

STAGE 1. TEST QUALIFICATION

Parameters of calcium and phosphate metabolism were assessed:
- in serum: Creatinine, Ca, P, Mg, Na, Ua, ALP, PTH, eGFR;
- in urine (24-hour collection): Creatinine, Ca, P, Mg, Na, Uric acid;
- in urine (second morning urine sample): urinalysis and urine culture.

STAGE 2. DECISION TO SUPPLEMENT

Examination:
- in serum: vitamin D (25 (OH) D) concentration;
- in urine (both 24-h samples, and second morning urine sample): Ca;
- abdominal ultrasound.

STAGE 3. VITAMIN D SUPPLEMENTATION
- children with moderate deficiency received 800 IU / day;
- children with a suboptimal concentration of 400jm / day.

STAGE 4. CONTROL VISITS

Every 3 months:
- in 24-hour urine collection: Ca excretion and calcium-creatinine indicator (Ca / Kr);
- in second morning urine sample, the calcium-creatinine ratio (Ca / Kr);
- in serum: concentration 25 (OH) D and Ca;
- abdominal ultrasound.

STAGE 5.
After 12 and 24 months of vitamin D supplementation, whole body densitometry was performed.

Figure 1. Study stages.

2.3. Biochemical Parameters

Parameters, others than calcium, creatinine and 25(OH)D, examined during Stage 1 has been used to confirm diagnosis of idiopathic hypercalciuria.

Blood was collected from cubital vein to biochemical tubes (BD Falcon, Warsaw, Poland), and serum was obtained by the centrifugation method (20 min., 4 °C, 2000× g).

24-h and second morning urine samples were collected to the sterile container, and urinalysis and urine culture were performed. The urine samples were centrifuged (20 min., 4 °C, 2000× g) and the supernatant was collected for biochemical analysis. The concentration of calcium, phosphorus, magnesium, and sodium was measured by the photometric absorption method in Cobas 6000 analyzer (Roche Diagnostics, Warsaw, Poland). Creatinine and urea concentration in serum and urine were evaluated by the enzymatic method in Cobas 6000 analyzer. eGFR (estimated glomerular filtration rate was calculated using the Schwartz formula (0.413 × height (cm)/serum creatinine (mg/dL)). A result above 90 mL/min/1.73 m^2 was considered as normal.

The Dia-Sorin LIAISON® analyzer (Dia-Sorin, Saluggia, Italy) and chemiluminescent immunoassays (CLIA) were used to determine the concentration of total 25-hydroxy-vitamin D in serum and plasma. The values below 30 ng/mL indicated 25(OH)D deficiency.

Calciuria was assessed on the basis of calcium excretion in a 24-h urine sample (urine calcium concentration (mg/dL) × body weight (kg)/collection volume (dL)) and calcium/creatinine ratio (Ca/Cr) calculated from the second morning urine sample (urine calcium (mg/dL)/ urine creatinine (mg/dL). Calciuria was defined as calcium excretion above 4 mg/kg/day, the values of calcium-creatinine index indicating hypercalciuria depending on age (Table 1).

Table 1. Values of the calcium-creatinine index in children, indicative of hypercalciuria.

Age	mg Calcium/mg Creatinine
<1 year	<0.81
1–3 years	<0.53
3–5 years	<0.39
5–7 years	<0.28
>7 years	<0.21

2.4. Ultrasonography and Densitometry

Abdominal ultrasound examinations were performed with the use of GE Logiq 5 Expert (Warsaw, Poland) and Philips EPIQ 5G (Warsaw, Poland) equipment. In all children, the abdominal ultrasound examination was performed according to the same examination protocol assessing the length and echogenicity of the kidneys, the presence/absence of dilatation of the calico-pelvic systems, and the presence/absence of urinary tract stones.

The densitometry was performed with the HOLOGIC model Delphi W (S/N 70608) in the Whole Body projection.

2.5. Statistical Analysis

Statistical evaluation of the results was performed using T-tests and one-way ANOVA with Bonferroni correction (in the case of a normal distribution) or non-parametric Kruskal–Wallis and Mann–Whitney U tests (in the case of an abnormal distribution). The data distribution was evaluated using the Shapiro–Wilk test. The percentile data were analyzed by the χ^2 tests with modifications or the Fischer test, depending on the size of the subgroups. Correlation analysis and the related regression analysis were performed for variables whose relationships could have medical significance. The Statistica software (version 13.1; StatSoft, Cracov, Poland)) was used. The $p < 0.05$ was considered as statistically significant.

3. Results

3.1. Study Population

36 children (18 boys, 18 girls) aged 5–16 (mean 10.47 ± 3.41) were examined. Seven patients were followed for one year, the rest (29 children) for 2 years. Vitamin D deficiency (concentration < 30 ng/mL) was observed in all children (Table 2). At the beginning of the study, 13 children had stones in the urinary tract visible on ultrasound.

Table 2. Mean values of the assessed parameters at the beginning of the study.

Parameter	N	Mean ± SD	Units	Median (q25–q75)
25-hydroxy-vitamin D	35	20.02 ± 8.52	ng/mL	20.2 (11.8–25.00)
Ca	35	9.72 ± 1.19	mg/dL	9.8 (9.6–10.20)
Calciuria	36	4.28 ± 1.85	mg/kg/24 h	4.515 (2.94–5.37)
Ca/Creatinine	33	0.19 ± 0.16	mg/mg	0.198 (0.13–0.26)
Z-score	36	−0.73 ± 0.87	-	−0.855 ((−)1.26–(−)0.36)

3.2. Vitamin D Level

The vitamin D 25 (OH) D concentration in the serum determined after 3, 6, 9, 12, 15, 18, 21, and 24 months showed a statistically significant increase. We did not observe significant changes in the serum calcium concentrations or urinary calcium excretion (measured in mg/kg/24 h and with the use of calcium-creatinine ratio) (Figure 2 and Table 3). There were no significant changes in bones density measured by the Z-score after 12 or 24 months of supplementation (Figure 3).

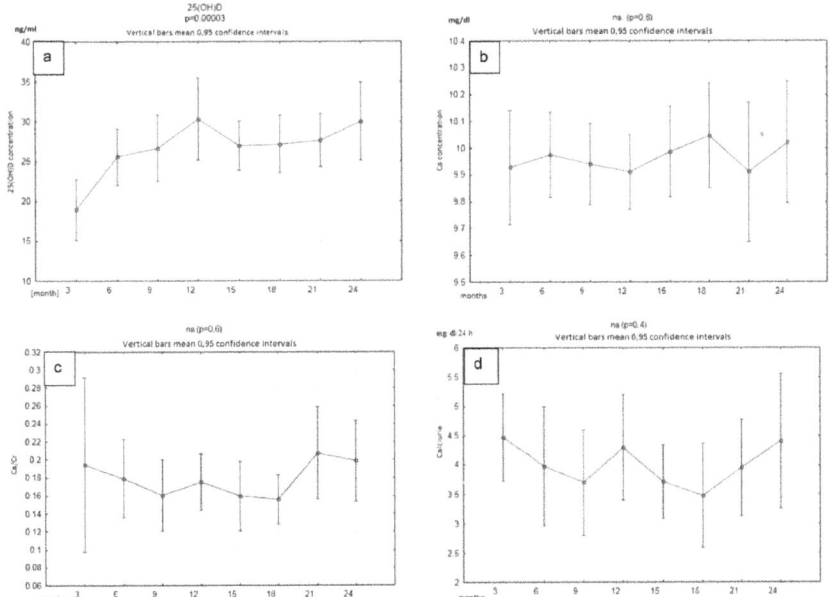

Figure 2. Time-dependent serum concentrations of vitamin D (**a**), calcium (**b**), and Ca/Creatinine (**c**), determined in the second morning urine sample, converted to creatinine ratio, and calciuria (**d**) determined in 24 h urine collection, in patients receiving vitamin D supplementation.

Table 3. The mean values of the assessed parameters after 24 months of vitamin D supplementation.

Parameter	N	Mean ± SD	Units	Median (q25–q75)
25-hydroxy-vitamin D	22	29.85 ± 9.65	ng/mL	29.25 (21.5–35.5)
Ca	21	10.02 ± 0.41	mg/dL	9.9 (9.8–10.20)
Calciuria	21	4.5 ± 2.24	mg/kg/24h	4.06 (3.30–5.43)
Ca/Creatinine	22	0.2 ± 0.09	mg/mg	0.185 (0.13–0.26)
Z-score	23	−1.05 ± 0.77	-	−0.96 ((−)1.7–(−)0.56)

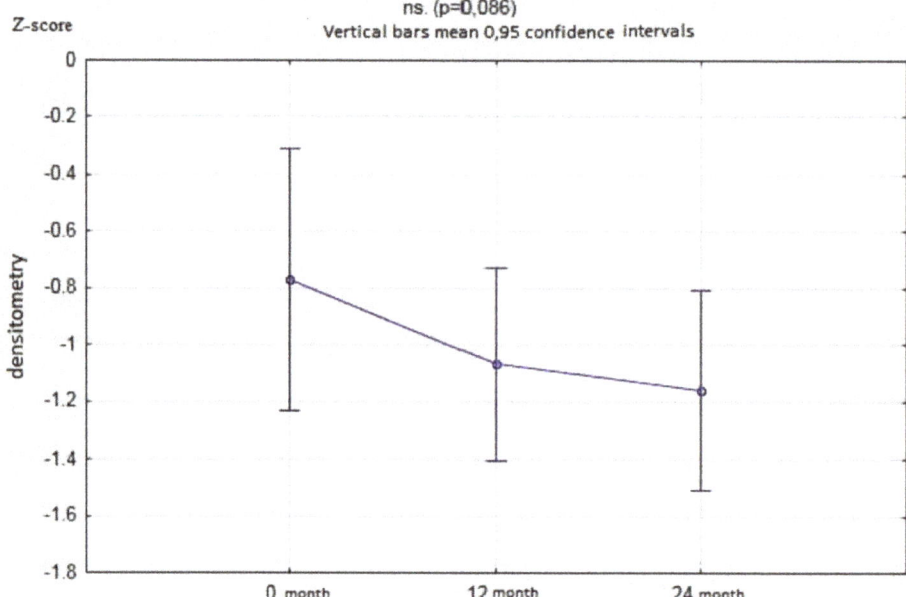

Figure 3. Z-score values in patients who received 12 or 24 months of vitamin D supplementation.

3.3. Correlations

A statistically significant correlation was found between vitamin D concentration and calcium concentration in the serum after 3 and 21 months of vitamin D supplementation. The average calcium concentration increased from 9.72 ± 1.19 to 10.06 ± 0.38 mg/dLwhich was still in the normal range), and the vitamin D concentration increased from 20.02 ± 8.52 to 27.89 ± 6.24 ng/mL. There was no statistically significant correlation between vitamin D and calcium concentration in the serum at other time points (Table 4, Figure 4). There was also no statistically significant correlation between vitamin D concentration and calcium excretion (in daily urine collection and in second morning urine sample, assessed by creatinine level) as well as between vitamin D concentration and Z-score assessed by densitometry (Table 4). The formation of new stones in the urinary system or enlargement of existing stones was not observed in the ultrasound examination performed during each follow-up visit (every 3 months) in children supplemented with vitamin D (Table 5).

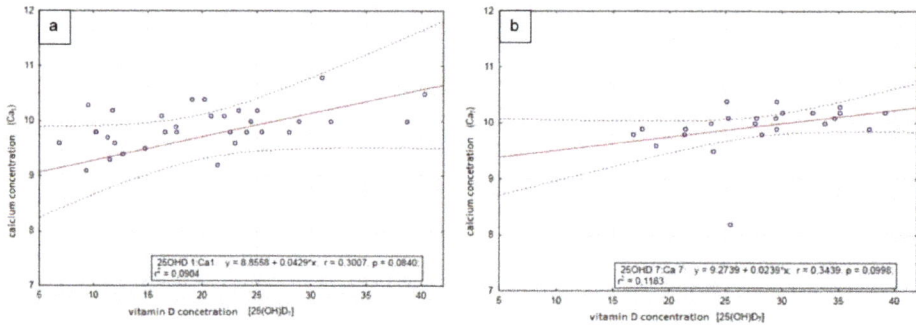

Figure 4. Dependence of serum calcium concentration on vitamin D concentration at 3 (**a**) and 21 (**b**) months after starting vitamin D administration..

Table 4. Correlations between vitamin D and calcium concentration in the serum, and calcium excretion (in the 24-h and the second morning urine sample, assessed by creatinine level) at different time points. The statistically significant values are marked in bold.

Variables	Time	R Spearman	p
25-hydroxy-vitamin D and calcium (Ca)	3 months	0.451871	0.007301
	6 months	0.215881	0.220112
	9 months	0.216470	0.226283
	12 months	0.037120	0.834899
	15 months	0.297773	0.103748
	18 months	0.068840	0.743692
	21 months	0.560887	0.004355
	24 months	0.237260	0.300404
25-hydroxy-vitamin D and calciuria	3 months	0.093781	0.592064
	6 months	−0.040049	0.822074
	9 months	−0.016993	0.921642
	12 months	0.223403	0.204067
	15 months	0.059459	0.754959
	18 months	0.087581	0.670520
	21 months	−0.142049	0.507896
	24 months	−0.059740	0.797001
25-hydroxy-vitamin D and Ca/creatinine ratio	3 months	−0.039043	0.831986
	6 months	−0.040196	0.821432
	9 months	−0.006245	0.971165
	12 months	−0.133705	0.450932
	15 months	0.176983	0.332539
	18 months	−0.098432	0.647248
	21 months	−0.235857	0.267205
	24 months	−0.206331	0.356917
25-hydroxy-vitamin D and densitometry	12 months	0.104499	0.575855
	24 months	−0.314512	0.153997

Table 5. The relationship between vitamin D concentration and urolithiasis activity after 3, 12, and 24 months of vitamin D supplementation.

	Time	p Value	Odds Ratio	Confidence OR −95%	Confidence OR +95%
25-hydroxy-vitamin D and urolithiasis activity	3 months	0.761	0.987	0.909	1.072
	12 months	0.498	1.027	0.952	1.108
	24 months	0.509	1.039	0.927	1.164

4. Discussion

Interest in vitamin D and its properties has increased significantly over the past two decades. Numerous studies conducted in various regions of the world indicate that vitamin D deficiencies occur in all countries, regardless of the latitude and age [15–18]. This is also true for Polish children. In a multicentre study of the pediatric population, a clear deficiency of vitamin D was found in 75–80% of children [19].

Similar observations were made at the Department of Paediatrics, Nephrology, and Paediatric Allergology of Military Institute of Medicine, especially in children with idiopathic hypercalciuria and urolithiasis. These observations were the basis of the presented study. Vitamin D was administered to children with urolithiasis in the course of idiopathic hypercalciuria. This is one of the few studies on the use of vitamin D treatment in such group of patients. There is controversy on the effect of vitamin D administration on the urolithiasis activity. Earlier reports suggested the possibility of negative impact of vitamin D supplementation on the activity of urolithiasis, and vitamin D treatment in these patients was, therefore, contraindicated [20,21].

Despite physiological bases some authors have already demonstrated that vitamin D supplementation does not increase calciuria. Increased calcium reabsorption in the renal tubules, associated with increased serum vitamin D levels, should reduce urinary calcium excretion [1,4]. Therefore, we decided to use vitamin D in the doses lower than those normally used in the deficient population (ie. 400 IU/day or 800 IU/day). In case of a significant calciuria increase and/or increase in urolithiasis activity, the vitamin D administration was planned to be stopped. However, this problem did not occur in any of our study patients. The dose of vitamin D was determined based on serum 25(OH)D concentration. The dose of 400 IU/day of vitamin D was administered to patients with serum 25(OH)D concentrations > 20 ng/mL and a dose of 800 IU/day in patients with serum 25(OH)D < 20 ng/mL concentration. There are no clear recommendations in the world literature regarding the administration of vitamin D in patients with low bone density and idiopathic hypercalciuria [4,9,20]. All known studies were performed in adult population and results are often contradictory. The observations from our study confirmed the observations of Ticinesi et al. [22] showing the decreased serum vitamin D concentration in patients with urolithiasis. The authors reported the patients with urolithiasis had a lower concentration of vitamin D than the patients from the control group (without urinary problems). They even concluded that vitamin D deficiency (<20 ng/mL) increases the risk of calcium stones.

Many studies have been conducted to assess the safety of vitamin D supplements in healthy people. Most studies have shown no adverse effects, either with constant use or with single high dose of vitamin D [23–28]. However, most of the analyzed cases were postmenopausal women or people with accompanying chronic diseases, including lupus, renal failure, diabetes, multiple sclerosis, or respiratory diseases, the course of which may affect the results. None of such analyzes were performed in children. In the present study, we showed, that vitamin D administration correlated with a statistically significant increase in the serum concentration of the hepatic metabolite of vitamin D. This result was consistent with other studies [29–34]. We also showed that low doses of vitamin D (400 IU/day) in patients with D hypovitaminosis caused a significant increase in the concentration of 25(OH)D in the serum. We also showed that there was no significant effect of vitamin D administration on calciuria and there was no correlation between concentration of vitamin D and calciuria, which is in agreement with the study of Eisner et al. [31]. Similar results were also observed by other authors. Penntiston et al. [34] showed that supplementation with high doses of ergocalciferol (vitamin D2) in healthy postmenopausal women, including four postmenopausal women with hypercalciuria, did not increase calcium excretion in urine. Similar results were obtained by Leaf et al. (29) who showed that in adult population with urolithiasis there was no significant increase in calcium excretion, despite the use of high doses of ergocalciferol (50,000 IU per week) for 2 months. Also, Johri et al. (30) found no statistically significant increase in calcium excretion in urine after 2 months supplementation with vitamin D (20,000 IU per week) in adults with urolithiasis, and vitamin D deficiency (<12 ng/mL in serum). However, in the group of patients with a low level of calciuria, there was an increase of calcium excretion in urine, which could have been associated with latent idiopathic hypercalciuria, and mutation or polymorphism in CYP24A1 gene. Also, Letaverier et al. [33] found a higher level of calcium extraction in the urine of rats supplemented with vitamin D. The calciuria was enhanced by the administration of calcium [33].

In the present study, the children's diet contained a normal concentration of calcium, and children did not receive additional calcium supplementation. Their calcium serum concentration was within the normal range. We found a statistically significant correlation between the concentration of calcium and vitamin D in the serum after 3 and 21 months of vitamin D administration. We also found that there was no increase in the activity of urolithiasis (defined as the presence of new stones in the urinary tract), assessed by the ultrasound analysis performed every 3 months. Similar results were obtained by Ferraro et al. [35] who evaluated the influence of vitamin D treatment on the increased risk of urolithiasis in almost 200,000 medical professionals. They divided the study group based on the daily intake (from 100 to 1000 IU) of vitamin D [35]. They found that vitamin D supplementation did not increase the risk of kidney stones. However, a limitation of the study was the method of assessing the activity of urolithiasis, which was solely based on reported renal colic incidents. In contrast, Letavernier et al. [33] showed the higher activity of stone formation in the group receiving calcium with vitamin D compared to the group receiving calcium alone, vitamin D alone, or the control group.

Bone mass is built in the first three decades of life and after the reached peak, involution of bone mass begins. The size of bone peak mass is fundamental for the risk of developing osteoporosis in the future [36,37]. The correlation between hypercalciuria and urolithiasis and osteopenia and osteoporosis is well documented [31,38]. In children, it is probably associated with increased calcium resorption from bone and/or increased bone turnover [1]. However, there is still no clear opinion on the effect of vitamin D supplementation on bone density in children with urolithiasis and hypercalciuria. The studies of Garcia-Nieto et al. [39] on the population of children with idiopathic hypercalciuria found osteopenia in 30% of the respondents (22 out of 73 children). In children with reduced bone density, they observed lower excretion of citrates and higher excretion of uric acid, which could affect both the activity of urolithiasis and the bone calcification state [39]. A comparison of 88 children with idiopathic hypercalciuria with 29 healthy children by Penido et al. [40] showed reduced bone mineral density in the lumbar spine in 35% of children with idiopathic hypercalciuria. Schwaderer et al. [41] observed a higher risk of bone mineralization disorders in children with idiopathic hypercalciuria and active urolithiasis than in children with idiopathic hypercalciuria alone. They also noted that such disorders more often affected boys with an increased Body Mass Index (BMI). On the other hand, Artemiuk et al. [42] showed a correlation between low vitamin D concentrations and reduced bone density in the lumbar spine of children. They also drew attention to the more frequent occurrence of bone mass reduction in older children compared to the younger group (mean age 11 vs. 8.5 years). In the present study, there was no improvement in bone density parameters in a densitometric examination, measured with Z-score, after 12 and 24 months supplementation with vitamin D.

Adequate dietary calcium intake is important for both urolithiasis course and bone density. Both too little and too much calcium supply in the diet favors the formation of stones in the urinary tract. According to the current opinion, patients diagnosed with idiopathic hypercalciuria should be switched to the normocalcemic diet [43]. On the other hand, patients with low bone mass are recommended a high-calcium diet, which, as previously shown, may promote the greater activity of urolithiasis. In the present work, we showed that the supplementation with low doses of vitamin D for 24 months together with the normocalcium diet is insufficient to improve bone mass. The lack of improvement in bone mineral density parameters is probably related to too low doses of vitamin D or too short observation period. One of the most important conclusions from our work is that the administration of the 400 or 800 IU/day of vitamin D seems to be safe as it did not affect the severity of urolithiasis activity.

5. Limitation

We are aware, however, that our study had some limitation: 1. the size of the studied group of children was small, 2. we had not full control of the diet or 3. regular administration of vitamin D. In our opinion the study of a larger population of children with supplementation with higher doses of vitamin D should be performed. In other limitations, we assumed that a three-month biochemical evaluations of patients were sufficient to conclude that patients followed with the recommendations.

6. Conclusions

(1). Supplementation with low doses of vitamin D (400–800 IU/day) in children with idiopathic hypercalciuria significantly increases the concentration of 25OHD vitamin D in the serum and does not affect the level of calciuria. It does not increase the dynamics of stones formation in the urinary tract, but also does not improve bone density.

(2). The use of vitamin D preparations in these patients is safe, without a significant influence on the severity of disease activity.

(3). Children with idiopathic hypercalciuria should be advised to carefully monitor the parameters of calcium metabolism and the level of urolithiasis activity without giving up vitamin D supplementation.

Author Contributions: Conceptualization, J.M. and K.J.; methodology, A.W., K.J.; validation, J.M., A.L. and K.J.; formal analysis, M.M.-Ł., A.L.; investigation, J.M., K.J., A.W., B.K.; resources, M.M.-Ł.; data curation J.M., B.K.; writing—original draft preparation, J.M., A.L. and A.W.; writing—review and editing, A.L., K.J. and M.M.-Ł.; visualization, J.M.; supervision, K.J., B.K.; project administration, J.M.; funding acquisition, B.K. All authors have read and agreed to the published version of the manuscript.

Funding: The research was supported by the statutory grant of the Military Institute of Medicine, Warsaw, Poland—project no. 293 (1/8841).

Conflicts of Interest: The authors certify that there is no conflict of interest with any financial organization regarding the material discussed in the manuscript.

References

1. Zerwekh, J.E. Vitamin D Metabolism and Stones. In *Urinary Tract Stone Disease*; Rao, N.P., Preminger, G.M., Kavanagh, J.P., Eds.; Springer: London, UK, 2011; pp. 169–179. ISBN 978-1-84800-362-0.
2. Holick, M.F.; Chen, T.C.; Lu, Z.; Sauter, E. Vitamin D and skin physiology: A D-lightful story. *J. Bone Miner. Res. Off. J. Am. Soc. Bone Miner. Res.* **2007**, *22* (Suppl. 2), V28–V33. [CrossRef] [PubMed]
3. Wytyczne dla lekarzy rodzinnych dotyczące suplementacji witaminy D. Available online: https://www.tvmed.pl/tresci/layout_min/11431/Wytyczne-dla-lekarzy-rodzinnych-dotyczace-suplementacji-witaminy-D (accessed on 28 June 2020).
4. Zerwekh, J.E. Bone disease and hypercalciuria in children. *Pediatr. Nephrol. Berl. Ger.* **2010**, *25*, 395–401. [CrossRef] [PubMed]
5. Worcester, E.M.; Coe, F.L. New insights into the pathogenesis of idiopathic hypercalciuria. *Semin. Nephrol.* **2008**, *28*, 120–132. [CrossRef] [PubMed]
6. Kamińska, A.; Bieroza, I. Hiperkalciuria–najczęstsze zaburzenie metaboliczne u dzieci z kamicą nerkową. *Nowa Pediatria* **2011**, *2*, 49–52.
7. Milart, J.; Jobs, K.; Anna, J. Hiperkalciuria idiopatyczna. *Pediatr. Med. Rodz.* **2016**, *12*, 22–27. [CrossRef]
8. Kamica układu moczowego u dzieci/Urolithiasis in children-Standardy Medyczne. Available online: http://www.standardy.pl/artykuly/id/873 (accessed on 28 June 2020).
9. Jobs, K.; Jung, A. Gęstość kości u pacjentów z hiperkalciurią idiopatyczną–przegląd piśmiennictwa w aspekcie bezpieczeństwa stosowania witaminy D. *Pediatr. Med. Rodz.* **2013**, *9*, 245–249.
10. Rakowska, M.; Królikowska, K.; Jobs, K.; Placzyńska, M.; Kalicki, B. Pathophysiology and symptoms of renal colic in children-a case report. *Dev. Period Med.* **2018**, *22*, 265–269.
11. Jobs, K.; Rakowska, M.; Paturej, A. Urolithiasis in the pediatric population-current opinion on epidemiology, patophysiology, diagnostic evaluation and treatment. *Dev. Period Med.* **2018**, *22*, 201–208.
12. López, M.; Hoppe, B. History, epidemiology and regional diversities of urolithiasis. *Pediatr Nephrol.* **2010**, *25*, 49–59. [CrossRef]
13. Iwańczak, B.; Krzesiek, E.; Iwańczak, F. Osteoporoza i osteopenia u dzieci i młodzieży–przyczyny, diagnostyka i leczenie. *Adv. Clin. Exp. Med.* **2004**, *13*, 177–184.
14. Arrabal-Polo, M.Á.; Sierra Girón-Prieto, M.; Orgaz-Molina, J.; Zuluaga-Gómez, A.; Arias-Santiago, S.; Arrabal-Martín, M. Calcium renal lithiasis and bone mineral density. Importance of bone metabolism in urinary lithiasis. *Actas Urol. Esp.* **2013**, *37*, 362–367. [CrossRef] [PubMed]
15. Cediel, G.; Pacheco-Acosta, J.; CastiUo-Durdn, C. Vitamin D deficiency in pediatric clinical practice. *Arch. Argent. Pediatr.* **2018**, *116*, e75–e81. [CrossRef] [PubMed]
16. Povoroznyuk, V.V.; Balatska, N.I.; Muts, V.Y.; Klymovytsky, F.V.; Synenky, O.V. Vitamin D deficiency in Ukraine: A demographic and seasonal analysis. *Gerontologija* **2012**, *13*, 191–198.
17. Zakharova, I.N.; Mal'tsev, S.V.; Borovik, T.E.; Yatsyk, G.V.; Malyavskaya, S.I.; Vakhlova, I.V.; Shumatova, T.A.; Romantsova, Y.B.; Romanyuk, F.P.; Klimov, L.Y.; et al. Vitamin d Insufficiency in Children of Tender years in Russia: The Results of a Multi-Centre Cohort Study Rodnichok (2013–2014). Available online: https://vsp.spr-journal.ru/jour/article/view/98 (accessed on 21 July 2020).

18. Vitamin D Deficiency/Insufficiency from Childhood to Adulthood: Insights from a Sunny Country. Available online: https://www.ncbi.nlm.nih.gov/pmc/articles/PMC5296623/ (accessed on 21 July 2020).
19. Wrzosek, M.; Woźniak, J.; Kozioł-Kaczorek, D.; Włodarek, D. The Assessment of the Supply of Calcium and Vitamin D in the Diet of Women Regularly Practicing Sport. *J. Osteoporos.* **2019**, *2019*. [CrossRef] [PubMed]
20. Tang, J.; Chonchol, M.B. Vitamin D and kidney stone disease. *Curr. Opin. Nephrol. Hypertens.* **2013**, *22*, 383–389. [CrossRef] [PubMed]
21. Taheri, M.; Tavasoli, S.; Shokrzadeh, F.; Amiri, F.B.; Basiri, A.; Taheri, M.; Tavasoli, S.; Shokrzadeh, F.; Amiri, F.B.; Basiri, A. Effect of vitamin D supplementation on 24-hour urine calcium in patients with calcium Urolithiasis and vitamin D deficiency. *Int. Braz. J. Urol.* **2019**, *45*, 340–346. [CrossRef] [PubMed]
22. Ticinesi, A.; Nouvenne, A.; Ferraro, P.M.; Folesani, G.; Lauretani, F.; Allegri, F.; Guerra, A.; Cerundolo, N.; Aloe, R.; Lippi, G.; et al. Idiopathic Calcium Nephrolithiasis and Hypovitaminosis D: A Case-control Study. *Urology* **2016**, *87*, 40–45. [CrossRef]
23. Malihi, Z.; Wu, Z.; Stewart, A.W.; Lawes, C.M.; Scragg, R. Hypercalcemia, hypercalciuria, and kidney stones in long-term studies of vitamin D supplementation: A systematic review and meta-analysis. *Am. J. Clin. Nutr.* **2016**, *104*, 1039–1051. [CrossRef]
24. Cranney, A.; Horsley, T.; O'Donnell, S.; Weiler, H.; Puil, L.; Ooi, D.; Atkinson, S.; Ward, L.; Moher, D.; Hanley, D.; et al. Effectiveness and Safety of Vitamin D in Relation to Bone Health. *Evid. Rep. Technol. Assess (Full Rep).* **2007**, *158*, 1–235.
25. Avenell, A.; Mak, J.C.S.; O'Connell, D. Vitamin D and vitamin D analogues for preventing fractures in post-menopausal women and older men. *Cochrane Database Syst. Rev.* **2014**, CD000227. [CrossRef]
26. Bjelakovic, G.; Gluud, L.L.; Nikolova, D.; Whitfield, K.; Wetterslev, J.; Simonetti, R.G.; Bjelakovic, M.; Gluud, C. Vitamin D supplementation for prevention of mortality in adults. *Cochrane Database Syst. Rev.* **2011**, CD007470. [CrossRef]
27. Bjelakovic, G.; Gluud, L.L.; Nikolova, D.; Whitfield, K.; Krstic, G.; Wetterslev, J.; Gluud, C. Vitamin D supplementation for prevention of cancer in adults. *Cochrane Database Syst. Rev.* **2014**, CD007469. [CrossRef] [PubMed]
28. Kearns, M.D.; Alvarez, J.A.; Tangpricha, V. Large, single-dose, oral vitamin D supplementation in adult populations: A systematic review. *Endocr. Pract. Off. J. Am. Coll. Endocrinol. Am. Assoc. Clin. Endocrinol.* **2014**, *20*, 341–351. [CrossRef] [PubMed]
29. Leaf, D.E.; Korets, R.; Taylor, E.N.; Tang, J.; Asplin, J.R.; Goldfarb, D.S.; Gupta, M.; Curhan, G.C. Effect of vitamin D repletion on urinary calcium excretion among kidney stone formers. *Clin. J. Am. Soc. Nephrol. CJASN* **2012**, *7*, 829–834. [CrossRef]
30. Johri, N.; Jaeger, P.; Ferraro, P.M.; Shavit, L.; Nair, D.; Robertson, W.G.; Gambaro, G.; Unwin, R.J. Vitamin D deficiency is prevalent among idiopathic stone formers, but does correction pose any risk? *Urolithiasis* **2017**, *45*, 535–543. [CrossRef]
31. Eisner, B.H.; Thavaseelan, S.; Sheth, S.; Haleblian, G.; Pareek, G. Relationship Between Serum Vitamin D and 24-Hour Urine Calcium in Patients With Nephrolithiasis. *Urology* **2012**, *80*, 1007–1010. [CrossRef]
32. Sorkhi, H.; Aahmadi, M.H. Urinary calcium to creatinin ratio in children. *Indian J. Pediatr.* **2005**, *72*, 1055–1056. [CrossRef]
33. Letavernier, E.; Verrier, C.; Goussard, F.; Perez, J.; Huguet, L.; Haymann, J.-P.; Baud, L.; Bazin, D.; Daudon, M. Calcium and vitamin D have a synergistic role in a rat model of kidney stone disease. *Kidney Int.* **2016**, *90*, 809–817. [CrossRef]
34. Penniston, K.L.; Jones, A.N.; Nakada, S.Y.; Hansen, K.E. Vitamin D repletion does not alter urinary calcium excretion in healthy postmenopausal women. *BJU Int.* **2009**, *104*, 1512–1516. [CrossRef]
35. Ferraro, P.M.; Taylor, E.N.; Gambaro, G.; Curhan, G.C. Vitamin D Intake and the Risk of Incident Kidney Stones. *J. Urol.* **2017**, *197*, 405–410. [CrossRef]
36. Nieradko-Iwanicka, B.; Borzęcki, A. Osteoporoza jako problem pediatryczny. *Probl. Hig. Epidemiol.* **2009**, *90*, 27–31.
37. Lorenc, R.; Karczmarewicz, E. Znaczenie wapnia i witaminy D w optymalizacji masy kostnej oraz zapobieganiu i leczeniu osteoporozy u dzieci. *Pediat. Współcz.* **2001**, *3*, 105–109.
38. Pfau, A.; Knauf, F. Update on Nephrolithiasis: Core Curriculum 2016. *Am. J. Kidney Dis. Off. J. Natl. Kidney Found.* **2016**, *68*, 973–985. [CrossRef] [PubMed]

39. Moreira Guimarães Penido, M.G.; de Sousa Tavares, M.; Campos Linhares, M.; Silva Barbosa, A.C.; Cunha, M. Longitudinal study of bone mineral density in children with idiopathic hypercalciuria. *Pediatr. Nephrol.* **2012**, *27*, 123–130. [CrossRef]
40. Penido, M.-G.M.G.; Lima, E.M.; Souto, M.F.O.; Marino, V.S.P.; Tupinambá, A.-L.F.; França, A. Hypocitraturia: A risk factor for reduced bone mineral density in idiopathic hypercalciuria? *Pediatr. Nephrol. Berl. Ger.* **2006**, *21*, 74–78. [CrossRef]
41. Schwaderer, A.L.; Cronin, R.; Mahan, J.D.; Bates, C.M. Low bone density in children with hypercalciuria and/or nephrolithiasis. *Pediatr. Nephrol. Berl. Ger.* **2008**, *23*, 2209–2214. [CrossRef]
42. Artemiuk, I.; Pańczyk-Tomaszewska, M.; Adamczuk, D.; Przedlacki, J.; Roszkowska-Blaim, M. Bone mineral density in children with idiopathic hypercalciuria. *Dev. Period Med.* **2015**, *19*, 356–361.
43. Gambaro, G.; Croppi, E.; Coe, F.; Lingeman, J.; Moe, O.; Worcester, E.; Buchholz, N.; Bushinsky, D.; Curhan, G.C.; Ferraro, P.M.; et al. Metabolic diagnosis and medical prevention of calcium nephrolithiasis and its systemic manifestations: A consensus statement. *J. Nephrol.* **2016**, *29*, 715–734. [CrossRef]

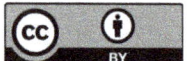

© 2020 by the authors. Licensee MDPI, Basel, Switzerland. This article is an open access article distributed under the terms and conditions of the Creative Commons Attribution (CC BY) license (http://creativecommons.org/licenses/by/4.0/).

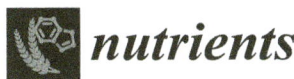

Article

Validation and Determination of 25(OH) Vitamin D and 3-Epi25(OH)D3 in Breastmilk and Maternal- and Infant Plasma during Breastfeeding

Jennifer Gjerde *, Marian Kjellevold, Lisbeth Dahl, Torill Berg, Annbjørg Bøkevoll and Maria Wik Markhus

Institute of Marine Research, P.O box 1870 Nordnes, 5817 Bergen, Norway; Marian.Kjellevold@hi.no (M.K.); Lisbeth.Dahl@hi.no (L.D.); Torill.Berg@hi.no (T.B.); Annbjorg.Bokevoll@hi.no (A.B.); Maria.Wik.Markhus@hi.no (M.W.M.)
* Correspondence: Jennifer.Gjerde@hi.no; Tel.: +4793652137

Received: 12 July 2020; Accepted: 27 July 2020; Published: 29 July 2020

Abstract: Vitamin D deficiency in pregnant women and their offspring may result in unfavorable health outcomes for both mother and infant. A 25hydroxyvitamin D (25(OH)D) level of at least 75 nmol/L is recommended by the Endocrine Society. Validated, automated sample preparation and liquid chromatography-tandem mass spectrometry (LC-MS/MS) methods were used to determine the vitamin D metabolites status in mother-infant pairs. Detection of 3-Epi25(OH)D3 prevented overestimation of 25(OH)D3 and misclassification of vitamin D status. Sixty-three percent of maternal 25(OH)D plasma levels were less than the recommended level of 25(OH)D at 3 months. Additionally, breastmilk levels of 25(OH)D decreased from 60.1 nmol/L to 50.0 nmol/L between six weeks and three months ($p < 0.01$). Furthermore, there was a positive correlation between mother and infant plasma levels ($p < 0.01$, r = 0.56) at 3 months. Accordingly, 31% of the infants were categorized as vitamin D deficient (25(OH)D < 50 nmol/L) compared to 25% if 3-Epi25(OH)D3 was not distinguished from 25(OH)D3. This study highlights the importance of accurate quantification of 25(OH)D. Monitoring vitamin D metabolites in infant, maternal plasma, and breastmilk may be needed to ensure adequate levels in both mother and infant in the first 6 months of infant life.

Keywords: breastmilk; infant; mother; plasma; vitamin D metabolites; 3-Epi25(OH)D3; 25-hydroxyvitamin

1. Introduction

Vitamin D plays an important role in bone metabolism. It regulates the calcium and phosphate in the body, making it important for muscle, tooth, and growth development [1]. It may also play an important role in immune system regulation [2,3]. The source of vitamin D in Norwegian diets is in the form of vitamin D2 (ergocalciferol) from plants and vitamin D3 (cholecalciferol) from fish, butter, and eggs [4]. Vitamin D2 and D3 bind to the Vitamin D carrier protein (DBP) before transported to the liver for hydroxylation, producing 25-hydroxyvitamin (25(OH)) D3 and 25(OH)D2. The 25(OH)D2 is derived solely from the diet/supplements and 25(OH)D3 is either derived from the diet/supplements or synthesized in the skin. The C3 epimer forms of vitamin D_3 have less affinity toward vitamin D protein and even lower affinity for vitamin D receptors compared to 25(OH)D3. The 3-Epi25(OH)D3 binds to vitamin D receptor (VDR) at 2–3% the affinity of 25(OH)D3 [5]. Studies have also shown reduced ability in inducing calcium transport and reduced gene expression in the human colonic carcinoma cell line, Caco-2 [6–8]. Determining the concentration of 25(OH)D3 and 3-Epi25(OH)D3 separately is therefore important due to possible difference of effectiveness. However, further studies on the function and source of 3-Epi25(OH)D3 in humans are warranted.

Vitamin D3 has a plasma half-life of 4 to 12 h [9,10] and a circulating half-life of 12 to 24 h [11]. On the other hand, 25(OH)D2 and 25(OH)D3 have longer half-lives, 13 and 15 to 25 days, respectively [12–15]. The 25(OH)D is further hydroxylated to 1,25-dihydroxyvitamin D (1,25(OH)2D), the most potent physiologically active metabolite with a relatively short half-life of 4 to 6 h [16]. This suggests that measurements of 25(OH)D, 25(OH)D2, and 25(OH)D3 are better indicators of vitamin D status in the blood. Holick et al. have published a set of guidelines for the evaluation of Vitamin D deficiencies [17]. Blood 25(OH)D levels < 50 nmol/L are considered 25(OH)D-deficient, levels between 50 and 75 nmol/L are considered 25(OH)D-insufficient, and >75 nmol/L are considered 25(OH)D-sufficient [17–20].

Methods which only measure 25(OH)D3 and not 3-Epi25(OH)D3 may cause overestimation of 25(OH)D3 because both analytes would be determined as 25(OH)D3. To obtain accurate measurements of vitamin D levels in mothers and infants, a highly selective and sensitive quantification method for measuring vitamin D metabolites in blood and breastmilk is needed [21]. Thus, in this study, simple, sensitive, and selective liquid chromatography-tandem mass spectrometric (LC-MS/MS) methods were used for determination of 25(OH)D2, 25(OH)D3, and 3-epi-25-hydroxyvitamin D3 (3-Epi25(OH)D3) in plasma, breastmilk, and infant formula. An automated sample preparation involving protein-crash and solid-phase extraction techniques was applied to ensure simple sample treatment, and reduced time and labor.

During pregnancy, the main source of vitamin D for the fetus is the mother, through the umbilical cord. Studies have reported correlation between maternal and infant cord blood 25(OH)D concentrations [22–25]. Thus, mothers with sufficient 25(OH)D during pregnancy can provide sufficient cord blood concentrations of 25(OH)D crossing the placenta [26,27]. However, vitamin D metabolites levels < 50 nmol/L have been observed in pregnant women and their offspring [28–30]. Pregnant women and infants are highly susceptible to vitamin D deficiency which has been associated with adverse health outcomes, such as pre-eclampsia, perinatal complications, postpartum depression, spontaneous abortion, emergency cesarean section delivery, oligohydramnios, polyhydramnios, and gestational diabetes [31,32]. As for the infants, vitamin D deficiency may cause a small-for-gestational age condition, preterm birth, low birth weight, stunting, impaired fetal bone formation, and rickets [31–35]. Accordingly, Norwegian maternal vitamin D < 30 nmol/L has been associated with lower offspring peak bone mass [36]. Personalized vitamin D supplementation during pregnancy and lactation has been suggested [37]. Monitoring vitamin D deficiency in Norwegian mother-infant pairs before and after childbirth is therefore of importance.

The aim of this study was to validate selective and sensitive LC-MS/MS methods for the analysis of vitamin D metabolites with automated sample preparation. These methods were applied to determine the concentration levels of Vitamin D metabolites in mother-infant pairs during the first six months of breastfeeding. Detection and quantification of 3-Epi25(OH)D3 allows evaluation of the impact of 3-Epi25(OH)D3 when assessing vitamin D metabolites status in plasma and breastmilk. The relationships between plasma vitamin D metabolites levels in mother-infant pairs and breastmilk levels were also examined.

2. Materials and Methods

2.1. Study Population and Design

From January 2016 until February 2017, pregnant women were recruited to participate in a two-armed randomized controlled intervention trial involving cod intake in pregnancy [38]. The study was registered on ClinicalTrials.gov (NCT02610959) in 17 November 2015. All participants were recruited through the womens' clinic at Haukeland University Hospital in Norway. A total of 137 pregnant women were included in this secondary analysis. Details regarding the main study have been described elsewhere [38].

2.2. Biological Samples and Laboratory Analysis

Blood samples were obtained from mother-infant pairs. The mothers were requested to provide a sample of breastmilk at six weeks and three months postpartum. Breastmilk was collected at the beginning, middle, and end of a chosen feed. The three samples were then stored in a freezer until pick-up by study investigators or submission during the third-month follow-up visit. Samples were placed in freezer packs during transport. Upon arrival in the laboratory, samples were stored at –80 °C until analyzed as a pooled sample. Meanwhile, blood sampling was conducted in mothers and infants at three and six months postpartum. Plasma samples from the participants were obtained by collecting blood into BD Vacutainer ® K2E 5.4 mg vials (Franklin Lakes, NJ, USA), centrifuged (1000–1300× g, 20 °C, 10 min) within 30 min, and the supernatant was stored at –80 °C until analyzed.

2.3. Laboratory Analysis

2.3.1. Chemical and Reagents

The standards 25(OH)D3, 25(OH)D2, 3-Epi25(OH)D3 and internal standard D_6-25(OH)D3-(26,26,26,27,27,27-D_6) were obtained from Cerilliant (Round Rock, TX, USA). The internal standards 25(OH)D2-(6,19,19-d_3) and 3-Epi25(OH)D3-(6,19,19-d_3), zink sulfate monohydrate, formic acid (analytical grade) and ammonium acetate were purchased from Sigma-Aldrich (St Louis, MO, USA).

2.3.2. Sample Preparation

All sample preparation and extraction process were performed using robotic a Dual Head MultiPurpose Sampler (MPS XL) equipped with an Anatune CF-100 Centrifuge Option, MicroLiter ITSP Option and Active WashStation [39,40] Using an automated system, samples were prepared by adding 80 µL of internal standards to aliquots of 200-µL samples. Protein-crash, centrifugation, and solid-phase extraction techniques were automated using MPS XL (Anatune, Cambridge, UK). The samples were precipitated with 200 µL zinc sulfate and 500 µL methanol. Samples were then vortexed and centrifuged for 5 min. An aliquot of 500 µL of supernatant was loaded for solid phase extraction and eluted with 40 µL methanol. High purity water (18.2 million ohms, MΩ x cm) was added to the eluted sample prior to LC-MS/MS injection.

2.3.3. LC-MS/MS Procedure

Waters Quattro Premier™/XE

LC-MS/MS conditions for the analysis of plasma samples were as follows. For chromatographic separation, acquity ultra performance liquid chromatography (UPLC) (Waters Corporation, Milford, MA, USA) was used. The system was equipped with a degasser, pump, a thermostated acquity sample manager and column oven. Twenty microliters of the sample was injected into the analytical column (Acquity UPLC, HSS PFP 1.8 µm, 2.1 × 100 mm, Waters, Milford, MA, USA). Two millimole per liter ammonium acetate with 0.1% formic acid was used as mobile phase A, while methanol with 0.3% formic acid was used as mobile phase B. The Waters binary solvent manager was programmed as follows: 0–3.0 min, 30% A and 70% B; 3.5–5.0 min, 25% A and 75% B; 5.5–6.0 min, 2% A and 98% B; 6.5–8.0 min, 30% A and 70% B. All gradient steps were linear. For sample detection, a triple-quadrupole mass spectrometry system from Waters Quattro Premier™/XE (Waters Corporation, Milford, MA, USA) was used, equipped with electrospray ion source. MS source parameters are as follows: capillary voltage, 3.0 kV; cone voltage, 15–20 V; source temperature, 120 °C; and cone gas flow rate, 15 L/h. Nitrogen and argon were used as the cone and collision gases, respectively. Parent and fragment ions were detected in multiple-reaction monitoring (MRM) mode and the respective collision energies are listed in Appendix A. Data acquisition for all experiments was carried out with Masslynx V4.1 software (Waters, Milford, USA).

Agilent MassHunter

LC-MS/MS conditions for the analysis of plasma, breastmilk, and infant formula samples were as follows: For chromatographic separation, an Agilent 1290 UPLC (Agilent Technologies, Palo Alto, CA, USA) was used. The system was equipped with a degasser, pump, a thermostated autosampler, and column oven. Fifteen microliters of the sample was injected to the analytical column (Acquity UPLC, HSS PFP 1.8 µm, 2.1 × 100 mm, Waters, Milford, MA, USA). Two millimole ammonium acetate with 0.1% formic acid was used as mobile phase A, while methanol with 0.3% formic acid was used as mobile phase B. The Agilent 1290 pump was programmed as follows: 0–3.0 min, 35% A and 65% B; 3.5–4.5 min, 30% A and 70% B; 5.0–6.4 min, 25% A and 75% B; 6.5–8.0 min, 2% A and 98% B; 8.1–9.5 min, 35% A and 65% B. All gradient steps were linear. For sample detection, a triple-quadrupole mass spectrometry system from Agilent 6495B (Agilent Technologies, Santa Clara, CA, USA) was used, equipped with jet stream electrospray ion source. Nitrogen was used as the drying gas, sheath gas, nebulizing gas, and collision gas. The drying and sheath gas temperatures were 200 °C and 300 °C, respectively. The following settings were used: drying gas flow 13 L/min and sheath gas flow: 10 L/min, nebulizer pressure: 40 psi, capillary voltage: 5000 V, and nozzle voltage: 2000 V. Parent and fragment ions were detected in multiple-reaction monitoring (MRM) mode and the respective collision energies are listed in Appendix A. The Agilent MassHunter Workstation software version B.08.00. (Agilent Technologies, Santa Clara, CA, USA) was used to control the LC-MS system, peak integration, quantitation, and calculation.

2.4. LC-MS/MS Assay Validation. Linearity, Sensitivity, Precision, Accuracy, and Recovery

Method validation was performed according to bioanalytical method guidelines for biological samples and industry [41,42]. The linearity of the two methods were assessed using six concentration levels of 25(OH)D2, 25(OH)D3, and 3-Epi25(OH)D3, analyzed for ten consecutive days. Sensitivity was determined by calculating the lower limit of detection (LOD) and lower limit of quantification (LOQ). The LOD was determined using the concentration of the lowest diluted sample with signal-to-noise ratio at approximately three. The LOQ was set as the concentration of the lowest standard.

Precision and accuracy were determined by an intra-day and inter-day analysis of in-house quality control samples. Precision was calculated as relative standard deviation (RSD) of experimental concentrations, and the criteria for acceptability was 15% RSD, except for the LOQ where it should not have exceeded 20%. Accuracy was calculated as the comparison between the measured values and nominal sample concentrations. The criteria for acceptability were 15% and 20% (at LOQ) deviation from the nominal values. An in-house quality control plasma sample consisting of 25(OH)D3 at a medium level was used to estimate intra-assay and inter-assay precision and accuracy of 25(OH)D3 for the Waters Quattro PremierTM/XE method. For the Agilent 6495B method, three concentration levels (low, medium, and high) of in-house quality control samples were prepared in plasma, breastmilk, and infant formula. The baseline concentrations of 25(OH)D2, 25(OH)D3, and 3-Epi25(OH)D3 were measured prior to addition of the standard solutions. The 25(OH)D2, 25(OH)D3, and 3-Epi25(OH)D3 were then assayed for intra-assay precision and accuracy for ten consecutive days. The inter-assay precision was evaluated for 25(OH)D2, 25(OH)D3, and 3-Epi25(OH)D3. Accuracy was determined using commercial quality control (QC) plasma samples; standard reference materials (SRM) 972a-C level 1, SRM 972a-C level 2, SRM 972a-C level 3, and SRM 972a-C level 4 Vitamin D Metabolites in frozen human serum. SRM 1950 metabolites in frozen human plasma were also used. In addition, QC serum samples were also included (SRM 972 level 2, SRM 1950, and SRM 2972). The recovery of the analytes was studied by spiking the samples (plasma, breastmilk, and infant formula) with standard solutions at three levels. Recovery was evaluated by comparing the baseline (unspiked) and spiked samples at three levels (low, medium, and high). Recovery was then calculated by comparing the measured concentration of the prepared samples with the nominal value (baseline and spiked concentration) representing 100% recovery.

2.5. Data Analysis and Statistical Analyses

LC-MS/MS data were analyzed by Agilent MassHunter 8.0 Quan Browser (Agilent Technologies, Santa Clara, CA, USA). The levels of vitamin D metabolites are presented as mean and standard deviation (SD). To examine differences between status and categories paired Student's t-test was used. Pearson's correlation coefficients were used to assess associations between continuous variables. A 2-sided p-value of <0.05 was considered significant. All statistical analyses were performed using IBM SPSS Statistics 26 (IBM Corp., Armonk, NY, USA).

3. Results

3.1. Evaluation of the LC-MS/MS Assay

The LC MS/MS methods for the determination of 25(OH)D2, 25(OH)D3, and 3-Epi25(OH)D3 using Waters Quattro Premier^{TM}/XE, and 25(OH)D2, 25(OH)D3, and 3-Epi25(OH)D3 using Agilent 6495B were developed and validated. The base peak ions and fragments of 25(OH)D2, 25(OH)D3, and 3-Epi25(OH)D3 ([M + H]$^+$) are shown in Appendix A. The Waters Quattro Premier^{TM}/XE is equipped with an electrospray ion source and Agilent 6495B is equipped with a jet stream electrospray ion source. The selected reaction monitoring was based on the mass-to-charge ratio (m/z). The Agilent 6495B MRM chromatograms of the analytes are shown in the Supplementary Material Figure S1. It provided separation between metabolites, with 25(OH)D3, 25(OH)D2, and 3-Epi25(OH)D3 eluting at 6.95, 7.18, and 7.19 min, respectively. The same was observed using Waters Quattro Premier^{TM}/XE with the mass-to-charge ratio (m/z) and fragmentations distinguished for Waters Quattro Premier^{TM}/XE (data not shown).

The Waters Quattro Premier^{TM}/XE method was linear for 25(OH)D3, 25(OH)D2, and 3-Epi25(OH)D3 as shown in Table 1, and the best fits were indicated by a correlation coefficient (r) of 0.99 for 25(OH)D3, 25(OH)D2, and 3-Epi25(OH)D3. The Agilent 6495B method was linear for 25(OH)D3, 25(OH)D2, and 3-Epi25(OH)D3 with correlation coefficients $\geq$ 0.999. The standard curves are considered acceptable when r is >0.99. The limit of detection (LOD) and limit of quantification (LOQ) were determined to evaluate sensitivity of the method and are shown in Table 1a for Quattro Premier^{TM}/XE and Table 1b for Agilent 6495B.

Table 1. Linearity, limit of quantification, and limit of detection of vitamin D metabolites measured by (a) Waters Quattro Premier^{TM}/XE and (b) Agilent 6495B.

	Linearity	r	LOQ	LOD
a. Waters Quattro Premier^{TM}/XE	nmol/L		nmol/L	nmol/L
25(OH)D2	7.6–242.3	0.9969	7.6	2.3
25(OH)D3	7.8–249.6	0.9985	7.8	2.34
3-Epi25(OH)D3	7.8–249.6	0.9986	7.8	2.3
b. Agilent 6495B				
25(OH)D2	7.0–335	0.9999	7.0	2.1
25(OH)D3	4.3–270	0.9998	4.3	1.3
3-Epi25(OH)D3	1.7–137	0.9999	1.7	0.5

Limit of quantification (LOQ), limit of detection (LOD).

The intra-assay and inter-assay precision and accuracy are summarized in Tables 2 and 3. Relative standard deviation (RSD) values for quality control (QC) plasma, breastmilk, and infant formula samples measured with Waters Quattro Premier^{TM}/XE and with Agilent 6495B were below 20% for 25(OH)D2, 25(OH)D3, and 3-Epi25(OH)D3, respectively. For low concentration levels, RSD value for breastmilk was 30% for 3-Epi25(OH)D3. The methods showed accuracy within 20%, as shown in Appendix B. The recoveries of the analytes obtained with the use of automated solid phase extraction and filtration autosampler, Gerstel multi-purpose sampler, ranged from 88% to 120%, 72% to 103% and 81% to 129% for plasma, breastmilk, and infant formula, respectively as shown in Appendix C.

Table 2. Intra-day (*n*) of vitamin D metabolites in plasma, breastmilk, and infant formula samples measured by (a) Waters Quattro Premier™/XE and (b) Agilent 6495B.

Intra-Day Precision	Vitamin D Metabolites		
a. Waters Quattro Premier™/XE			
Plasma (*n* = 6)	25(OH)D2	25(OH)D3	3-Epi25(OH)D3
Medium1			
Average (nmol/L)	-	55.7 ± 4.8	-
RSD (%)		8	
b. Agilent 6495B			
Plasma (*n* = 10)	25(OH)D2	25(OH)D3	3-Epi25(OH)D3
Low2			
Average (nmol/L)	31.5 ± 4.4	46.1 ± 2.8	34.6 ± 2.7
RSD (%)	14	6	8
Medium2			
Average (nmol/L)	76.2 ± 7.5	111.0 ± 3.9	49.3 ± 3.5
RSD (%)	10	3	7
High2			
Average (nmol/L)	120.3 ± 8.9	177.9 ± 14.6	105.6 ± 5.6
RSD (%)	7	8	5
Breastmilk (*n* = 10)	25(OH)D2	25(OH)D3	3-Epi25(OH)D3
Low3			
Average (nmol/L)	<LOQ	11.7 ± 1.9	6.8 ± 1.0
RSD (%)		16	14
Medium3			
Average (nmol/L)	47.8 ± 3.0	71.6 ± 2.5	51.7 ± 2.3
RSD (%)	6	4	4
High3			
Average (nmol/L)	103.1 ± 4.4	126.8 ± 9.4	96.7 ± 4.6
RSD (%)	4	7	5
Infant formula (*n* = 10)	25(OH)D2	25(OH)D3	3-Epi25(OH)D3
Low4			
Average (nmol/L)	<7.6	<7.8	<7.8
RSD (%)			
Medium4			
Average (nmol/L)	18.1 ± 3.0	75.3 ± 6.6	31.1 ± 1.7
RSD (%)	17	9	5
High4			
Average (nmol/L)	88.5 ± 8.0	119.2 ± 6.1	109 ± 3.3
RSD (%)	9	5	3

Relative standard deviation (RSD %).

Table 3. Inter-day precision (n) of vitamin D metabolites in plasma, breastmilk, and infant formula samples measured by (**a**) Waters Quattro Premier^{TM}/XE and (**b**) Agilent 6495B.

	Analyte		
a. Waters Quattro Premier^{TM}/XE			
Plasma ($n = 10$)	25(OH)D2	25(OH)D3	3-Epi25(OH)D3
Medium1			
Average (nmol/L)	-	55.5 ± 5.2	-
RSD (%)		9	
b. Agilent 6495B			
Plasma ($n = 10$)	25(OH)D2	25(OH)D3	3-Epi25(OH)D3
Low2			
Average (nmol/L)	30.2 ± 2.7	42.9 ± 3.4	34.5 ± 2.2
RSD (%)	9	8	6
Medium2			
Average (nmol/L)	71.2 ± 4.2	102.6 ± 5.6	48.2 ± 3.6
RSD (%)	6	5	7
High2			
Average (nmol/L)	115.3 ± 8.9	162.7 ± 9.0	99.9 ± 5.6
RSD (%)	8	6	6
Breastmilk ($n = 10$)	25(OH)D2	25(OH)D3	3-Epi25(OH)D3
Low3			
Average (nmol/L)	<7	12.0 ± 2	5.8 ± 1.7
RSD (%)		17	30
Medium3			
Average (nmol/L)	39.9 ± 2.7	65.0 ± 5.2	45.7 ± 2.6
RSD (%)	7	8	6
High3			
Average (nmol/L)	97.9 ± 4.6	114.8 ± 8	92.0 ± 9
RSD (%)	5	7	10
Infant formula ($n = 10$)	25(OH)D2	25(OH)D3	3-Epi25(OH)D3
Low4			
Average (nmol/L)	<7	<4.3	<1.7
SD			
RSD (%)			
Medium4			
Average (nmol/L)	21.4 ± 2.3	66.6 ± 2.7	32.2 ± 1.8
RSD (%)	11	4	6
High4			
Average (nmol/L)	93.2 ± 8.7	112.1 ± 4.1	107.1 ± 3.6
RSD (%)	9	4	3

3.2. Vitamin D Levels at Each Time-Point for Maternal and Infant Plasma Samples

Table 4 shows the number of samples collected. The samples were divided into 3 diagnostic categories according to 25(OH)D status: deficient (25(OH)D < 50 nmol/L), insufficient (50 nmol/L < 25(OH)D < 75 nmol/L), and sufficient (25(OH)D ≥ 75 nmol/L). The 3-Epi25(OH)D3 was not included in the calculations. Eighteen percent and 30.6% of the measured breastmilk samples had 25(OH)D levels lower than 50 nmol/L, 39.3% and 40% had levels between 50 and 75 nmol/L, and 42.7% and 29.4% had levels equal to or more than 75 nmol/L at 6 weeks and 3 months, respectively. Prevalence of 25(OH)D deficiency was determined in mother-infant pairs (Table 4). At 3 months, 63% of maternal 25(OH)D plasma levels were less than 75 nmol/L 25(OH)D. Accordingly, 31% of the infants were categorized as vitamin D deficient (25(OH)D < 50 nmol/L).

Table 4. Distribution of vitamin D status at each time-point (6 weeks, 3, and 6 months) for maternal and infant samples.

		Weeks	Months	
		6	3	6
Mothers				
Breastmilk	n [1]	89 (%)	85 (%)	
Deficient	<50 nmol/L	16 (18.0)	26 (30.6)	
Insufficient	50–74 nmol/L	35 (39.3)	34 (40.0)	
Sufficient	≥75 nmol/L	38 (42.7)	25 (29.4)	
Plasma	n [1]		87 (%)	84 (%)
Deficient	<50 nmol/L		11 (12.6)	12 (14.3)
Insufficient	50–74 nmol/L		44 (50.6)	40 (47.6)
Sufficient	≥75 nmol/L		32 (36.8)	32 (38.1)
Infants				
Plasma	Total		52 (%)	48 (%)
Deficient	<50 nmol/L		16 (30.8)	4 (8.3)
Insufficient	50–74 nmol/L		15 (28.8)	23 (47.9)
Sufficient	≥75 nmol/L		21 (40.4)	21 (43.8)

[1] number of samples (n).

3.3. Maternal and Infant Plasma Vitamin D Metabolites Concentration at 3 and 6 Months

The 25(OH)D2, 25(OH)D3, and 3-Epi25(OH)D3 plasma levels of the mothers and their infants, and the breastmilk levels of vitamin D metabolites at 6 weeks and 3 months are presented in Table 5. At 3 months, the concentration of 3-Epi25(OH)D3 contributed 11% and 24% of the total 25(OH)D3 in infants' plasma and breastmilk, respectively.

Table 5. Concentration levels of 25(OH)D2, 25(OH)D3, and 3-Epi25(OH)D3 at 6 weeks, 3, and 6 months among mother and infant. Paired samples tests.

		Weeks	Months		p Value [1]
		6	3	6	
Mothers		nmol/L	nmol/L		
Breastmilk	25(OH)D2	12.8 ± 6.7	12.7 ± 7.1	-	0.728
	25(OH)D3	60.1 ± 24.8	50.0 ± 23.4	-	0.001
	3-Epi25(OH)D3	19.7 ± 8.7	18.6 ± 9.0	-	0.327
			nmol/L	nmol/L	
Plasma	25(OH)D2		<7.6 [2]	<7.6	
	25(OH)D3		69.6 ± 16.3	69.6 ± 19.0	0.526
	3-Epi25(OH)D3		<7.8	<7.8	
Infants					
Plasma	25(OH)D2		<7.6	<7.6	
	25(OH)D3		64.6 ± 29.1	83.1 ± 27	0.001
	3-Epi25(OH)D3		7.8 ± 4.8	<7.6	

[1] Paired samples test. [2] The number of breastmilk samples below limit of quantification (LOQ) were 31 and 32 for 25(OH)D2, 0 and 2 for 25(OH)D3, and 1 and 3 for 3-Epi25(OH)D3 at 6 weeks and 3 months, respectively. The number of infant plasma samples below LOQ were 19 and 20 for 3-Epi25(OH)D3 at 3 and 6 months, respectively.

3.4. Correlation between Vitamin D Metabolites and Mother and Infant Levels of Vitamin D Metabolites

At 6 weeks, a positive association between breastmilk concentration of 25(OH)D3 and 3-Epi25(OH)D3 ($p < 0.01$; r = 0.711, Figure 1a) was observed. The same was seen at 3 months ($p < 0.01$; r = 0.805, Figure 1b). There was also a positive association observed between the infant's plasma levels of 25(OH)D3 and 3-Epi25(OH)D3 ($p < 0.01$, r = 0.678) at 3 months. A positive association between mother and infant plasma levels of 25(OH)D3 was observed ($p < 0.01$; r = 0.555, Figure 2).

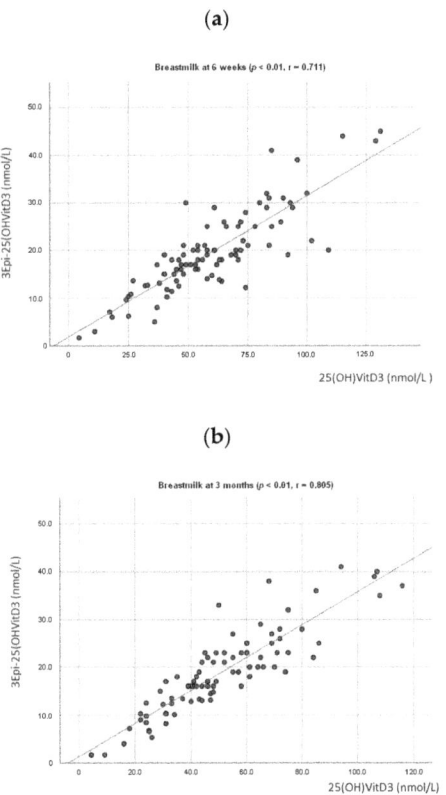

Figure 1. Association between mother's breastmilk concentration level of 25(OH)D3 and 3-Epi25(OH)D3 at 6 weeks postpartum (**a**) and 3 months postpartum (**b**).

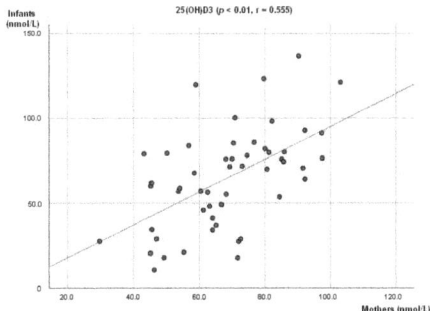

Figure 2. Association between mother's and infant concentration level of 25(OH)D3.

4. Discussion

In this study, a robotic autosampler was used to automate sample preparation prior to LC-MS/MS analysis which included protein-crash, solid-phase extraction techniques and dilution. This ensured reproducibility, simple sample treatment, and reduced time and labor and costs. Two simple, sensitive, and selective LC-MS/MS methods were then used to separate and detect 25(OH)D2, 25(OH)D3, and 3-Epi25(OH)D3. The concentrations of 25(OH)D2, 25(OH)D3, and 3-Epi25(OH)D3 in plasma were measured with Waters Quattro PremierTM/XE. Breastmilk samples were measured with

Agilent 6495B which resulted in an improved detection limit. Both LC-MS/MS methods separated 3-Epi25(OH)D3 from 25(OH)D3 for accurate detection and measurement of 25(OH)D3. Our validation showed a concentration-response relationship fitted with a simple regression model. The accuracy and inter-precision were within the acceptable criteria of RSD at 15% for 25(OH)D2, 25(OH)D3, and 3-Epi25(OH)D3 in plasma, breastmilk, and infant formula [42] with an exception of the measured inter-precision RSD for 25(OH)D2 in infant formula (17%.) At LOQ levels, the 25(OH)D2, 25(OH)D3, and 3-Epi25(OH)D3 were also within the acceptable criteria of 20% RSD. The intra-precision was within acceptable criteria of 15% RSD. This also applies at LOQ levels with an exception for 3-Epi25(OH)D3 in breastmilk with an RSD of 30%. These two LC-MS/MS methods were used to determine the vitamin D status in Norwegian mother-infant pairs.

The LC-MS/MS methods presented in this study distinguished between 25(OH)D3 and 3-Epi25(OH)D3. At 3 months, the C-3 epimer contributed 11% of the total 25(OH)D in infants' plasma. Thus, if 3-Epi25(OH)D3 was not distinguished from 25(OH)D3, only 25% of the infants are categorized as vitamin D deficient instead of 31%. The observed positive correlation between infants' 25(OH)D3 and 3-Epi25(OH)D3 at 3 months suggests possible overestimation of 25(OH)D3 and more likely, misclassification of vitamin D in studies using methods that only measure 25(OH)D3 [43]. In breastmilk, at 3 and 6 months, the 3-Epi25(OH)D3 contributed 24% and 27% of the total 25(OH)D, respectively. In addition, positive associations were also observed between 25(OH)D3 and 3-Epi25(OH)D3 in breastmilk at 6 weeks and 3 months. Accordingly, studies have shown positive correlation between 25(OH)D3 and 3-Epi25(OH)D3 in both maternal and cord blood [43,44]. This may imply maternal cord blood and breastmilk as a possible source of 3-Epi25(OH)D3 in infants. Studies on epimers function and source are warranted.

Infants are highly dependent on their mother's cord 25(OH)D concentrations, which is usually 60–80% of maternal values at delivery [45,46]. A survey of 25(OH)D levels in pregnant Black South Africans gave a mean of 57.0 nmol/L, while 41.9 nmol/L was found in the cord blood [47]. On the other hand, the measured concentrations of 25(OH)D in light-skinned pregnant women at northern latitudes was 71.4 nmol/L, while 39.2 nmol/L was recorded for cord blood [48]. Another study observed that in pregnant women, the mean 25(OH)D concentrations were 41 nmol/L and 50.7 nmol/L during the first trimester and in the umbilical cord, respectively [49]. Meanwhile, vitamin D deficiency appears to be common in mothers and their infants in New Zealand, with mean cord blood 25(OH)D value of 41 nmol/L [50]. In general, studies suggest that low levels of 25(OH)D in mothers are likely to be reflected in their infants. In this study, maternal plasma levels, at 3 and 6 months, 13% and 14% of mothers were categorized as deficient (25(OH)D < 50 nmol/L), 51% and 48% as insufficient (50 nmol/L < 25(OH)D < 75 nmol/L), and 37% and 38% as sufficient (25(OH)D ≥ 75 nmol/L), respectively. However, 31% and 29% of the infants had deficient and insufficient 25(OH)D status at 3 months, respectively. Vitamin D body stored in infants can decline by 50% over less than a month, hence without another source of vitamin D, vitamin D deficiency can develop [51]. This may explain the higher prevalence of 25(OH)D deficiency in infants compared with mothers.

A positive association between maternal 25(OH)D plasma levels and infant 25(OH)D plasma levels at 3 months was observed. The maternal and infant 25(OH)D3 plasma concentrations were 69.6 (±16.3) nmol/L and 64.9 (±29.1) nmol/L, respectively. Hence, measured infant plasma level of 25(OH)D at 3 months may reflect the 25(OH)D transferred from mother to infant during pregnancy and start of vitamin D supplement. There was a rise of infant plasma 25(OH)D concentration observed from 3 months to 6 months. Accordingly, a positive correlation between maternal and infant plasma was no longer observed suggesting an increase in 25(OH)D level as a possible result of vitamin D supplementation and start of fortified complementary feeding. In Norway, vitamin D supplements, such as vitamin D drops or cod liver oil, are recommended for all infants from the age of four weeks. A Norwegian population study showed that 92% of the children at age 9-16 months were given vitamin D containing supplements [30]. Here, results showed decreased prevalence of 25(OH)D deficiency in infants, from 3 months (31%) to 6 months (8%). Even with the decrease in vitamin D deficiency prevalence at 6 months, vitamin D deficiency originating in the intrauterine period or immediately after birth to 3 months may still result in adverse effects on skeletal development [49,52]. Correspondingly, in vitamin D-deficient infants, rickets usually develops between the age of 6 months and 2 years [53]. Interestingly, the prevalence of infants categorized as 25(OH)D sufficient at 3 and 6 months had a minor change: 40% and 44%, respectively.

The WHO's recommendation of exclusive breastfeeding for 6 months may further lead to vitamin D deficiency among infants [54,55]. Although breastmilk is rich in essential nutrients for the earliest life stage, it contains about three-times-less vitamin D than the maternal circulating concentration [56]. A study showed that during the third trimester of pregnancy, maternal 25(OH)D was 60 nmol/L, and the breastmilk level at delivery was 1.26 nmol/L [57]. As for non-Vitamin-D-supplemented Norwegian mothers and infants, a study reported no change in mother's plasma levels of 25(OH)D (58 to 42 nmol/L) between 4 days and 6 weeks after birth. However, infant's plasma levels dropped from 26 to 15 nmol/L, thus, suggesting that Norwegian mothers have insufficient 25(OH)D, and therefore that breastmilk is inadequate as a lone source of vitamin D, and supplementation of 10 µg per day is recommended [18,58,59].

There was no observed change in maternal 25(OH)D plasma levels between 3 and 6 months. The prevalence of maternal vitamin D deficiency at 3 and 6 months was almost the same. Likewise, another study showed that the measured 25(OH)D3 of 67 nmol/L did not change between 2 weeks and 12 months postpartum [60]. Thus, maternal vitamin status was maintained through 6 months of breastfeeding and possibly just enough for their own needs. These results do not support the theory that maternal vitamin D status decreases due to a transfer of vitamin D from the mother to infant through breastmilk [61]. Accordingly, breastmilk 25(OH)D2 remained unchanged between 6 weeks and 3 months. In contrast, breastmilk concentration of 25(OH)D3 decreased from 6 weeks to 3 months. Thus, decreased level of 25(OH)D3 in breastmilk suggests that transfer of 25(OH)D3 to breastmilk production was not prioritized. Studies have shown that vitamin D is readily transferred into breastmilk, while 25(OH)D is transferred very poorly, and 1,25 (OH)2D is not transferred at all [62]. This may explain the lack of association between maternal plasma and breastmilk 25(OH)D3 concentration. Thus, 25(OH)D in the blood may not be a good reflection of the available amount of vitamin D that can be transferred to infants through breastfeeding. Accordingly, studies have also reported that UV exposure and increased maternal vitamin D supplementation showed minimal changes in 25(OH)D concentrations but a profound increase in breastmilk concentration of vitamin D was observed [56,63]. Thus, measurement of vitamin D3 and vitamin D2 in breastmilk and plasma samples in this study population is warranted.

In this study, an automated robust sample preparation was used. The methods distinguished between 25(OH)D3 and 3 epimer of 25(OH)D3, 3-Epi25(OH)D3 preventing overestimation of 25(OH)D3 and misclassification of vitamin D status. However, a limitation in this study is that two different LC-MS/MS methods were used, resulting in different validation parameters and LOD. Anyhow, the challenge with the overestimation of 25(OH)D3 has been addressed and managed resulting in a reliable quantification of 25(OH)D. Here, we provided novel results of 25(OH)D status in Norwegian mother-infant pairs during the first 6 months of breast feeding. A possible source of 3-epi-25(OH)2D3 was also discussed. Prevalence of vitamin D deficiency (25(OH)D < 50 nmol/L) among Norwegian mother-infant pairs was determined. Surprisingly, a prevalence of 31% 25(OH)D deficiency was observed among infants at three months. Studies suggest the importance of vitamin D supplementation during pregnancy, and the breastfeeding period to ensure the achievement of the recommended 25(OH)D level of at least 75 nmol/L in mothers and their infants [17,20,34,64,65]. Vitamin D supplementation in pregnant women seems to reduce the risk of pre-eclampsia, gestational diabetes, low birthweight, and severe postpartum hemorrhage [66]. Wide ranges of vitamin D doses, from 400 to 2000 IU have been recommended [17,67–69]. However, some doses may not result in optimal 25(OH)D levels during pregnancy. This may be due to interindividual variability in vitamin D metabolism and other factors [70,71]. Thus, establishing a personalized dosing regimen has been suggested [37].

5. Conclusions

In summary, two simple, sensitive, and selective LC-MS/MS methods enable reliable quantification of 25(OH)D2, 25(OH)D3, and 3-Epi25(OH)D3. The automated sample preparation makes it suitable for routine laboratory analysis of plasma, breastmilk, and infant formula. This study demonstrated the importance of separating 3-Epi25(OH)D3 from 25(OH)D3 to prevent overestimation of 25(OH)D3 and misclassification of vitamin D status. Accordingly, at 3 months, 13% and 31% of the mothers and infants were categorized as vitamin D deficient (25(OH)D < 50 nmol/L), respectively. Thus, we suggest monitoring vitamin D metabolites in infant, maternal plasma, and breastmilk to ensure adequate levels in both mother and infant in the first 6 months of infant life. Further studies on personalized supplementation with vitamin D during pregnancy and breastfeeding are warranted.

Supplementary Materials: The following are available online at http://www.mdpi.com/2072-6643/12/8/2271/s1, Figure S1. Representative chromatograms of 25(OH)D3 and 3-Epi25(OH)D3 8(a.) and 25(OH)D2 (b.).

Author Contributions: M.K., L.D. and M.W.M. study design, sample collection and conducted research; J.G. and T.B. LC-MS analyzes and data acquisition; A.B., M.K. and M.W.M. project administration; M.K., M.W.M. and J.G. analyzed data or performed statistical analysis; J.G. original draft preparation and writing. All authors have read and agreed to the published version of the manuscript.

Funding: The Mommy's Food study is financially supported by The Norwegian Seafood Research Fund (http://www.fhf.no/). The funder had no role in the design or the decision to publish this protocol.

Acknowledgments: We thank Elisabeth Ødegård for technical support and Zylla Marie Oane for proofreading the manuscript. We also thank Jojo Tibon for comments and feedback on the manuscript.

Conflicts of Interest: The authors declare no conflict of interest.

Appendix A

Table A1. Multiple-reaction monitoring (MRM) mode and the respective dwell time, cone voltage, and collision energy used in Waters Quattro Premier^{TM}/XE (**a**) and in Agilent 6495B (**b**).

Analytes	Parention [1]	Daughterion [1]	Dwell Time [2]	Cone	Collision Energy [3]
a. Waters Quattro Premier^{TM}/XE					
25(OH) D$_3$/3-Epi25(OH)D3	401.35	159.10	0.05	20	28
25(OH) D$_3$/3-Epi25(OH)D3	401.35	383.20	0.05	20	9
d3-3-Epi25(OH)D3	404.36	162.10	0.05	25	22
d6-25(OH)D$_3$	407.36	159.10	0.05	20	26
25(OH)D$_2$	413.35	159.00	0.05	20	26
25(OH)D$_2$	413.35	395.20	0.05	20	10
d3-25(OH)D$_2$	416.30	162.00	0.05	20	26
1.25(OH)D$_3$	434.30	399.30	0.05	15	10
d6-1.25(OH)D$_3$	440.3	405.30	0.05	15	10
b. Agilent 6495B					
25(OH) D$_3$/3-Epi25(OH)D3	401.3	365.4	25	5	5
25(OH) D$_3$/3-Epi25(OH)D3	401.3	383.4	25	5	5
d3-3-Epi25(OH)D3	404.4	368.4	25	5	5
d3-3-Epi25(OH)D3	404.4	386.4	25	5	5
d6-25(OH)D$_3$	407.4	371.4	25	5	5
d6-25(OH)D$_3$	407.4	389.4	25	5	5
25(OH)D$_2$	413.3	395.3	25	5	5
25(OH)D$_2$	413.3	355.4	25	5	5
d3-25(OH)D$_2$	416.4	398.3	25	5	5
d3-25(OH)D$_2$	416.4	358.5	25	5	5
1.25(OH)D$_3$	434.6	399.4	25	5	8
1.25(OH)D$_3$	434.6	381.7	25	5	8
d6-1.25(OH)D$_3$	440.6	405.7	25	5	5
d6-1.25(OH)D$_3$	440.6	387.5	25	5	5

[1] m/z; [2] ms; [3] volts.

Appendix B

Table A2. Accuracy for the analysis of 25(OH)D2, 25(OH)D3, and 3-Epi25(OH)D3 in plasma and serum using (**a**) Waters Quattro Premier™/XE and (**b**) Agilent 6495B.

Samples	Analytes			
	a. Waters Quattro Premier™/XE			
Serum (n = 3)	1,25(OH)2D3	25(OH)D2	25(OH)D3	3-Epi25(OH)D3
SRM 972a-C Level 2				
Concentration (nmol/L)	-	-	30.8	-
Accuracy (%)			106	
SRM 972a-C Level 3				
Concentration (nmol/L)	-	32.3	49.4	-
Accuracy (%)		101	110	
SRM 972a-C Level 4				
Concentration (nmol/L)	-	-	73.4	65.8
Accuracy (%)			111	101
SRM 1950				
Concentration (nmol/L)	-	-	61.8	-
Accuracy (%)			108	
SRM 2972				
Concentration (nmol/L)	-	-	835.6	-
Accuracy (%)			106	
	b. Agilent 6495B			
Plasma (n = 2)	1,25(OH)2D3	25(OH)D2	25(OH)D3	3-Epi25(OH)D3
SRM 1950 Level 2				
Concentration (nmol/L)	-	-	61.8	-
Accuracy (%)			104	
Serum (n = 2)	1,25(OH)2D3	25(OH)D2	25(OH)D3	3-Epi25(OH)D3
SRM 972a-C Level 1				
Concentration (nmol/L)	-	-	71.8	4.5
Accuracy (%)			102	103
SRM 972a-C Level 2				
Concentration (nmol/L)	-	-	45.1	3.2
Accuracy (%)			113	106
SRM 972a-C Level 3				
Concentration (nmol/L)	-	32.3	49.5	2.9
Accuracy (%)		100	97	99
SRM 972a-C Level 4				
Concentration (nmol/L)	-	-	73.4	64.8
Accuracy (%)			102	108

Each value is presented as mean.

Appendix C

Table A3. Recovery (n = 10) of vitamin D metabolites in plasma, breastmilk, and infant formula at inter-day.

Samples	Analytes		
Plasma (n = 10)	25(OH)D2	25(OH)D3	3-Epi25(OH)D3
Low			
Added (nmol/L)	26.47	46.36	27.96
Measured (nmol/L)	30.22 ± 2.66	42.93 ± 3.41	34.50 ± 2.18
Recovery (%)	114	93	128
Medium			
Added (nmol/L)	74.94	96.28	51.92
Measured (nmol/L)	71.19 ± 4.19	102.63 ± 5.59	48.18 ± 3.59
Recovery (%)	95	107	93
High			
Added (nmol/L)	121.17	146.20	101.84
Measured (nmol/L)	115.33 ± 8.95	162.75 ± 8.99	99.94 ± 5.59
Recovery (%)	95	111	98

Table A3. Cont.

Samples	Analytes		
Breastmilk (n = 10)	25(OH)D2	25(OH)D3	3-Epi25(OH)D3
Low			
Added (nmol/L)	<LOQ	15.18	8.07
Measured (nmol/L)		12.04 ± 2.04	5.83 ± 1.73
Recovery (%)		79	72
Medium			
Added (nmol/L)	48.74	65.10	57.99
Measured (nmol/L)	39.89 ± 2.75	65.01 ± 5.19	45.74 ± 2.64
Recovery (%)	82	100	79
High			
Added (nmol/L)	97.20	111.50	107.91
Measured (nmol/L)	97.88 ± 4.63	114.80 ± 7.98	91.98 ± 8.98
Recovery (%)	101	103	85
Infant formula (n = 10)	25(OH)D2	25(OH)D3	3-Epi25(OH)D3
Low			
Added (nmol/L)	<LOQ	<LOQ	<LOQ
Measured (nmol/L)			
Recovery (%)			
Medium			
Added (nmol/L)	26.48	51.53	24.96
Measured (nmol/L)	21.37 ± 2.35	66.63 ± 2.71	32.22 ± 1.80
Recovery (%)	81	129	129
High			
Added (nmol/L)	99.18	101.45	99.84
Measured (nmol/L)	93.17 ± 8.67	112.08 ± 4.15	107.10 ± 3.61
Recovery (%)	94	110	107

Recovery (%) = 100 × measured concentration/amount added.

References

1. Dhamo, B.; Miliku, K.; Voortman, T.; Tiemeier, H.; Jaddoe, V.W.; Wolvius, E.B.; Ongkosuwito, E.M. The Associations of Maternal and Neonatal Vitamin D with Dental Development in Childhood. *Curr. Dev. Nutr.* **2019**, *3*, nzy100. [CrossRef] [PubMed]
2. van Halteren, A.G.; van Etten, E.; de Jong, E.C.; Bouillon, R.; Roep, B.O.; Mathieu, C. Redirection of human autoreactive T-cells Upon interaction with dendritic cells modulated by TX527, an analog of 1,25 dihydroxyvitamin D(3). *Diabetes* **2002**, *51*, 2119–2125. [CrossRef]
3. Gonzalez-Gross, M.; Valtuena, J.; Breidenassel, C.; Moreno, L.A.; Ferrari, M.; Kersting, M.; De Henauw, S.; Gottrand, F.; Azzini, E.; Widhalm, K.; et al. Vitamin D status among adolescents in Europe: The Healthy Lifestyle in Europe by Nutrition in Adolescence study. *Br. J. Nutr.* **2012**, *107*, 755–764. [CrossRef] [PubMed]
4. Totland, T.H.; Melnæs, B.K.; Lundberg-Hallen, N.; Helland-Kigen, K.M.; Lund-Blix, N.A.; Myhre, J.B.; Johansen, A.M.W.; Løken, E.B.; Andersen, L.F. Norkost 3 En landsomfattende kostholdsundersøkelse blant menn og kvinner i Norge i alderen 18-70 år, 2010–11. *Oslo Helsedir.* **2012**, *67*, 25–33.
5. Kamao, M.; Tatematsu, S.; Hatakeyama, S.; Sakaki, T.; Sawada, N.; Inouye, K.; Ozono, K.; Kubodera, N.; Reddy, G.S.; Okano, T. C-3 epimerization of vitamin D_3 metabolites and further metabolism of C-3 epimers: 25-hydroxyvitamin D_3 is metabolized to 3-epi-25-hydroxyvitamin D_3 and subsequently metabolized through C-1alpha or C-24 hydroxylation. *J. Biol. Chem.* **2004**, *279*, 15897–15907. [CrossRef]
6. Bianchini, C.; Lavery, P.; Agellon, S.; Weiler, H.A. The generation of C-3alpha epimer of 25-hydroxyvitamin D and its biological effects on bone mineral density in adult rodents. *Calcif. Tissue Int.* **2015**, *96*, 453–464. [CrossRef]
7. Fleet, J.C.; Bradley, J.; Reddy, G.S.; Ray, R.; Wood, R.J. 1α, 25-(OH)$_2$-vitamin D_3 analogs with minimal in vivo calcemic activity can stimulate significant transepithelial calcium transport and mRNA expression in vitro. *Arch. Biochem. Biophys.* **1996**, *329*, 228–234. [CrossRef]
8. Al-Zohily, B.; Al-Menhali, A.; Gariballa, S.; Haq, A.; Shah, I. Epimers of Vitamin D: A Review. *Int. J. Mol. Sci.* **2020**, *21*, 470. [CrossRef]
9. Mawer, E.B.; Lumb, G.A.; Schaefer, K.; Stanbury, S.W. Metabolism of Isotopically Labelled Vitamin-D_3 in Man—Influence of State of Vitamin-D Nutrition. *Clin. Sci.* **1971**, *40*, 39–53. [CrossRef]

10. Smith, J.E.; Goodman, D.W.S. The turnover and transport of vitamin D and of a polar metabolite with the properties of 25-hydroxycholecalciferol in human plasma. *J. Clin. Investig.* **1971**, *50*, A86. [CrossRef]
11. Clemens, T.L.; Adams, J.S.; Nolan, J.M.; Holick, M.F. Measurement of Circulating Vitamin-D in Man. *Clin. Chim. Acta* **1982**, *121*, 301–308. [CrossRef]
12. Jones, G. Pharmacokinetics of vitamin D toxicity. *Am. J. Clin. Nutr.* **2008**, *88*, 582S–586S. [CrossRef]
13. Jones, K.S.; Assar, S.; Harnpanich, D.; Bouillon, R.; Lambrechts, D.; Prentice, A.; Schoenmakers, I. 25(OH)D$_2$ Half-Life Is Shorter Than 25(OH)D$_3$ Half-Life and Is Influenced by DBP Concentration and Genotype. *J. Clin. Endocrinol. Metab.* **2014**, *99*, 3373–3381. [CrossRef] [PubMed]
14. Oliveri, B.; Mastaglia, S.R.; Brito, G.M.; Seijo, M.; Keller, G.A.; Somoza, J.; Diez, R.A.; Di Girolamo, G. Vitamin D$_3$ seems more appropriate than D$_2$ to sustain adequate levels of 25OHD: A pharmacokinetic approach. *Eur. J. Clin. Nutr.* **2015**, *69*, 697–702. [CrossRef] [PubMed]
15. Lips, P. Relative value of 25(OH)D and 1,25(OH)$_2$D measurements. *J. Bone Miner. Res.* **2007**, *22*, 1668–1671. [CrossRef] [PubMed]
16. Kumar, R. The metabolism and mechanism of action of 1,25-dihydroxyvitamin D$_3$. *Kidney Int.* **1986**, *30*, 793–803. [CrossRef]
17. Holick, M.F.; Binkley, N.C.; Bischoff-Ferrari, H.A.; Gordon, C.M.; Hanley, D.A.; Heaney, R.P.; Murad, M.H.; Weaver, C.M.; Endocrine, S. Evaluation, treatment, and prevention of vitamin D deficiency: An Endocrine Society clinical practice guideline. *J. Clin. Endocrinol. Metab.* **2011**, *96*, 1911–1930. [CrossRef]
18. Vitamin D in Norway: Need for Measures to Ensure Good Vitamin D Status? 2018. Available online: https://www.helsedirektoratet.no/rapporter/vitamin-d-i-norge-behov-for-tiltak-for-a-sikre-god-vitamin-d-status/Vitamin%20D%20i%20Norge%20--%20Behov%20for%20tiltak%20for%20å%20sikre%20god%20vitamin%20D-status.pdf/_/attachment/inline/b307f785-c4cc-4fde-aec1-ebc86fdd0b4f:829f3ad84cbdf0322f46b3f44d1c6fc14f151a97/Vitamin%20D%20i%20Norge%20--%20Behov%20for%20tiltak%20for%20å%20sikre%20god%20vitamin%20D-status.pdf (accessed on 14 April 2020).
19. Nordic Nutrition Recommendations 2012. Available online: https://www.norden.org/en/publication/nordic-nutrition-recommendations-2012 (accessed on 14 April 2020).
20. Lips, P. Which circulating level of 25-hydroxyvitamin D is appropriate? *J. Steroid. Biochem. Mol. Biol.* **2004**, *89*, 611–614. [CrossRef]
21. van den Ouweland, J.M.; Beijers, A.M.; van Daal, H. Overestimation of 25-hydroxyvitamin D$_3$ by increased ionisation efficiency of 3-epi-25-hydroxyvitamin D$_3$ in LC-MS/MS methods not separating both metabolites as determined by an LC-MS/MS method for separate quantification of 25-hydroxyvitamin D$_3$, 3-epi-25-hydroxyvitamin D$_3$ and 25-hydroxyvitamin D$_2$ in human serum. *J. Chromatogr. B Anal. Technol. Biomed. Life Sci.* **2014**, *967*, 195–202. [CrossRef]
22. Bouillon, R.; Van Baelen, H.; De Moor, P. 25-hydroxyvitamin D and its binding protein in maternal and cord serum. *J. Clin. Endocrinol. Metab.* **1977**, *45*, 679–684. [CrossRef]
23. Bouillon, R.; Van Assche, F.A.; Van Baelen, H.; Heyns, W.; De Moor, P. Influence of the vitamin D-binding protein on the serum concentration of 1,25-dihydroxyvitamin D$_3$. Significance of the free 1,25-dihydroxyvitamin D$_3$ concentration. *J. Clin. Investig.* **1981**, *67*, 589–596. [CrossRef] [PubMed]
24. Markestad, T.; Aksnes, L.; Ulstein, M.; Aarskog, D. 25-Hydroxyvitamin D and 1,25-dihydroxyvitamin D of D$_2$ and D$_3$ origin in maternal and umbilical cord serum after vitamin D$_2$ supplementation in human pregnancy. *Am. J. Clin. Nutr.* **1984**, *40*, 1057–1063. [CrossRef] [PubMed]
25. Hollis, B.W.; Johnson, D.; Hulsey, T.C.; Ebeling, M.; Wagner, C.L. Vitamin D supplementation during pregnancy: Double-blind, randomized clinical trial of safety and effectiveness. *J. Bone Miner. Res.* **2011**, *26*, 2341–2357. [CrossRef] [PubMed]
26. Hillman, L.S.; Haddad, J.G. Human perinatal vitamin D metabolism. I. 25-Hydroxyvitamin D in maternal and cord blood. *J. Pediatr.* **1974**, *84*, 742–749. [CrossRef]
27. Kovacs, C.S. Vitamin D in pregnancy and lactation: Maternal, fetal, and neonatal outcomes from human and animal studies. *Am. J. Clin. Nutr.* **2008**, *88*, 520S–528S. [CrossRef]
28. Abbasian, M.; Chaman, R.; Amiri, M.; Ajami, M.E.; Jafari-Koshki, T.; Rohani, H.; Taghavi-Shahri, S.M.; Sadeghi, E.; Raei, M. Vitamin D Deficiency in Pregnant Women and Their Neonates. *Glob. J. Health Sci.* **2016**, *8*, 83. [CrossRef]

29. Lips, P.; Cashman, K.D.; Lamberg-Allardt, C.; Bischoff-Ferrari, H.A.; Obermayer-Pietsch, B.R.; Bianchi, M.; Stepan, J.; El-Hajj Fuleihan, G.; Bouillon, R. Management of Endocrine Disease: Current vitamin D status in European and Middle East countries and strategies to prevent vitamin D deficiency; a position statement of the European Calcified Tissue Society. *Eur. J. Endocrinol.* **2019**, *180*, 23–54. [CrossRef]

30. Madar, A.A.; Gundersen, T.E.; Haug, A.M.; Meyer, H.E. Vitamin D supplementation and vitamin D status in children of immigrant background in Norway. *Public Health Nutr.* **2017**, *20*, 2887–2892. [CrossRef]

31. van der Pligt, P.; Willcox, J.; Szymlek-Gay, E.A.; Murray, E.; Worsley, A.; Daly, R.M. Associations of Maternal Vitamin D Deficiency with Pregnancy and Neonatal Complications in Developing Countries: A Systematic Review. *Nutrients* **2018**, *10*, 640. [CrossRef]

32. Palacios, C.; Trak-Fellermeier, M.A.; Martinez, R.X.; Lopez-Perez, L.; Lips, P.; Salisi, J.A.; John, J.C.; Pena-Rosas, J.P. Regimens of vitamin D supplementation for women during pregnancy. *Cochrane Database Syst. Rev.* **2019**, *10*, 30. [CrossRef]

33. Cashman, K.D. Vitamin D in childhood and adolescence. *Postgrad. Med. J.* **2007**, *83*, 230–235. [CrossRef] [PubMed]

34. Wagner, C.L.; Greer, F.R. American Academy of Pediatrics Section on B., American Academy of Pediatrics Committee on N. Prevention of rickets and vitamin D deficiency in infants, children, and adolescents. *Pediatrics* **2008**, *122*, 1142–1152. [CrossRef]

35. Mahon, P.; Harvey, N.; Crozier, S.; Inskip, H.; Robinson, S.; Arden, N.; Swaminathan, R.; Cooper, C.; Godfrey, K.; Group, S.W.S.S. Low maternal vitamin D status and fetal bone development: Cohort study. *J. Bone Miner. Res.* **2010**, *25*, 14–19. [CrossRef] [PubMed]

36. Gustafsson, M.K.; Romundstad, P.R.; Stafne, S.N.; Helvik, A.S.; Stunes, A.K.; Morkved, S.; Salvesen, K.A.; Thorsby, P.M.; Syversen, U. Alterations in the vitamin D endocrine system during pregnancy: A longitudinal study of 855 healthy Norwegian women. *PLoS ONE* **2018**, *13*, e0195041. [CrossRef] [PubMed]

37. Moon, R.J.; Davies, J.H.; Cooper, C.; Harvey, N.C. Vitamin D, and Maternal and Child Health. *Calcif. Tissue Int.* **2020**, *106*, 30–46. [CrossRef]

38. Markhus, M.W.; Kvestad, I.; Midtbo, L.K.; Nerhus, I.; Odegaard, E.R.; Graff, I.E.; Lie, O.; Dahl, L.; Hysing, M.; Kjellevold, M. Effects of cod intake in pregnancy on iodine nutrition and infant development: Study protocol for Mommy's Food—A randomized controlled trial. *BMC Nutr.* **2018**, *4*, 7. [CrossRef]

39. Roberts, P.H. Online Automated Protein Crash, Solid Phase Extraction and Analysis of Vitamin D in Serum Using Instrument Top Sample Prep (ITSP), Gerstel Multi Purpose Sampler and Agilent LC-MS/MS. Available online: https://www.itspsolutions.com/sites/default/files/Anatune%20Vitamin%20D%20in%20Serum.pdf (accessed on 3 April 2020).

40. Foster, D.; Cabrices, O.; Pfannkoch, E.A.; Roberts, P. Automated Extraction of Vitamin D Metabolites from Serum. Available online: https://grupobiomaster.com/wp-content/uploads/2015/01/162.pdf (accessed on 3 April 2020).

41. Guideline on Bioanalytical Method Validation. Available online: https://www.ema.europa.eu/en/documents/scientific-guideline/guideline-bioanalytical-method-validation_en.pdf (accessed on 3 April 2020).

42. US Department of Health and Human Services. Bioanalytical Method Validation Guidance for Industry. Available online: https://www.fda.gov/files/drugs/published/Bioanalytical-Method-Validation-Guidance-for-Industry.pdf (accessed on 3 April 2020).

43. Aghajafari, F.; Field, C.J.; Rabi, D.; Kaplan, B.J.; Maggiore, J.A.; O'Beirne, M.; Hanley, D.A.; Eliasziw, M.; Dewey, D.; Ross, S.; et al. Plasma 3-Epi-25-Hydroxycholecalciferol Can Alter the Assessment of Vitamin D Status Using the Current Reference Ranges for Pregnant Women and Their Newborns. *J. Nutr.* **2016**, *146*, 70–75. [CrossRef]

44. Kiely, M.; O'Donovan, S.M.; Kenny, L.C.; Hourihane, J.O.; Irvine, A.D.; Murray, D.M. Vitamin D metabolite concentrations in umbilical cord blood serum and associations with clinical characteristics in a large prospective mother-infant cohort in Ireland. *J. Steroid. Biochem. Mol. Biol.* **2017**, *167*, 162–168. [CrossRef]

45. Hollis, B.W.; Pittard, W.B. Evaluation of the Total Fetomaternal Vitamin-D Relationships at Term—Evidence for Racial-Differences. *J. Clin. Endocrinol. Metab.* **1984**, *59*, 652–657. [CrossRef]

46. Streym, S.V.; Moller, U.K.; Rejnmark, L.; Heickendorff, L.; Mosekilde, L.; Vestergaard, P. Maternal and infant vitamin D status during the first 9 months of infant life-a cohort study. *Eur. J. Clin. Nutr.* **2013**, *67*, 1022–1028. [CrossRef]

47. Velaphi, S.C.; Izu, A.; Madhi, S.A.; Pettifor, J.M. Maternal and neonatal vitamin D status at birth in black South Africans. *S. Afr. Med. J.* **2019**, *109*, 807–813. [CrossRef]
48. O'Callaghan, K.M.; Hennessy, A.; Hull, G.L.J.; Healy, K.; Ritz, C.; Kenny, L.C.; Cashman, K.D.; Kiely, M.E. Estimation of the maternal vitamin D intake that maintains circulating 25-hydroxyvitamin D in late gestation at a concentration sufficient to keep umbilical cord sera >/= 25–30 nmol/L: A dose-response, double-blind, randomized placebo-controlled trial in pregnant women at northern latitude. *Am. J. Clin. Nutr.* **2018**, *108*, 77–91. [CrossRef]
49. Viljakainen, H.T.; Saarnio, E.; Hytinantti, T.; Miettinen, M.; Surcel, H.; Makitie, O.; Andersson, S.; Laitinen, K.; Lamberg-Allardt, C. Maternal vitamin D status determines bone variables in the newborn. *J. Clin. Endocrinol. Metab.* **2010**, *95*, 1749–1757. [CrossRef] [PubMed]
50. Wheeler, B.J.; Taylor, B.J.; de Lange, M.; Harper, M.J.; Jones, S.; Mekhail, A.; Houghton, L.A. A Longitudinal Study of 25-Hydroxy Vitamin D and Parathyroid Hormone Status throughout Pregnancy and Exclusive Lactation in New Zealand Mothers and Their Infants at 45° S. *Nutrients* **2018**, *10*, 86. [CrossRef] [PubMed]
51. Pietrek, J.; Otto-Buczkowska, E.; Kokot, F.; Karpiel, R.; Cekanski, A. Concentration of 25-hydroxyvitamin D in serum of infants under the intermittent high-dose vitamin D_3 prophylactic treatment. *Arch. Immunol. Ther. Exp. Warsz.* **1980**, *28*, 805–814. [PubMed]
52. Cooper, C.; Javaid, K.; Westlake, S.; Harvey, N.; Dennison, E. Developmental origins of osteoporotic fracture: The role of maternal vitamin D insufficiency. *J. Nutr.* **2005**, *135*, 2728S–2734S. [CrossRef] [PubMed]
53. Molgaard, C.; Michaelsen, K.F. Vitamin D and bone health in early life. *Proc. Nutr. Soc.* **2003**, *62*, 823–828. [CrossRef] [PubMed]
54. Kramer, M.S.; Kakuma, R. Optimal duration of exclusive breastfeeding. *Cochrane Database Syst. Rev.* **2002**, *1*, 11. [CrossRef]
55. Kramer, M.S.; Kakuma, R. Optimal duration of exclusive breastfeeding. *Cochrane Database Syst. Rev.* **2012**, *8*, 10. [CrossRef]
56. Greer, F.R.; Hollis, B.W.; Napoli, J.L. High concentrations of vitamin D_2 in human milk associated with pharmacologic doses of vitamin D_2. *J. Pediatr.* **1984**, *105*, 61–64. [CrossRef]
57. Mohamed, H.J.J.; Rowan, A.; Fong, B.; Loy, S.L. Maternal serum and breast milk vitamin D levels: Findings from the Universiti Sains Malaysia Pregnancy Cohort Study. *PLoS ONE* **2014**, *9*, e100705. [CrossRef]
58. Markestad, T. Plasma concentrations of vitamin D metabolites in unsupplemented breast-fed infants. *Eur. J. Pediatr.* **1983**, *141*, 77–80. [CrossRef]
59. Madar, A.A.; Klepp, K.I.; Meyer, H.E. Effect of free vitamin D_2 drops on serum 25-hydroxyvitamin D in infants with immigrant origin: A cluster randomized controlled trial. *Eur. J. Clin. Nutr.* **2009**, *63*, 478–484. [CrossRef]
60. Brembeck, P.; Winkvist, A.; Baath, M.; Barebring, L.; Augustin, H. Determinants of changes in vitamin D status postpartum in Swedish women. *Br. J. Nutr.* **2016**, *115*, 422–430. [CrossRef] [PubMed]
61. Narchi, H.; Kochiyil, J.; Zayed, R.; Abdulrazzak, W.; Agarwal, M. Maternal vitamin D status throughout and after pregnancy. *J. Obstet. Gynaecol.* **2010**, *30*, 137–142. [CrossRef] [PubMed]
62. Kovacs, C.S.; Kronenberg, H.M. Maternal-fetal calcium and bone metabolism during pregnancy, puerperium, and lactation. *Endocr. Rev.* **1997**, *18*, 832–872. [CrossRef] [PubMed]
63. Greer, F.R.; Hollis, B.W.; Cripps, D.J.; Tsang, R.C. Effects of maternal ultraviolet B irradiation on vitamin D content of human milk. *J. Pediatr.* **1984**, *105*, 431–433. [CrossRef]
64. Salle, B.L.; Glorieux, F.H.; Lapillone, A. Vitamin D status in breastfed term babies. *Acta Paediatr.* **1998**, *87*, 726–727. [CrossRef]
65. Aly, H.; Abdel-Hady, H. Vitamin D and the Neonate: An Update. *J. Clin. Neonatol.* **2015**, *4*, 1–7. [CrossRef]
66. Palacios, C.; Kostiuk, L.K.; Pena-Rosas, J.P. Vitamin D supplementation for women during pregnancy. *Cochrane Database Syst. Rev.* **2019**, *7*, CD008873. [CrossRef]
67. Ross, A.C.; Manson, J.E.; Abrams, S.A.; Aloia, J.F.; Brannon, P.M.; Clinton, S.K.; Durazo-Arvizu, R.A.; Gallagher, J.C.; Gallo, R.L.; Jones, G.; et al. The 2011 report on dietary reference intakes for calcium and vitamin D from the Institute of Medicine: What clinicians need to know. *J. Clin. Endocrinol. Metab.* **2011**, *96*, 53–58. [CrossRef] [PubMed]
68. Yesiltepe Mutlu, G.; Ozsu, E.; Kalaca, S.; Yuksel, A.; Pehlevan, Y.; Cizmecioglu, F.; Hatun, S. Evaluation of vitamin D supplementation doses during pregnancy in a population at high risk for deficiency. *Horm. Res. Paediatr.* **2014**, *81*, 402–408. [CrossRef]

69. Munns, C.F.; Shaw, N.; Kiely, M.; Specker, B.L.; Thacher, T.D.; Ozono, K.; Michigami, T.; Tiosano, D.; Mughal, M.Z.; Makitie, O.; et al. Global Consensus Recommendations on Prevention and Management of Nutritional Rickets. *J. Clin. Endocrinol. Metab.* **2016**, *101*, 394–415. [CrossRef]
70. Hu, Z.; Tao, S.; Liu, H.; Pan, G.; Li, B.; Zhang, Z. The Association between Polymorphisms of Vitamin D Metabolic-Related Genes and Vitamin D_3 Supplementation in Type 2 Diabetic Patients. *J. Diabetes. Res.* **2019**, *2019*, 8289741. [CrossRef] [PubMed]
71. Mazahery, H.; von Hurst, P.R. Factors Affecting 25-Hydroxyvitamin D Concentration in Response to Vitamin D Supplementation. *Nutrients* **2015**, *7*, 5111–5142. [CrossRef] [PubMed]

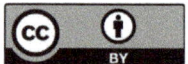

© 2020 by the authors. Licensee MDPI, Basel, Switzerland. This article is an open access article distributed under the terms and conditions of the Creative Commons Attribution (CC BY) license (http://creativecommons.org/licenses/by/4.0/).

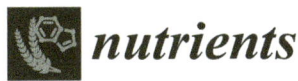

Article

Vitamin-D Receptor-Gene Polymorphisms Affect Quality of Life in Patients with Autoimmune Liver Diseases

Agnieszka Kempinska-Podhorodecka [1],*, Monika Adamowicz [1], Mateusz Chmielarz [1], Maciej K. Janik [2], Piotr Milkiewicz [2,3] and Malgorzata Milkiewicz [1]

1. Department of Medical Biology, Pomeranian Medical University, 70-111 Szczecin, Poland; monikadamowicz@gmail.com (M.A.); ch.mateusz94@gmail.com (M.C.); milkiewm@pum.edu.pl (M.M.)
2. Liver and Internal Medicine Unit, Medical University of Warsaw, 02-097 Warsaw, Poland; mjanik24@gmail.com (M.K.J.); p.milkiewicz@wp.pl (P.M.)
3. Translational Medicine Group, Pomeranian Medical University, 70-111 Szczecin, Poland
* Correspondence: agnieszkakempinska@interia.eu; Tel.: +48-91-466-18-66; Fax: +48-91-466-17-88

Received: 20 June 2020; Accepted: 23 July 2020; Published: 27 July 2020

Abstract: Vitamin D deficiency has been associated with depressive symptoms and reduced physical functioning. The aim of the study was to characterize the relationship between polymorphisms of the vitamin D receptor (VDR) gene and the quality of life in patients with autoimmune hepatitis (AIH) and primary biliary cholangitis (PBC). Three polymorphisms of the *VDR* gene (*TaqI*-rs731236, *BsmI*-rs1544410, and *ApaI*-rs7975232) were analyzed in patients with AIH (n = 142) and PBC (n = 230) and in healthy individuals (n = 376). Patient quality of life was assessed by validated questionnaires such as Medical Outcomes Study Short-Form 36 (SF-36), State Trait Anxiety Inventory (STAI), Modified Fatigue-Impact Scale (MFIS), Patient-Health Questionnaire 9 (PHQ-9), and PBC-40. The *TaqI* C and *ApaI* A alleles are risk alleles in both AIH and PBC, and a significant dominance of the A allele in *BsmI* was observed in AIH patients. In terms of quality of life, the presence of the CC or CT *TaqI* genotype was associated with emotional reactions, including the fatigue and the cognitive skills of patients with PBC, whereas in the group of AIH patients, homozygotes CC of *TaqI*, AA of *BsmI*, and AA of *ApaI* had worse physical, social, emotional, and mental function. The genetic variations of *VDR* gene can influence individual susceptibility to develop chronic autoimmune liver diseases such as AIH and PBC and affect quality of life.

Keywords: autoimmune hepatitis; primary biliary cholangitis; vitamin D; health-related quality of life; mental well-being

1. Introduction

Autoimmune liver diseases, such as primary biliary cholangitis (PBC) and autoimmune hepatitis (AIH), have complex etiologies and are characterized by the progressive destruction of liver structures through autoimmunity mechanisms [1,2]. The vast majority of patients with PBC (80%–90%) are women [3]. The reaction between antimitochondrial antibodies (AMA) and pyruvate dehydrogenase complex-E2 (PDC-E2), located in the inner mitochondrial membrane, underlies the pathogenesis of PBC [4]. The most common clinical symptoms are persistent pruritus and chronic fatigue; however, a substantial percentage of patients may experience no symptoms of liver disease [1]. In biochemistry, elevated alkaline phosphatase and gamma-glutamyltranspeptidase activity, hypercholesterolemia, and often an increase in IgM level are observed. Histologically, the disease is characterized by bile-duct damage leading to chronic cholestasis, progressive fibrosis, and liver cirrhosis [3].

AIH is a disease that affects women more often than men regardless of age or ethnicity [5]. Biochemically, it is characterized by elevated transaminases and hypergammaglobulinemia. It can be divided into two types depending on autoantibodies; Type 1 is the most common and confirmed by the presence of an antinuclear antibody (ANA) or anti-smooth muscle antibody (ASMA). Histologically, AIH is marked by interface hepatitis, emperipolesis, and hepatocyte rosettes [6].

A substantial impairment of health-related quality of life (HRQoL) was reported in both PBC and AIH, with chronic fatigue and depression occurring in a significant proportion of patients with both diseases and pruritus affecting patients with PBC [7,8].

Vitamin D3 inhibits parathyroid-hormone secretion, cell proliferation, and adaptive immunity [9]. The activity of autoimmune diseases is influenced by vitamin-D3 deficiency [10], and this nonclassical effect of vitamin D is associated with the presence of the vitamin-D receptor (VDR) on numerous cells in the immune system. It was demonstrated that vitamin D has an impact on the Th1 lymphocytes responsible for the production of interleukin 2, tumor necrosis factor-alpha (TNA-α), and interferon gamma (IFNγ) [11]. The secretion of these cytokines can inhibit calcitriol ($1.25(OH)_2D_3$—the active metabolite of vitamin D), which translates into the alleviation of the inflammatory reaction. This substance also has a promoting effect on T regulatory cells that are also responsible for turning off the immune-system response, which may be crucial in the treatment of autoimmune diseases associated with excessive responses by the immune system [12]. Furthermore, the presence of VDR was observed on Th2 cells that, after activation, produce interleukins 4 and 10 [13]. Vitamin D enhances the diversification of macrophages and their bactericidal effect; it also inhibits the maturation of dendritic cells, which is essential in autoimmune diseases [14]. Consequently, attempts were made to use vitamin D_3 as a biopreparate capable of treating humans through the immunomodulation of the immune system [15].

Recent studies showed that vitamin D is also involved in neurotransmission and neuroprotection, and its receptor (VDR) is present in brain tissue, like glial cells, hippocampus, thalamus, or neurons [16]. In turn, the polymorphism of the *VDR* gene modulates *VDR* expression that can affect the vitamin D_3 signaling cascade [17,18]. A combination of these factors may suggest the impact of polymorphisms of the *VDR* gene on cognitive dysfunction, thus reducing the quality of life of patients with PBC and AIH.

Therefore, bearing in mind the results of our own study regarding the reduced expression of *VDR* in patients with PBC [19], the clinical symptoms of patients with PBC and AIH (including chronic fatigue and insomnia) [20,21], and reports on the protective effect of vitamin D on vessels and nerves, the aims of this study were characterizing the relationship between *VDR* gene polymorphisms (*BsmI and ApaI*, located in an intron between exons 8 and 9, and *TaqI* C > T located in exon 9) and the HRQoL in patients with a clinical diagnosis of PBC and AIH using validated scale tools and clinical-data forms.

2. Materials and Methods

2.1. Patients

Two-hundred-and-thirty patients with PBC (213 females and 17 males; median age at diagnosis 55; range 28–90 years) and 142 patients with AIH (111 females and 31 males; median age at diagnosis 32; range 24–64 years) were include into this study. Vitamin D supplementation was recommended in all patients with PBC. Main laboratory and demographic data of the included patients are presented at Table 1.

All patients with PBC met The European Association for the Study of the Liver (EASL) criteria for the diagnosis of PBC [22]. One-hundred-and-fifty-eight (68.7%) patients who had histological/clinical/imaging features consistent with liver cirrhosis AIH were diagnosed according EASL's Clinical Practice Guideline [2] for this condition and sixty-five (45.8%) of them had features of liver cirrhosis in histology.

Table 1. Demographic data of analyzed subjects.

Feature	PBC (n = 230)	AIH (n = 142)	Controls (n = 376)
Age (years)	55 (28–90)	32 (24–64)	28 (18–66)
Gender (F/M)	213/17	111/31	344/32
ALT (IU/L) (normal: 5–35)	47.0 (10.0–987.0)	113.8 (1.0–1542.0)	W.N.R.
ALP (IU/L) (normal: 40–120)	286.0 (37.0–1344.0)	100.1 (23.0–344.0)	W.N.R.
GGT, IU/L (normal: 5–35)	177.0 (11.0–1932.0)	102.9 (8.0–766.0)	W.N.R.
Bilirubin (mg/dL) (normal: 0.2–1.0)	0.9 (0.2–45.0)	1.6 (0.2–34.1)	N.D.
Albumin (g/dL) (normal: 3.5–4.5)	4.0 (2.1–5.8)	4.0 (2.0–5.0)	N.D.
Cholesterol (mg/dL) (normal: <190)	217.0 (50.0–1096.0)	182.0 (53.0–319.0)	N.D.
TG (mg/dL) (normal: <150)	105.0 (47.0–681.0)	91.0 (27.0–252.0)	N.D.

PBC: primary biliary cholangitis; AIH: autoimmune; ALT: alanine aminotransferase; ALP: alkaline phosphatase; GGT: gamma-glutamyl transferase; TG: triglycerides; W.N.R.: within normal range; N.D. not done.

A control group of 376 blood donors from the Regional Blood Donor Center in Szczecin (Poland), (344 females and 32 males; median age at enrollment 28; range 18–66 years) was investigated. All participants had a medical check-up. A good state of health was a prerequisite to qualify for blood donation. Each participant provided their written informed consent. All materials were deposited in the Department of Medical Biology, Pomeranian Medical University in Szczecin.

The study was approved by the Bioethical Committee of the Pomeranian Medical University in Szczecin, 2011, no. KB-0012/57/11.

2.2. VDR Genotyping

DNA was extracted from peripheral blood mononuclear cells using the DNeasy Blood and Tissue Kit (Qiagen, Hilden, Germany). Genotyping of three variants of *VDR* gene polymorphism (*TaqI-rs731236, BsmI-rs1544410, ApaI-rs7975232*) was carried out using real-time polymerase chain reaction using TaqMan probes (Applied Biosystems, Foster City, CA, Country; assay ID: C_2404008_10, C_8716062_10, C_28977635_10, respectively). Fluorescence analysis was conducted with Allelic Discrimination 7500 software v.2.0.2.

2.3. Health-Related Quality-of-Life Tools

Medical Outcomes Study Short Form 36 version 1.0 (*SF-36v1*, license no. QM011392-QualityMetric CT133208/OP018661) is a standardized questionnaire that contains 36 questions in 8 domains related to physical health (Physical Functioning, Role-Physical, Bodily Pain, General Health) and psychological well-being (Vitality, Social Functioning, Role-Emotional, Mental Health), which can be calculated in addition to two summary parameters: Physical-Component Summary and Mental-Component Summary [23].

PBC-40 was developed in 2005 and focuses on PBC [24]. The questionnaire consists of 40 questions related to the various aspects of chronic cholestatic liver disease: the worsening of chronic fatigue syndrome; feeling of health; skin pruritus; and cognitive, emotional, and social functions.

The Polish version of the Modified Fatigue-Impact Scale (MFIS) was used to assess the impact of fatigue on AIH patients' life [25]. It is a modified form of the original Fatigue-Impact Scale. The questionnaire that included 21 items and a total MFIS score (range 0–84) is based on three subscales: physical (9 items, score range 0–36), cognitive (10 items, score range 0–40), and psychical (2 items, score range 0–8).

State Trait Anxiety Inventory (STAI) is a tool designed to measure the levels of state and trait anxiety [25]. The Polish version of this questionnaire was used in this study. This 40-item scale includes two subscales, state anxiety (1–20 items) and trait anxiety (20–40 items). Each item is given a weighted score of 1 to 4. Higher score suggests elevated levels of anxiety. Therefore, 0–20 results from both subscales represent no anxiety, a 41–60 score indicates midlevel anxiety, and results from 61 to 80 indicate severe anxiety.

Patient-Health Questionnaire 9 (PHQ-9) is a self-administered screening tool that is used to monitor the severity of depressive symptoms [26]. A questionnaire was validated for Polish population. PHQ-9 scores of 5–9, 10–14, 15–19, and 20–27 are the ranges for mild, moderate, moderately severe, and severe depression, respectively.

In patients with PBC, two questionnaires were used, SF-36 and PBC-40. In patients with AIH, SF-36, MFIS, PHQ-9, and STAI were applied.

2.4. Statistical Analysis

All statistical analyses were carried out using StatView version 5 software (SAS Institute Inc., Carry, NC, USA). The genotype and allelic frequencies were compared using a chi-squared test of association (Pearson). The odds ratio (OR) and 95% confidence interval (CI) for each variable were also estimated. Analysis of genotype frequency in regard to the clinical characteristics and HRQoL assessment of PBC and AIH patients was performed using ANOVA with Fisher's protected least significant difference (PLSD). Data are shown as medians (and ranges) for demographic data, and as means and standard deviations (SD) for continuous variables of assessing HRQoL. p-values of less than 0.05 were considered to be statistically significant.

3. Results

The frequencies of all three *VDR* polymorphisms investigated in patients with PBC or AIH showed significant differences in comparison to the control group. The odds ratios (ORs) observed for the presence of these polymorphisms in the diseases and control groups are summarized in Table 2.

Table 2. Genotype counts for vitamin-D receptor (*VDR*) polymorphisms (rs731236, rs1544410, rs7975232) in PBC, AIH, and control subjects.

Frequencies	Controls (%) $n = 376$	PBC (%) $n = 230$	p * PBC vs. Control	X^2	OR (95% CI)	AIH (%) $n = 142$	p * AIH vs. Control	X^2	OR (95% CI)
				TaqI (rs731236)					
TT (TT)	172 (45.7%)	28 (12.2%)	<0.001	72.7	0.2 (0.1–0.3)	48 (33.8%)	0.01	6.0	0.6 (0.4–0.9)
CT (tT)	160 (42.6%)	118 (51.3%)	0.04	4.4	1.4 (1.0–2.0)	62 (43.7%)	0.8	0.05	1.0 (0.7–1.5)
CC (tt)	44 (11.7%)	84 (36.5%)	<0.001	52.8	4.3 (2.9–6.6)	32 (22.5%)	0.002	9.7	2.2 (1.3–3.6)
				BsmI (rs1544410)					
AA (BB)	52 (13.8%)	25 (10.9%)	0.3	1.1	0.8 (0.5–1.3)	34 (23.9%)	0.006	7.6	2.0 (1.2–3.2)
GA (bB)	173 (46%)	109 (47.4%)	0.7	0.1	1.1 (0.8–1.5)	60 (42.3%)	0.4	0.6	0.9 (0.6–1.3)
GG (bb)	151 (40.2%)	96 (41.7%)	0.7	0.1	1.1 (0.8–1.5)	48 (33.8%)	0.2	1.76	0.8 (0.5–1.1)
				ApaI (rs7975232)					
AA (AA)	74 (19.7%)	63 (27.4%)	0.03	4.8	1.5 (1.0–2.3)	46 (32.4%)	0.002	9.4	2.0 (1.3–3.0)
CA (aA)	196 (52.1%)	111 (48.2%)	0.3	0.8	0.9 (0.6–1.2)	61 (43.0%)	0.06	3.5	0.7 (0.5–1.0)
CC (aa)	106 (28.2%)	56 (24.4%)	0.3	1.0	0.8 (0.6–1.2)	35 (24.6%)	0.4	0.6	0.8 (0.5–1.3)

* Chi-squared test of association (Pearson); PBC: primary biliary cholangitis; AIH: autoimmune hepatitis; OR: odds ratio; CI: confidence interval. Bold font indicates statistical significance.

In PBC patients, the *TaqI* CC and CT genotypes were more prevalent in comparison to controls (36.5% vs. 11.7%, $p < 0.001$, and 51.3% vs. 42.6%, $p = 0.04$, respectively), whereas the TT genotype of *TaqI* was considerably less frequent than in the controls (12.2% vs. 45.7%, $p < 0.001$; Table 2). Similarly, in AIH patients, the *TaqI* CC genotype appeared more often than in the control group (22.5% vs. 11.7%, $p = 0.002$), while the TT was less frequent than in the controls (33.8% vs. 45.7%, $p = 0.01$; Table 2).

Regarding *BsmI* polymorphism, the frequency of the AA genotype was substantially higher in patients with AIH compared to controls (23.9% vs. 13.8%, $p = 0.006$; Table 2). The results of *ApaI* genotyping showed that the AA genotype occurred more frequently in both patients with PBC and AIH (27.4% vs. 19.7% in controls, $p = 0.03$, and 32.4% vs. 19.7% in controls; $p = 0.002$, respectively; Table 2).

Furthermore, analyses of frequencies of each allele in the three polymorphic sites clearly demonstrated that the *TaqI* C and *ApaI* A alleles were more prevalent in both PBC and AIH compared to in healthy individuals. Thus, the distribution of the *TaqI* C allele was 62.0% in PBC and 44.4% in AIH vs. 33.0% in controls (both $p < 0.001$); for the *ApaI* A allele, 51.4% in PBC and 54% in AIH vs. 45.7% in controls, $p = 0.05$ and $p = 0.02$, respectively. Additionally, 45.0% of AIH patients were carriers of the *BsmI* A allele in comparison to 36.8% controls, $p = 0.02$ (Table 3).

Table 3. Allele association for VDR in PBC, AIH, and control subjects.

SNP	Allele	Controls n = 376 (%)	PBC n = 230 (%)	p * PBC vs. Control	X²	OR (95%CI)	AIH n = 142 (%)	p * AIH vs. Control	X²	OR (95%CI)
TaqI rs731236	T/C (T/t)	504/248 (67.0/33.0)	174/286 (38.0/62.0)	<0.001	98.7	3.3 (2.6–4.3)	158/126 (55.6/44.4)	<0.001	11.6	1.6 (1.3–2.1)
BsmI rs1544410	A/G (B/b)	277/475 (36.8/63.2)	159/301 (34.6/65.4)	0.4	0.6	1.1 (0.9–1.4)	128/156 (45.0/55.0)	0.02	5.9	1.4 (1.1–1.9)
ApaI rs7975232	A/C (A/a)	344/408 (45.7/54.3)	237/223 (51.4/48.6)	0.05	3.8	0.8 (0.6–1.0)	153/131 (54.0/46.0)	0.02	5.4	1.4 (1.1–1.8)

* Chi-squared test of association (Pearson); PSC: primary biliary cholangitis; AIH: Autoimmune hepatitis; OR: odds ratio; CI: confidence interval. Bold font indicates statistical significance.

In addition, the clinical status and biochemical findings of the patients were examined in relation to *VDR* polymorphism. In PBC patients, *TaqI* and *BsmI* variants were associated with the histological features of cirrhosis regardless of cholestasis and autoimmune parameters in PBC. Thus, in patients with PBC who were cirrhotic at the diagnosis, 52.8% were *TaqI* CC, 39% were CT and 7.5% were TT genotype carriers ($p < 0.0001$ vs. *CC*). Similarly, in *BmsI* variant, 56.6% of cirrhotics were GG homozygous, 33.9% were GA heterozygous ($p = 0.03$ vs. *GG*), and 9.4% were AA homozygotes genotype ($p < 0.0001$ vs. *GG*). Other laboratory markers of the disease severity and enhanced level of AMAs, Gp210, and Sp100 antibodies failed to have any association to the analyzed polymorphisms. In contrast, in the group of AIH patients, the presence of the *VDR* polymorphisms did not correlate with the examined clinical and biochemical features (data not shown).

Regarding the quality of life of PBC patients, several domains of SF-36 and PBC-40 questionnaires were correlated only with the *TaqI* variant of *VDR* polymorphisms. The SF-36 general questionnaire demonstrated that PBC patients with CC and CT genotypes of *TaqI* variants had lower scores for Vitality ($p = 0.01$, and $p = 0.04$, respectively) and Role-Emotional ($p = 0.03$ and $p = 0.04$, respectively) than TT homozygotes did. The results of the PBC-40 questionnaires showed that carriers of CC and CT genotypes had significant cognitive impairment versus the TT genotype ($p = 0.04$ and $p = 0.04$, respectively). Furthermore, PBC patients with the *TaqI* CT genotype suffer from greater fatigue than patients with TT do ($p = 0.04$; Table 4).

In view of the fact that the *TaqI* C allele was associated with the increased risk of cirrhosis as well as reduced quality of life, we did an additional sub-group analysis corresponding to the presence of cirrhosis. We looked at features which came out significant, i.e., vitality and role emotional from SF-36 and cognitive function from PBC40. No significant differences between cirrhotic and non-cirrhotic patients were found, which may suggest that the allele itself, but not the presence of cirrhosis, exerts its negative effect on patients QoL.

Among patients with AIH, health-related quality of life was evaluated by the SF-36, STAI, MFIS, and PHQ-9 questionnaires. Differences between patients in relation to variants of *VDR* polymorphisms were observed only in SF-36 domains. The *TaqI* CC homozygotes scored fewer points for Role-Physical ($p = 0.04$) than the CT heterozygotes did, which, in turn, scored higher than TT homozygotes on Social-Functioning ($p = 0.03$; Table 5).

Table 4. Relationship between *TaqI* polymorphism and features of quality-of-life scales in PBC group.

Domain	TaqI (rs731236 T/C)					
	CC (tt)	CT (tT)	TT (TT)	*p* * CC vs CT	*p* * CC vs TT	*p* * TT vs CT
SF-36						
Physical Functioning	57.0 ± 3.2	59.5 ± 2.3	67.0 ± 5.3	0.5	0.09	0.2
Role-Physical	36.5 ± 4.3	34.0 ± 3.7	50.0 ± 8.3	0.6	0.1	0.05
Bodily Pain	54.4 ± 3.2	55.4 ± 2.4	61.0 ± 5.8	0.8	0.3	0.3
General Health	43.4 ± 1.9	43.6 ± 1.7	45.1 ± 3.4	0.9	0.7	0.7
Vitality	44.5 ± 2.4	47.5 ± 1.9	57.0 ± 4.8	0.3	**0.01**	**0.04**
Social Functioning	59.2 ± 3.0	61.2 ± 2.3	69.0 ± 5.3	0.6	0.08	0.1
Role-Emotional	47.4 ± 5.0	49.7 ± 4.2	69.0 ± 7.8	0.7	**0.03**	**0.04**
Mental Health	59.0 ± 2.0	59.9 ± 1.9	67.2 ± 4.3	0.7	0.06	0.09
Physical Component Summary	47.8 ± 2.6	47.8 ± 2.0	55.0 ± 4.7	0.8	0.1	0.1
Mental Component Summary	52.2 ± 2.5	54.4 ± 2.1	65.0 ± 5.0	0.5	0.2	0.4
PBC-40						
Other Symptom	17.0 ± 0.6	17.3 ± 0.5	16.1 ± 1.0	0.6	0.4	0.2
Itch	6.0 ± 0.5	5.4 ± 0.4	5.0 ± 0.9	0.4	0.3	0.6
Fatigue	29.6 ± 1.2	30.4 ± 1.0	26.1 ± 1.8	0.6	0.1	**0.04**
Cognitive function	14.2 ± 0.7	14.1 ± 0.5	11.7 ± 1.0	0.8	**0.04**	**0.04**
Social and Emotional function	31.5 ± 10.7	31.6 ±11.5	28.0 ±11.0	0.9	0.1	0.08

* ANOVA with Fisher's protected least significant difference (PLSD). Letters enclosed in brackets represent previously described nomenclature derived from restriction-fragment length polymorphism (RFLP) analysis. Bold font indicates statistical significance.

Table 5. Relationship between *TaqI* polymorphism and features of quality-of-life scales in AIH group.

Domain	TaqI (rs731236 T/C)					
	CC (tt)	CT (tT)	TT (TT)	*p* * CC vs CT	*p* * CC vs TT	*p* * TT vs CT
SF-36						
Physical Functioning	73.0 ± 4.6	79.0 ± 2.8	73.6 ± 3.4	0.2	0.9	0.2
Role-Physical	47.7 ± 7.6	66.1 ± 5.5	55.7 ± 5.8	**0.04**	0.4	0.2
Bodily Pain	67.4 ± 5.2	74.2 ± 3.1	69.4 ± 4.1	0.3	0.7	0.3
General Health	47.5 ± 3.5	49.9 ± 2.5	47.5 ± 3.5	0.6	0.9	0.6
Vitality	53.3 ± 3.5	54.3 ± 2.5	51.6 ± 2.8	0.8	0.7	0.5
Social Functioning	67.2 ± 4.1	75.4 ± 3.2	65.1 ± 3.7	0.1	0.7	**0.03**
Role-Emotional	59.4 ± 7.3	74.7 ± 4.8	68.1 ± 5.8	0.08	0.3	0.4
Mental Health	63.5 ± 2.9	66.3 ± 2.6	61.3 ± 2.5	0.5	0.6	0.2
Physical Component Summary	58.9 ± 4.2	67.3 ± 2.7	61.6 ± 3.5	0.09	0.6	0.2
Mental Component Summary	60.8 ± 3.8	67.7 ± 2.8	61.5 ± 3.0	0.1	0.9	0.1
STAI						
STAI1	47.4 ± 0.8	45.9 ± 0.8	46.2 ± 0.8	0.2	0.4	0.8
STAI2	45.1 ± 0.9	45.3 ± 0.7	46.0 ± 0.8	0.9	0.5	0.5
MFIS						
Physical	13.7 ± 1.6	14.1 ± 1.0	14.1 ± 1.1	0.8	0.9	0.9
Cognitive	13.2 ± 1.6	11.7 ± 0.9	12.2 ± 1.0	0.4	0.6	0.7
Psychosocial	2.8 ± 0.4	2.5 ± 0.2	3.0 ± 0.3	0.4	0.7	0.2
MFIS Score	13.7 ± 1.6	14.1 ± 1.0	14.1 ± 1.1	0.8	0.9	0.9
PHQ-9						
PHQ-9	7.2 ± 0.8	6.0 ± 0.6	7.7 ± 0.8	0.3	0.6	0.08

* ANOVA with Fisher's protected least significant difference (PLSD); The letters enclosed in square brackets represent previously described nomenclature derived from a restriction-fragment length polymorphism (RFLP) analysis. Bold font indicates statistical significance.

The *BsmI* AA homozygotes had lower scores for Physical-Component Summary than the GA heterozygotes did ($p = 0.04$; Table 6).

Table 6. Relationship between *BsmI* polymorphism and features of quality-of-life scales in AIH group.

Domain	BsmI (rs1544410 A/G)					
	GG (bb)	GA (bB)	AA (BB)	*p* * GG vs GA	*p* * GG vs AA	*p* * AA vs GA
SF-36						
Physical Functioning	73.9 ± 3.4	80.5 ± 2.5	72.3 ± 4.9	0.1	0.8	0.1
Role-Physical	56.2 ± 5.7	66.7 ± 5.4	49.3 ± 7.6	0.2	0.5	0.05
Bodily Pain	70.3 ± 4.1	73.5 ± 2.9	65.1 ± 5.2	0.5	0.4	0.1
General Health	48.9 ± 3.4	51.0 ± 2.5	46.2 ± 3.7	0.6	0.6	0.3
Vitality	53.3 ± 2.6	54.5 ± 2.4	52.0 ± 3.7	0.7	0.8	0.5
Social Functioning	65.8 ± 3.7	75.2 ± 3.0	67.0 ± 4.2	0.05	0.8	0.1
Role-Emotional	68.7 ± 5.9	75.5 ± 4.7	60.8 ± 7.2	0.4	0.4	0.08
Mental Health	63.5 ± 2.4	67.1 ± 2.4	61.9 ± 3.2	0.3	0.7	0.2
Physical Component Summary	62.3 ± 3.3	67.9 ± 2.5	58.2 ± 4.4	0.2	0.4	**0.04**
Mental Component Summary	62.9 ± 3.0	68.1 ± 2.6	60.4 ± 4.0	0.2	0.6	0.09
STAI						
STAI1	47.1 ± 0.8	45.6 ± 0.8	46.9 ± 0.8	0.1	0.8	0.3
STAI2	46.2 ± 0.8	45.3 ± 0.8	44.7 ± 0.8	0.4	0.2	0.6
MFIS						
Physical	14.0 ± 1.0	14.1 ± 1.0	14.2 ± 1.6	0.9	0.9	0.9
Cognitive	12.4 ± 1.0	11.4 ± 0.8	13.0 ± 1.5	0.5	0.7	0.3
Psychosocial	3.0 ± 0.3	2.6 ± 0.2	2.9 ± 0.4	0.4	0.8	0.6
MFIS Score	29.4 ± 2.0	28.2 ± 1.9	30.1 ± 3.3	0.7	0.9	0.6
PHQ-9						
PHQ-9	7.0 ± 0.8	6.2 ± 0.6	7.4 ± 0.8	0.4	0.7	0.2

* ANOVA with Fisher's protected least-significant difference (PLSD). Letters enclosed in brackets represent previously described nomenclature derived from restriction-fragment length polymorphism (RFLP) analysis. Bold font indicates statistical significance.

The most noticeable differences in quality of life measured by the generic SF-36 were observed in *ApaI* variants of *VDR* polymorphism. *ApaI* AA homozygotes had lower scores for 6 out of 10 factors, namely, Role-Physical ($p = 0.02$), Social Functioning ($p = 0.04$), Role-Emotional ($p = 0.003$), Mental Health ($p = 0.04$), Physical-Component Summary ($p = 0.04$), and Mental-Component Summary ($p = 0.04$) compared to CA heterozygotes (Table 7). Additionally, CA heterozygotes scored more points for Social Functioning ($p = 0.01$) than CC individuals did (Table 7).

Table 7. Relationship between *ApaI* polymorphism and features of quality-of-life scales in AIH group.

Domain	ApaI (rs7975232 C/A)					
	CC (aa)	CA (aA)	AA (AA)	*p* * CC vs CA	*p* * CC vs AA	*p* * AA vs CA
SF-36						
Physical Functioning	73.6 ± 4.0	80.5 ± 2.3	74.0 ± 3.9	0.1	0.9	0.1
Role-Physical	56.1 ± 6.9	68.1 ± 5.0	49.5 ± 6.3	0.2	0.5	**0.02**
Bodily Pain	71.7 ± 4.9	72.7 ± 3.1	67.8 ± 4.1	0.8	0.5	0.3
General Health	47.3 ± 3.8	51.5 ± 2.5	47.5 ± 3.1	0.3	0.9	0.3
Vitality	52.2 ± 3.1	56.5 ± 2.3	50.4 ± 2.8	0.3	0.7	0.09
Social Functioning	63.8 ± 3.9	76.4 ± 2.8	66.6 ± 3.9	**0.01**	0.6	**0.04**
Role-Emotional	64.7 ± 6.9	80.6 ± 4.2	58.5 ± 6.1	0.05	0.4	**0.003**
Mental Health	62.5 ± 2.7	67.8 ± 2.2	60.9 ± 2.9	0.2	0.7	**0.04**
Physical Component Summary	62.5 ± 2.7	67.9 ± 2.2	60.9 ± 2.9	0.2	0.7	**0.04**
Mental Component Summary	62.2 ± 3.9	68.2 ± 2.5	58.7 ± 3.5	0.2	0.6	**0.04**
STAI						
STAI1	46.5 ± 1.0	45.7 ± 0.7	46.9 ± 0.8	0.5	0.7	0.2
STAI2	46.3 ± 0.9	45.2 ± 0.6	45.0 ± 0.8	0.4	0.3	0.8

Table 7. Cont.

Domain	ApaI (rs7975232 C/A)					
	CC (aa)	CA (aA)	AA (AA)	p * CC vs CA	p * CC vs AA	p * AA vs CA
MFIS						
Physical	13.2 ± 1.2	14.8 ± 1.0	13.9 ± 1.2	0.3	0.7	0.6
Cognitive	11.5 ± 1.1	12.6 ± 0.9	12.3 ± 1.2	0.5	0.3	0.8
Psychosocial	2.8 ± 0.3	3.0 ± 0.2	2.6 ± 0.3	0.6	0.7	0.3
MFIS Score	27.4 ± 2.4	30.4 ± 1.9	28.8 ± 2.6	0.4	0.8	0.6
PHQ-9						
PHQ-9	7.1 ± 0.9	6.6 ± 0.6	6.9 ± 0.7	0.7	0.8	0.8

* ANOVA with Fisher's protected least-significant difference (PLSD). Letters enclosed in brackets represent previously described nomenclature derived from restriction-fragment length polymorphism (RFLP) analysis. Bold font indicates statistical significance.

4. Discussion

In this study, we analyzed the prevalence of three common *VDR* polymorphisms (*TaqI-rs731236*, *BsmI-rs1544410*, and *ApaI-rs7975232*) and investigated their potential relationships with the quality of life in a well-characterized cohort of Polish patients with PBC and AIH.

Calcium and vitamin-D supplementation (400–800 IU/day) is recommended to both patients with AIH, who are frequently on long-term steroids, and with PBC, who in their majority are postmenopausal females prone to osteoporosis and impaired vitamin-D absorption secondary to cholestasis. Vitamin D, operating through a nuclear receptor (VDR), is an important modulator of immune processes that adjust both types of immune response [27] by strengthening innate immunity and suppressing acquired immunity reactions [9].

Interestingly, in our study, in the two examined autoimmune liver diseases, both the CC *TaqI* and the AA *ApaI* genotype occurred more frequently than in the controls, and both the C allele of *TaqI* and the A allele of *ApaI* were risk alleles for PBC and AIH. Our results are in contrast to a study in which a significant association of the *TaqI* but not the *ApaI* polymorphism within German AIH patients was reported [28]. However, results from the study that included both patients with AIH and patients with PBC in one merged group showed an increased incidence of the A allele of *ApaI* [29]. These findings may be explained by the genetic heterogeneity that exists in different populations. For instance, the distribution of *BsmI*, *ApaI*, and *TaqI* gene variants was reported to be dissimilar in healthy Chinese controls as compared to healthy Caucasian controls [30]. In our patients with AIH, the A allele and AA genotype of the *BsmI* variant were more prevalent compared to the controls. These results are in a line with reports showing the link between *VDR* polymorphisms and autoimmunity. Thus, the *TaqI*, *BsmI*, and *ApaI* polymorphisms of *VDR* gene are the most widely reported as being closely linked with a high risk of autoimmune diseases including PBC [31], multiple sclerosis (*BsmI* AA) [32], Type 1 diabetes (*TaqI* T [33] or *BsmI* AA [34]), and systemic lupus erythematosus (*BsmI* AA) [35,36]. The functional consequence of these *VDR* polymorphisms is important in determining the potential effect on inflammatory mediators in autoimmune diseases. Vitamin D stimulates the development of Th2 cells and the production of anti-inflammatory interleukins. Therefore, reduced signal transduction due to polymorphic variants of the *VDR* gene might skew the immune response to the Th1 pathway that was implicated in the progress of organ-specific autoimmune diseases. *ApaI* and the *BsmI* polymorphisms do not change the amino acid sequence of the VDR protein but may affect gene expression through the alteration of mRNA stability (the disruption of splice sites for mRNA transcription or a change in intronic regulatory elements) [28], and it was demonstrated that the ApaI variant was positively associated with the serum concentration of 25 $(OH)_2D_3$ [37]. Moreover, IFN gamma production upon anti-CD3 stimulation in the AA [BB] genotype of *BsmI* was significantly higher than that in the AG (Bb) and GG (bb) genotype groups, which showed that the polyclonal T-cell response in BB genotype patients was Th1-dominant [34]. In turn, the *TaqI* polymorphism is involved in the regulation of the stability of VDR mRNA, and the TT genotype modulates VDR expression and confers protection against multiple sclerosis [17,28,38].

Our previous report, on a smaller group of PBC patients (n = 143), showed that there is an association between the *TaqI* and *BsmI*, a predisposition to earlier onset of liver damage and a more severe manifestation of disease [39]. In this study on a larger group of PBC patients (n = 230), it was confirmed that the *TaqI* CC and *BsmI* GG genotypes are related to the degree of liver morphologic damage, as assessed by severity of liver fibrosis (Stage IV on histology). On the basis of the results of this study, we validated our previous conclusion that these variants of the *VDR* gene may prompt more severe liver injury and a worse course of primary biliary cholangitis. However, the interpretation of the role of *TaqI* and *BsmI* variants in the development of liver fibrosis is hindered because only limited information is available on the functional changes induced by these variants of the *VDR* gene.

In general, little is known about the impact of *VDR* polymorphisms on the quality of patients' life since previous studies mostly focused on the prevalence of each polymorphism in autoimmune diseases but not on their relation with the clinical course of the disease [29]. Most studies on the quality of life in patients with PBC or AIH addressed relations between specific aspects of disease, such as fatigue, pruritus, depression, and quality of life after liver transplantation [7,40–49] but not the impact of *VDR* gene polymorphisms.

In this present study, we showed that there is an association between the *TaqI* variant of the *VDR* gene and impaired well-being of patients with PBC, as measured with general and disease-specific questionnaires. The CC of *TaqI* was associated with worse health-related quality of life, as measured by the generic SF-36. This was mainly due to the decrease in subscores of energy and emotional reactions, both associated with fatigue and significant cognitive impairment. Moreover, our analysis of the PBC-40 domains showed that PBC patients' quality of life was significantly impaired in the carriers of CC and CT genotype of *TaqI*, and fatigue and cognitive function were the most affected domains. In contrast to patients with PBC, among AIH patients, all three variants of *VDR* polymorphism, i.e., *TaqI*, *BsmI*, and *ApaI*, affected health-related quality of life. We observed that the CC and CT of *TaqI* were associated with worse physical and social functioning, while the AA genotype of *BsmI* had physical problems and worse overall health. Interestingly, *ApaI* was the polymorphic variant that mostly affected the quality of life of AIH patients. Our study clearly indicated that the AA homozygotes of *ApaI* variant had disturbed or maladaptive emotional responses and mental disorders, while the CC homozygotes scored fewer points for social functioning. We observed a similar phenomenon in patients with another liver disease of presumed autoimmune background, namely, primary sclerosing cholangitis (PSC) [19]. In that group of patients, the SF-36 questionnaire showed that the C allele of *ApaI* was associated with a reduction of physical, emotional, and mental function and worse overall health. Furthermore, the PBC-40 and PBC-27 questionnaires confirmed that the C allele was associated with itching, fatigue, and the impairment of cognitive functions. Correspondingly, individuals who were AA homozygotes (noncarriers of the C allele of *ApaI*) had higher summary scores for the physical and mental disorders measured with SF-36; they suffered less from itching or fatigue and did not have significant cognitive impairment [19]. The observed association between *VDR* polymorphisms and quality of life is of importance to daily clinical practice because patients with AIH struggle with serious symptoms that significantly affect their well-being, including mood disturbance, cognitive dysfunction, chronic fatigue, decreased physical activity, and a high rate of previously unrecognized severe symptoms of depression and anxiety [7,50]; thus, the presence of the CC *ApaI* variant may result in those symptoms worsening.

Perhaps the major limitation of this study, related to its retrospective nature, is the lack of data on Vitamin D serum levels in analyzed patients and thus the inability to correlate these levels with analyzed polymorphisms. This problem has also been noted in other, similar studies. Serum levels of Vitamin D depend not only on whether patient supplements it but also on patient's diet and several other factors. Therefore, normal serum levels of Vitamin D could be related to its regular intake, and this would certainly be independent of the presence of VDR polymorphisms. Judgement based on information provided by the patient regarding Vitamin D/calcium supplementation can also be inaccurate in view of widely reported non-adherence to drugs, which do not directly relieve symptoms such as Vitamin D deficiency or hypertension. Thus, in a real-world situation, it is very difficult to reliably assess relationship between real serum Vitamin D levels and VDR polymorphisms. For the same reason, we were not able to study a direct effect of serum Vitamin D levels on patients QoL.

5. Conclusions

We observed a significant dominance of the CC *TaqI* and AA *ApaI* genotypes in patients with PBC and AIH. Moreover, the impaired quality of life in patients with AIH was significantly associated with the presence of the AA *ApaI* variant of the *VDR* gene. Awareness of this association can contribute to a deeper understanding of the mechanisms responsible for the occurrence of symptoms associated with poorer quality of life, thereby offering the chance to improve the care of AIH patients.

Author Contributions: Conceptualization, A.K.-P. and M.M.; methodology, A.K.-P., M.A., M.C., and M.K.J.; validation, A.K.-P., M.M., and M.K.J.; formal analysis, A.K.-P., M.A., M.C., and M.M.; investigation, P.M.; resources, A.K.-P., M.M., and P.M.; data curation, A.K.-P., M.A., M.K.J., and M.C.; writing—original-draft preparation, A.K.-P. and M.M.; writing—review and editing, all authors; visualization, A.K.-P. and M.A.; supervision, M.M. and P.M.; project administration, A.K.-P., M.M., M.K.J., and P.M.; funding acquisition, A.K.-P., M.M., and P.M. All authors have read and agreed to the published version of the manuscript.

Funding: This research received no external funding.

Conflicts of Interest: The authors declare no conflict of interest.

References

1. Hirschfield, G.M.; Dyson, J.K.; Alexander, G.J.M.; Chapman, M.H.; Collier, J.; Hübscher, S.; Pereira, S.P.; Thain, C.; Thorburn, D.; Tiniakos, D.; et al. Primary biliary cholangitis treatment and management guidelines. *Gut* **2018**, *67*, 1568–1594. [CrossRef]
2. Lohse, A.W.; Chazouillères, O.; Dalekos, G.; Drenth, J.; Heneghan, M.; Hofer, H.; Lammert, F.; Lenzi, M. EASL clinical practice guidelines: Autoimmune hepatitis. *J. Hepatol.* **2015**, *63*, 971–1004. [CrossRef]
3. Onofrio, F.Q.; Hirschfield, G.M.; Gulamhusein, A.F. A practical review of primary biliary cholangitis for the gastroenterologist. *Gastroenterol. Hepatol. (NY)* **2019**, *15*, 145–154.
4. Hisamoto, S.; Shimoda, S.; Harada, K.; Iwasaka, S.; Onohara, S.; Chong, Y.; Nakamura, M.; Bekki, Y.; Yoshizumi, T.; Ikegami, T.; et al. Hydrophobic bile acids suppress expression of AE2 in biliary epithelial cells and induce bile duct inflammation in primary biliary cholangitis. *J. Autoimmun.* **2016**, *75*, 150–160. [CrossRef] [PubMed]
5. Puustinen, L.; Barner-Rasmussen, N.; Pukkala, E.; Färkkilä, M. Incidence, prevalence, and causes of death of patients with autoimmune hepatitis: A nationwide register-based cohort study in Finland. *Dig. Liver Dis.* **2019**, *51*, 1294–1299. [CrossRef]
6. Linzay, C.D.; Sharma, B.; Pandit, S. Autoimmune Hepatitis. Available online: https://www.ncbi.nlm.nih.gov/books/NBK459186/ (accessed on 25 July 2020).
7. Janik, M.K.; Wunsch, E.; Raszeja-Wyszomirska, J.; Moskwa, M.; Kruk, B.; Krawczyk, M.; Milkiewicz, P. Autoimmune hepatitis exerts a profound, negative effect on health-related quality of life: A prospective, single-centre study. *Liver Int.* **2019**, *39*, 215–221. [CrossRef]
8. Raszeja-Wyszomirska, J.; Wunsch, E.; Krawczyk, M.; Rigopoulou, E.I.; Kostrzewa, K.; Norman, G.L.; Bogdanos, D.P.; Milkiewicz, P. Assessment of health related quality of life in Polish patients with primary biliary cirrhosis. *Clin. Res. Hepatol. Gastroenterol.* **2016**, *40*, 471–479. [CrossRef]
9. Di Rosa, M.; Malaguarnera, M.; Nicoletti, F.; Malaguarnera, L. Vitamin D3: A helpful immuno-modulator. *Immunology* **2011**, *134*, 123–139. [CrossRef] [PubMed]
10. Gil, Á.; Plaza-Diaz, J.; Mesa, M.D. Vitamin D: Classic and novel actions: Vdre deviation repression. *Ann. Nutr. Metab.* **2018**, *72*, 87–95. [CrossRef] [PubMed]
11. Lemire, J.M.; Archer, D.C.; Beck, L.; Spiegelberg, H.L. Immunosuppressive actions of 1,25-dihydroxyvitamin D3: Preferential inhibition of Th1 functions. *J. Nutr.* **1995**, *125*, 1704S–1708S. [CrossRef] [PubMed]

12. Cantorna, M.T.; Snyder, L.; Lin, Y.D.; Yang, L. Vitamin D and 1,25(OH)2D regulation of t cells. *Nutrients* **2015**, *7*, 3011–3021. [CrossRef] [PubMed]
13. Lemire, J.M.; Adams, J.S.; Kermani-Arab, V.; Bakke, A.C.; Sakai, R.; Jordan, S.C. 1,25-dihydroxyvitamin D3 suppresses human T helper/inducer lymphocyte activity in vitro. *J. Immunol.* **1985**, *134*, 3032–3035. [PubMed]
14. Abbas, A.K.; Murphy, K.M.; Sher, A. Functional diversity of helper T lymphocytes. *Nature* **1996**, *383*, 787–793. [CrossRef] [PubMed]
15. Barchetta, I. Could vitamin D supplementation benefit patients with chronic liver disease? *Gastroenterol. Hepatol. (NY)* **2012**, *8*, 755–757.
16. Cui, X.; Gooch, H.; Petty, A.; McGrath, J.J.; Eyles, D. Vitamin D and the brain: Genomic and non-genomic actions. *Mol. Cell. Endocrinol.* **2017**, *453*, 131–143. [CrossRef]
17. Agliardi, C.; Guerini, F.R.; Saresella, M.; Caputo, D.; Leone, M.A.; Zanzottera, M.; Bolognesi, E.; Marventano, I.; Barizzone, N.; Fasano, M.E.; et al. Vitamin D receptor (VDR) gene SNPs influence VDR expression and modulate protection from multiple sclerosis in HLA-DRB1 * 15-positive individuals. *Brain. Behav. Immun.* **2011**, *25*, 1460–1467. [CrossRef] [PubMed]
18. Mahajan, M.; Sharma, R. Current understanding of role of vitamin D in Type 2 diabetes mellitus. *Int. J. Recent Sci. Res.* **2015**, *6*, 2602–2604.
19. Kempinska-Podhorodecka, A.; Milkiewicz, M.; Jabłonski, D.; Milkiewicz, P.; Wunsch, E. ApaI polymorphism of vitamin D receptor affects health-related quality of life in patients with primary sclerosing cholangitis. *PLoS ONE* **2017**, *12*, e0176264. [CrossRef]
20. Zhao, X.; Wong, P. Managing sleep disturbances in cirrhosis. *Scientifica (Cairo)* **2016**, *2016*, 5. [CrossRef]
21. Purohit, T.; Cappell, M.S. Primary biliary cirrhosis: Pathophysiology, clinical presentation and therapy. *World J. Hepatol.* **2015**, *7*, 926–941. [CrossRef]
22. Hirschfield, G.M.; Beuers, U.; Corpechot, C.; Invernizzi, P.; Jones, D.; Marzioni, M.; Schramm, C. EASL clinical practice guidelines: The diagnosis and management of patients with primary biliary cholangitis. *J. Hepatol.* **2017**, *67*, 145–172. [CrossRef]
23. Ware, J.E.; Sherbourne, C.D. The MOS 36-item short form health status survey (SF-36). *Med. Care* **1992**, *30*, 473–483. [CrossRef] [PubMed]
24. Jacoby, A.; Rannard, A.; Buck, D.; Bhala, N.; Newton, J.L.; James, O.F.W.; Jones, D.E.J. Development, validation, and evaluation of the PBC-40, a disease specific health related quality of life measure for primary biliary cirrhosis. *Gut* **2005**, *54*, 1622–1629. [CrossRef] [PubMed]
25. Fisk, J.D.; Ritvo, P.G.; Ross, L.; Haase, D.A.; Marrie, T.J.; Schlech, W.F. Measuring the functional impact of fatigue: Initial validation of the fatigue impact scale. *Clin. Infect. Dis.* **1994**, *18*, 79–83. [CrossRef]
26. Kroenke, K.; Spitzer, R.L.; Williams, J.B.W. The PHQ-9: Validity of a brief depression severity measure. *J. Gen. Intern. Med.* **2001**, *16*, 606–613. [CrossRef] [PubMed]
27. Yang, C.Y.; Leung, P.S.C.; Adamopoulos, I.E.; Gershwin, M.E. The implication of vitamin D and autoimmunity: A comprehensive review. *Clin. Rev. Allergy Immunol.* **2013**, *45*, 217–226. [CrossRef]
28. Vogel, A.; Strassburg, C.P.; Manns, M.P. Genetic association of vitamin D receptor polymorphisms with primary biliary cirrhosis and autoimmune hepatitis. *Hepatology* **2002**, *35*, 126–131. [CrossRef]
29. Zhong, Z.-X. Polymorphisms in the vitamin D receptor gene and risk of autoimmune liver Diseases: A meta-analysis. *Biomed. J. Sci. Tech. Res.* **2018**, *9*, 1–8. [CrossRef]
30. Fan, L.; Tu, X.; Zhu, Y.; Zhou, L.; Pfeiffer, T.; Feltens, R.; Stoecker, W.; Zhong, R. Genetic association of vitamin D receptor polymorphisms with autoimmune hepatitis and primary biliary cirrhosis in the Chinese. *J. Gastroenterol. Hepatol.* **2005**, *20*, 249–255. [CrossRef]
31. Tanaka, A.; Nezu, S.; Uegaki, S.; Kikuchi, K.; Shibuya, A.; Miyakawa, H.; Takahashi, S.-I.; Bianchi, I.; Zermiani, P.; Podda, M.; et al. Vitamin D receptor polymorphisms are associated with increased susceptibility to primary biliary cirrhosis in Japanese and Italian populations. *J. Hepatol.* **2009**, *50*, 1202–1209. [CrossRef]
32. Niino, M.; Fukazawa, T.; Yabe, I.; Kikuchi, S.; Sasaki, H.; Tashiro, K. Vitamin D receptor gene polymorphisms in multiple sclerosis and the association with HLA class II alleles. *J. Neurol. Sci.* **2000**, *177*, 65–71. [CrossRef]
33. Mohammadnejad, Z.; Ghanbari, M.; Ganjali, R.; Afshari, J.T.; Heydarpour, M.; Taghavi, S.M.; Fatemi, S.; Rafatpanah, H. Association between vitamin D receptor gene polymorphisms and type 1 diabetes mellitus in Iranian population. *Mol. Biol. Rep.* **2012**, *39*, 831–837. [CrossRef] [PubMed]

34. Shimada, A.; Kanazawa, Y.; Motohashi, Y.; Yamada, S.; Maruyama, T.; Ikegami, H.; Awata, T.; Kawasaki, E.; Kobayashi, T.; Nakanishi, K.; et al. Evidence for association between vitamin D receptor bsmi polymorphism and type 1 diabetes in Japanese. *J. Autoimmun.* **2008**, *30*, 207–211. [CrossRef] [PubMed]
35. Ozaki, Y.; Nomura, S.; Nagahama, M.; Yoshimura, C.; Kagawa, H.; Fukuhara, S. Vitamin-D receptor genotype and renal disorder in Japanese patients with systemic lupus erythematosus. *Nephron* **2000**, *85*, 86–91. [CrossRef] [PubMed]
36. Huang, C.M.; Wu, M.C.; Wu, J.Y.; Tsai, F.J. Association of vitamin D receptor gene bsmi polymorphisms in Chinese patients with systemic lupus erythematosus. *Lupus* **2002**, *11*, 31–34. [CrossRef]
37. Zhang, J.Z.; Wang, M.; Ding, Y.; Gao, F.; Feng, Y.Y.; Yakeya, B.; Wang, P.; Wu, X.J.; Hu, F.X.; Xian, J.; et al. Vitamin D receptor gene polymorphism, serum 25-hydroxyvitamin D levels, and risk of vitiligo: A meta-analysis. *Medicine* **2018**, *97*, e11506. [CrossRef]
38. Wang, X.; Cheng, W.; Ma, Y.; Zhu, J. Vitamin D receptor gene FokI but not TaqI, ApaI, BsmI polymorphism is associated with hashimoto's thyroiditis: A meta-analysis. *Sci. Rep.* **2017**, *7*, 1–11. [CrossRef]
39. Kempińska-Podhorecka, A.; Wunsch, E.; Jarowicz, T.; Raszeja-Wyszomirska, J.; Loniewska, B.; Kaczmarczyk, M.; Milkiewicz, M.; Milkiewicz, P. Vitamin D receptor polymorphisms predispose to primary biliary cirrhosis and severity of the disease in Polish population. *Gastroenterol. Res. Pract.* **2012**, *2012*, 8. [CrossRef]
40. Huet, P.M.; Deslauriers, J.; Tran, A.; Faucher, C.; Charbonneau, J. Impact of fatigue on the quality of life of patients with primary biliary cirrhosis. *Am. J. Gastroenterol.* **2000**, *95*, 760–767. [CrossRef]
41. Goldblatt, J.; Taylor, P.J.S.; Lipman, T.; Prince, M.I.; Baragiotta, A.; Bassendine, M.F.; James, O.F.W.; Jones, D.E.J. The true impact of fatigue in primary biliary cirrhosis: A population study. *Gastroenterology* **2002**, *122*, 1235–1241. [CrossRef]
42. Navasa, M.; Forns, X.; Sánchez, V.; Andreu, H.; Marcos, V.; Borràs, J.M.; Rimola, A.; Grande, L.; García-Valdecasas, J.C.; Granados, A.; et al. Quality of life, major medical complications and hospital service utilization in patients with primary biliary cirrhosis after liver transplantation. *J. Hepatol.* **1996**, *25*, 129–134. [CrossRef]
43. Younossi, Z.M.; Kiwi, M.L.; Boparai, N.; Price, L.L.; Guyatt, G. Cholestatic liver diseases and health-related quality of life. *Am. J. Gastroenterol.* **2000**, *95*, 497–502. [CrossRef] [PubMed]
44. Kotarska, K.; Wunsch, E.; Kempińska-Podhorodecka, A.; Raszeja-Wyszomirska, J.; Bogdanos, D.P.; Wójcicki, M.; Milkiewicz, P. Factors affecting health-related quality of life and physical activity after liver transplantation for autoimmune and nonautoimmune liver diseases: A prospective, single centre study. *J. Immunol. Res.* **2014**, *2014*, 9. [CrossRef] [PubMed]
45. Janik, M.K.; Wunsch, E.; Raszeja-Wyszomirska, J.; Krawczyk, M.; Milkiewicz, P. Depression: An overlooked villain in autoimmune hepatitis? *Hepatology* **2019**, *70*, 2232–2233. [CrossRef] [PubMed]
46. Milkiewicz, P.; Heathcote, E.J. Fatigue in chronic cholestasis. *Gut* **2004**, *53*, 475–477. [CrossRef]
47. Krawczyk, M.; Koźma, M.; Szymańska, A.; Leszko, K.; Przedniczek, M.; Mucha, K.; Foroncewicz, B.; Pączek, L.; Moszczuk, B.; Milkiewicz, P.; et al. Effects of liver transplantation on health-related quality of life in patients with primary biliary cholangitis. *Clin. Transplant.* **2018**, *32*, e13434. [CrossRef]
48. Raszeja-Wyszomirska, J.; Wunsch, E.; Krawczyk, M.; Rigopoulou, E.I.; Bogdanos, D.; Milkiewicz, P. Prospective evaluation of PBC-specific health-related quality of life questionnaires in patients with primary sclerosing cholangitis. *Liver Int.* **2015**, *35*, 1764–1771. [CrossRef]
49. Raszeja-Wyszomirska, J.; Wunsch, E.; Kempinska-Podhorodecka, A.; Smyk, D.S.; Bogdanos, D.P.; Milkiewicz, M.; Milkiewicz, P. TRAF1-C5 affects quality of life in patients with primary biliary cirrhosis. *Clin. Dev. Immunol.* **2013**, *2013*, 7. [CrossRef]
50. Schramm, C.; Wahl, I.; Weiler-Normann, C.; Voigt, K.; Wiegard, C.; Glaubke, C.; Brähler, E.; Löwe, B.; Lohse, A.W.; Rose, M. Health-related quality of life, depression, and anxiety in patients with autoimmune hepatitis. *J. Hepatol.* **2014**, *60*, 618–624. [CrossRef]

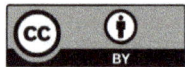

© 2020 by the authors. Licensee MDPI, Basel, Switzerland. This article is an open access article distributed under the terms and conditions of the Creative Commons Attribution (CC BY) license (http://creativecommons.org/licenses/by/4.0/).

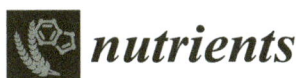

Article

Vitamin D Synthesis Following a Single Bout of Sun Exposure in Older and Younger Men and Women

Jenna R. Chalcraft [1,†], Linda M. Cardinal [2,†], Perry J. Wechsler [3], Bruce W. Hollis [4], Kenneth G. Gerow [5], Brenda M. Alexander [6], Jill F. Keith [1] and D. Enette Larson-Meyer [1,7,*]

1. Department of Family and Consumer Sciences, University of Wyoming, Laramie, WY 82071, USA; jchalcra@uwyo.edu (J.R.C.); jkeith5@uwyo.edu (J.F.K.)
2. Billings Clinic, Cody, WY 82414, USA; lcardinal06@gmail.com
3. Alpenglow Instruments, Laramie, WY 82072, USA; perrywechsler@alpenglowinstruments.com
4. Dr Bruce Hollis' Laboratory, Medical University of South Carolina, Charleston, SC 29425, USA; hollisb@musc.edu
5. Department of Mathematics & Statistics, University of Wyoming, Laramie WY 82071, USA; gerow@uwyo.edu
6. Department of Animal Sciences, University of Wyoming, Laramie, WY 82071, USA; balex@uwyo.edu
7. Department of Human Nutrition, Foods & Exercise, Virginia Tech, Blacksburg, VA 24061, USA
* Correspondence: enette@uwyo.edu; Tel.: +1-540-231-1025
† Designated shared first authorship.

Received: 30 May 2020; Accepted: 16 July 2020; Published: 27 July 2020

Abstract: Older adults are frequently cited as an at-risk population for vitamin D deficiency that may in part be due to decreased cutaneous synthesis, a potentially important source of cholecalciferol (vitamin D_3). Previous studies found that cutaneous D_3 production declines with age; however, most studies have been conducted ex vivo or in the photobiology lab. The purpose of this study was to characterize the response of vitamin D metabolites following a 30-min bout of sun exposure (15-min each to the dorsal and ventral sides) at close to solar noon in younger and older adults. Methods: 30 healthy individuals with skin type II/III were recruited; a younger cohort, aged 20–37 ($n = 18$) and an older cohort ($n = 12$), age 51–69 years. Exposure was at outer limits of sensible sun exposure designed to enhance vitamin D synthesis without increasing risk of photo ageing and non-melanoma skin cancer. Serum D_3 concentration was measured at baseline, 24, 48 and 72 h post-exposure. Serum 25(OH)D was measured at baseline and 72 h post-exposure plus 168 h post-exposure in the older cohort. Results: D_3 increased in response to sun exposure (time effect; $p = 0.002$) with a trend for a difference in D_3 between cohorts (time*group; $p = 0.09$). By regression modeling of continuous data, age accounted for 20% of the variation in D_3 production. D_3 production decreased by 13% per decade. Despite changes in D_3, however, serum 25(OH)D did not change from baseline to 72 or 168 h post exposure ($p > 0.10$). Conclusions: Serum D_3 concentration increased significantly in response to outdoor sun exposure in younger and older adults. While ageing may dampen cutaneous synthesis, sunlight exposure is still a significant source of vitamin D_3.

Keywords: ageing; older persons; sensible sun exposure; cutaneous synthesis; vitamin D_3; natural sunlight; serum 25(OH)D

1. Introduction

Accumulating evidence has documented that vitamin D deficiency is associated with the onset and progression of a variety of chronic diseases including cardiovascular disease, type 2 diabetes, immune system diseases, neuropsychiatric disorders and certain cancers [1]. Older adults are frequently cited as an at-risk population for vitamin D deficiency [2–4]. Population-based studies suggest a high prevalence of vitamin D deficiency (serum 25(OH)D <20 ng/mL) among older adults (>60 to 65 years) that varies by location and ethnicity, and ranges from 12.1% of individuals with mixed ancestry in Greater Toronto (43° N) [5] to 37.3% in Mexico (<32° N) [6] and 45% in the Netherlands (52° N) [7]. Recent analysis of data from the National Health and Nutrition Examination Survey (NHANES 2011–2014), however, found that while vitamin D status differed by age, the prevalence of at risk of deficiency or inadequacy (defined as serum 25(OH)D <20 and 50 nmol/L, respectively) was highest in adults aged 20–39 years (7.6 and 23.8%) compared to adults ages 40–59 years (5.7 and 18.6) and those 60 years or older (2.9 and 12.3) [8], with no differences between men and women. Indeed, all adults and children may be at risk for vitamin D deficiency, especially when living in high latitude regions (>35°) [9] or receiving limited sun exposure. Nonetheless, deficiency in older adults is most often a combination of age-related changes in vitamin D metabolism and lifestyle factors. Age-related alterations in vitamin D metabolism include decreased epidermal 7-dehydrocholesterol (DHC) concentration, reduced thickness of the epidermis [10,11], reduced dermal [12] (and epidermal) vitamin D production, increased adiposity [13] (fat sequestration), decreased renal 1,25(OH)$_2$D synthesis [14–16] and increased 1,25(OH)$_2$D catabolism [16]. The reduced dermal capacity to synthesize vitamin D at age 65 for example has been estimated to be ~25% of that of a 20–30-year-old exposed to the same amount of radiation [12,17]. Lifestyle factors associated with deficiency include poor appetite, low vitamin D intake, limited sun exposure/sun avoidance, increased clothing coverage/sunscreen use, reduced physical activity and financial constrains [3,9,14,18–20].

A number of studies in older adults, on the other hand, have demonstrated that exposure to ultraviolet B (UVB, 290–315 nm) radiation is an effective strategy for increasing serum 25(OH)D concentration [21–24]; this may suggest that sun avoidance rather than reduced synthesis per se is an important risk factor for suboptimal status in older individuals. Most of the aforementioned studies, except for that of Reid et al. [24], however, have been conducted in the photobiology lab following delivery of a measured dose of UVB. Further research using ambient sun exposure is necessary to continue to characterize the pattern of cutaneous vitamin D production in older versus younger adults in a natural environment (i.e., the sun is freely available) and determine the effectiveness of sun exposure therapy on vitamin D status.

Despite its potential benefit, however, sunlight exposure is considered a controversial way to maintain vitamin D status [25]. Many health authorities including the World Health Organization [26], the American Cancer Society [27] and the surgeon general [28] emphasize sun abstention, especially during mid-day when the sun's ultra-violet (UV) rays are the most potent. UV damage from too much sun exposure plays a role in the development of skin cancer and is considered a public health risk [25]. General public health efforts target sunscreen use, skin coverage with clothing and/or a sun hat and sun avoidance to reduce exposure to UVA and UVB radiation [3] and prevent cancer and photo ageing. While these public health efforts are understandable from the viewpoint of prevention of nonmelanoma skin cancer, they neglect the potential physiological benefits of mindful sunlight exposure that includes elevation of vitamin D status [25] and the potential influence of sun exposure and vitamin D on health in ageing individuals [29]. "Sensible sun exposure" is the practice of obtaining the minimum sun exposure required for adequate vitamin D synthesis followed by application of sunscreen or clothing coverage; and is often characterized as sun exposure of 5–30 min, two–three times per week to the arms, legs and torso during 10:00 h to 15:00 h [2,30]. The specific duration required within this time frame is dependent on skin type, previous tanning, latitude, season and environmental conditions. The minimal erythemal dose (MED), or the minimum quantity of UVB that induces a slight erythema 16–24 h post exposure, is a common dosage employed for sensible sun exposure guidelines [31]. The standard erythemal dose (SED) is a standardized method for quantifying erythemal UV radiation (UVR) dose and is becoming more commonly used because the MED varies from person to person even within the same skin type. The SED is defined as 100 J/m^2 [32]. For adults with a fair complexion, one MED is equal to about 10–12 min of full body exposure during peak summer sun for all skin types [33]. One MED may be considered equivalent to ~2.5 to 3.5 SEDs depending on skin type [34].

As "sensible sun exposure" may be a simple, cost effective method to obtain optimal 25(OH)D concentration and/or prevent deficiency in older populations, the purpose of this study was to characterize the response of vitamin D_3 and 25(OH)D to a single bout of outdoor sun exposure of 15 min to both the dorsal and ventral sides of the body (30 min total) in older and younger adults. We hypothesized, based on previous literature, that a single bout of sun exposure would be effective at increasing serum vitamin D_3 concentration but that older individuals would demonstrate a reduced response to natural sunlight exposure compared to younger individuals.

2. Materials and Methods

This study consisted of exposing younger (19–39 years) and older (51–69 years) adults to a 30-min bout of natural outdoor sunlight (15 min each on the dorsal and frontal sides of the body) at moderate-altitude (2194 m, 41.3° N) in late spring/early summer (close to the summer solstice). Both research procedures were reviewed and approved by the Institutional Review Board at the University of Wyoming (Protocols # 20150317EL 00717 and #20180219EL01882) and approved in April 2015 and April 2018, respectively. Volunteers provided written, informed consent before participation.

2.1. Participants

Young male and female volunteers (19–39 years of age) and healthy community-dwelling older adults (50–70 years) with skin type II or III were recruited from the local community in the spring (April–June) of 2015 (younger cohort) and spring of 2018 (older cohort) through advertisements posted on a university campus and in the local community. To be eligible, participants had to have skin type II or III and must not have a personal or family history of skin cancer or melanoma. Skin type was self-identified using the Fitzpatrick skin typing scale [35], which was read to potential participants. Those who self-identified as skin types II (white, fair; blond or red hair; blue, green or hazel eyes; usually burns, tans minimally) or III (cream white, fair with any hair or eye color; sometimes mild burn, tans uniformly) were permitted into the study. Exclusion criterion included: current vitamin D supplementation or supplementation one month before the study, current use of medications that have the potential to alter vitamin D status or photosensitivity, travel within three months to a sunny location close to the equator, appearing visibly tanned or the inability to either refrain from sunlight or artificial UV exposure from screening until the scheduled sun exposure session and for 3 days following this session or fully participate in the study due to work, school or personal scheduling constrains.

A total of 51 volunteers in the younger-aged cohort and 45 in the older-aged cohort responded to the advertisement. Interested volunteers were initially screened by phone and asked a series of questions about their general health, personal and family risk of skin cancer, use of supplements and perceived skin type. In the younger age cohort, five were unable to complete screening and 15 were unable to participate due to schedule conflicts. Thirteen were deemed ineligible for participation because they reported a family history of skin cancer, were taking vitamin D supplements, did not meet skin type guidelines or had travelled to a sunny location and/or spent a generous time outside without sunscreen in the previous three months. In the older-aged cohort, the majority of interested participants were not eligible due to either a personal or family history of melanoma or pre-cancerous skin lesions. Additional reasons for ineligibility included skin type, tanning bed use, recent travel to a sunny location or use of medications that might influence vitamin D status. Of the 51 and 45 individuals interviewed in the younger and older-age groups, 18 and 12 were both eligible and available to participate in the study.

2.2. Baseline Measurements

Baseline anthropometric measurements, which included height, weight, and body composition measured by dual energy x-ray absorptiometry (DXA) (Lunar Prodigy, GE Healthcare, Fairfield, CT, USA), were obtained on all participants. Height and weight were measured without shoes and in minimal clothing using a standing digital scale (Tanita, Tokyo, Japan) and stadiometer (Invicta Plastics,

Leicester, England). Body mass index (BMI) was calculated as weight divided by height in meters squared and body surface area (BSA) was calculated using the Mosteller equation [36]. Participants also completed a vitamin D-specific food frequency and lifestyle questionnaire (FFLQ) [37]. The FFLQ addresses questions about the frequency of consumption of vitamin D-containing foods, vitamin D supplementation, sun exposure and tanning bed usage.

2.3. Sunlight Exposure

Following the baseline visit, volunteers were scheduled to participate in one of several sunlight exposure sessions or test days. The exposure days had to meet certain criteria (cloudless sunny day with a minimum ambient temperature of 16 °C and a maximum of 32 °C) and were selected based on weather patterns, the university calendar and participant/research staff availability for the exposure day and for the 72 h (all participants) to 168 h period (older group only) following exposure. The period of April through June was selected to ensure that exposure occurred to early-season naive skin (i.e., skin that had not been recently tanned). On each test day, a sun exposure station was set up in a mostly sheltered outdoor environment at a local park (younger group) or landscaped courtyard (older group). Volunteers had pre-sun exposure (baseline) blood drawn for analysis of serum vitamin D_3 (cholecalciferol), vitamin D_2 (ergocalciferol) and 25-hydroxyvitamin D (25(OH)D) immediately before undergoing sunlight exposure that consisted of exactly 15 min of exposure to both the front and back sides of the body (30 min total) between 11:30 and 13:00 h standard time (12:30 to 14:00 h daylight saving time) while lying supine and prone, respectively, in shorts (men) or shorts and sports bra (women). The shorts worn had a 2- to 3-inch inseam or were cuffed to a similar length. This amount of skin exposure was estimated to be approximately 43% of BSA for men and 41% for women. A member of the research team closely monitored the sessions to ensure compliance with time and protocol and to watch for signs of notable erythema. Close to solar noon was selected because UVB is most intense during this time, which allowed for more efficient vitamin D synthesis and reduced risk for skin cancer [38,39]. Sunscreen (Equate Broad Spectrum SPF, Bentonville, AR) was applied to the face and sunglasses were provided to all participants who did not bring their own protective eyewear. Following carefully timed exposure, volunteers took immediate cover in a designated area indoors and were served a light lunch. Participants were asked to completely avoid outdoor sunlight for the next 72 h; if outdoor daytime exposure was unavoidable, participants were asked to cover up with full-body clothing and/or the provided sunscreen. 72 h was extended to 168 h in the older participants. To prevent the chance that some newly synthesized vitamin D was sloughed off with skin cells [40], volunteers were asked not to bath, shower or swim until after their 24-h blood draw.

2.4. Blood Draws and Analyses

Blood was drawn at baseline and approximately 24-, 48- and 72-h after initial exposure for the analysis of serum vitamin D_3, vitamin D_2 and 25(OH)D concentration. Blood was also obtained at 168 h post-exposure in the older group. Blood was allowed to coagulate at room temperature for 30-min and then centrifuged at 5800 rpm for 15 min (VWR Clinical 100, VWR International, Woodbridge, NJ). Serum was frozen until analysis. Vitamin D_3/D_2 was analyzed via liquid chromatography-mass spectrometry (LC/MS) by a commercial laboratory (Heartland Assays, Ames, IA). The intra- and inter assay coefficient for these assays is <3% and <6%, respectively. 25(OH)D concentration was analyzed via Diasorin 25(OH)D RIA (B.W. Hollis, Charleston, SC). The intra- and inter-assay coefficient for 25(OH) D assay is less than 10%.

2.5. Estimates of UV-Irradiance

UV irradiance was measured during sun exposure using a meteorological grade UV instrument (Total Ultraviolet Radiometer model 27901, The Eppley Laboratory, Inc. Newport, RI) and a logging data acquisition system (National Instruments, Austin, TX). UV data were measured in one-second intervals for all exposure days in the younger participants and for a single representative day in the older participants due to computer malfunction. Total UV exposure was calculated per participant from actual recorded start and stop times on the test day or the representative test day. Data from the Eppley radiometer is recorded in native units of volts and were then converted to irradiances using the device calibration coefficient of 1 mv = 2.28 mW/cm^2. The UVA/UVB ratio of 20:1 or 5% of the total UV irradiance was used to estimate UVB [41]. The sum of irradiances for 30 min (1800 s) were then calculated and subsequently converted to a standard erythemal dose (SED) using the conversion: 1 SED = 100 J/m^2 [32]. As participants were supine and prone during exposure, total exposure was divided by two to represent the exposure to each body side. Prior to data collection, baseline data (or calibration data) were measured by taking running averages of one-minute data segments with the radiometer shielded from any incident light; these data indicated that there was no significant offset to the total UV data collected.

2.6. Statistical Procedures

Statistical analyses were performed using IBM SPSS version 26.0 (Chicago, IL, USA) and Minitab version 19.0 (State College, Pennsylvania, USA). Independent Samples t-tests were used to test for differences between older and younger groups for baseline physical characteristics, baseline serum vitamin D metabolites, and sun exposure variables. To address our primary aim, Repeated Measures Analysis of Variance (ANOVA) was initially used to evaluate the effect of group (older vs. younger) by time (baseline, 24, 48 and 72 h) on serum D_3 concentration following sun exposure. Paired T-Tests with Bonferroni correction were then used post hoc to test for differences in serum vitamin D_3 from baseline to 24, 48 and 72 h, and to test for differences between serum 25(OH)D at baseline and 72 h (and baseline and 168 in the older group). A Fishers Exact Test was used to evaluate differences in timing of the peak serum D_3 concentration following sun exposure. ANOVA was also employed to evaluate sun exposure and UVB irradiance variables between and within studies on peak vitamin D_3 concentration following sun exposure including sun exposure day/year, temperature during sun exposure and estimated UVB dose (SED). The best subsets method was utilized to identify predictors of D_3 production from baseline to peak concentration that included important inter-subject characteristics and confounders (age, baseline serum vitamin D_3 concentration, fat mass, lean mass, reported baseline vitamin D intake and sun exposure history). A simple linear regression model for D_3 production was subsequently constructed to evaluate the relationship between age and D_3 production. Log transformation was performed to best quantify the relative relationship.

3. Results

3.1. Subject Characteristics

All participants (n = 30) were Caucasian who identified with having skin type II or III. The characteristics of the participants, including estimated vitamin D intake and reported sun exposure are summarized in Table 1. The older group was significantly shorter than the younger group but no other differences (other than age) were observed. There were no differences in average daily vitamin D intake over the past 3 months and average daily sun exposure between the older and younger groups (Table 1).

3.2. Sun Exposure and Estimates of UVB Irradiance

Weather conditions and participant availability allowed for three mostly cloudless, sun exposure days in the spring of 2015 and four similar days in the Spring of 2018. In 2015, days were 68, 19 and 4 days prior to the summer solstice (21 June) and had recorded temperatures (typically at 12:53 h) of 19.4°, 25° and 23.3 °C, respectively. In 2018, days were 35, 29, 17 and 9 days prior to the summer solstice, with recorded temperatures of 21.6°, 21.1°, 25.6° and 25.6 °C, respectively. Average body surface area exposed was estimated to be 0.78 m^2 ± 0.02 in the younger cohort and 0.73 m^2 ± 0.03 in the older cohort and average UVB radiant exposure estimated via the radiometer was 386.3 ± 9.2 mJ/cm^2

and the SED was 38.6 ± 0.92 for whole body (19.3 for the frontal and dorsal sides) for the younger group and was 377.3 ± 1.6 mJ/cm² with an average total SED of 37.7 ± 0.16 (18.85 for the frontal and dorsal sides). Neither BSA exposed nor SED differed between groups ($p > 0.10$).

Table 1. Participant Characteristics.

	Total Group	Younger Adults	Older Adults	p *
Sex (M/F)	11/19	9/9	2/10	—
Age (years)	38.4 ± 10.4 (20–69)	25.1 ± 4.8 (20–37)	58.3 ± 5.1 (50–69)	0.0001 *
Skin Type (II/III)	3/27	3/15	0/12	—
Hair (Bl/Br/R)	7/21/2	5/12/1	2/9/1	—
Mass (kg)	71.2 ± 15.2 (50.1–106.1)	71.8 ± 13.4 (54.2–102.1)	70.4 ± 18.2 (50.1–106)	0.816
Height (cm)	170.4 ± 7.9 (156.5–186.0)	173.3 ± 7.4 (156.5–186)	166.2 ± 6.8 (159.0–179)	0.013 *
BMI (kg/m²)	24.4 ± 4.5 (18.7–39.4)	23.8 ± 3.2 (20.0–30.0)	25.4 ± 6.1 (18.7–39.4)	0.34
Body Fat (%)	30.3 ± 10.3 (11.9–54.0)	28.8 ± 9.4 (11.9–47.7)	32.5 ± 11.5 (12.7–54.0)	0.35
Vitamin D Intake (IU)	187 ± 182 (20–828)	183.5 ± 167.4 (20–828)	151.3 ± 96.2 (64–385)	0.64
Sun Exposure (h/month)	14.5 ± 15.2 (0–60)	13.4 ± 17.4 (0–60)	16.2 ± 16.9 (2–60)	0.63
Baseline Serum D_3 (nmol/L)	15.0 ± 19.5 (3.7–110.1)	18.0 ± 24.2 (3.7–110.1)	10.7 ± 8.2 (3.7–30.0)	0.33
Baseline Serum D_2 (nmol/L)	<3.7	<3.7	<3.7	—
Baseline Serum 25(OH)D (nmol/L)	84.9 ± 26.0 (42.4–166.5)	86.6 ± 6.3 (56.7–166.5)	82.6 ± 7.5 (42.4–123.5)	0.69

Data are mean ± SD with ranges shown in parentheses. Bl, blond; Br, brown; R, red BMI, body mass index.
* Difference between older and younger cohorts via Independent Samples t-tests.

3.3. Impact of Sun Exposure on Serum D_3 and 25(OH)D

In the 24 h following sunlight exposure, only one participant (younger cohort) had observable signs of erythema. Following the single bout of sun exposure, serum vitamin D_3 concentration increased significantly in the 24 to 48 h post exposure (time effect; $p < 0.002$) with a trend for a difference in vitamin D_3 response between older and younger individuals (time*group; $p = 0.09$) and no group effect ($p = 0.21$) (Figure 1). The average increase was of 76.4 ± 83.7%, 88.1% ± 73.3 and 54.1 ± 52.5% at 24, 48 and 72 h, respectively, which were significantly greater than baseline at all points ($p < 0.017$). Peak concentration in serum D_3 were generally observed between 24 and 48 h with a few participants, all in the younger cohort, experiencing slight upward trends in D_3 concentration from 48 to 72 h. Overall there was a trend for older individuals to peak later (at 48 h) compared to younger individuals (at 24 h) ($p = 0.0875$), with one participant in the older cohort experiencing a peak at 24 h and nine at 48 h compared to seven participants in the younger cohort who peaked at 24 h and eight between 48 and 72 h. Two subjects in the older and three in the younger cohorts (16.7%) did not experience an increase in serum D_3 at any time point. The average increase in D_3 at peak was 9.8 ± 7.8 nmol/L (including the non-responders) and was not different between cohorts (7.7 ± 5.7 vs. 11.2 ± 8.8 nmol/L, older vs. younger, $p = 0.25$).

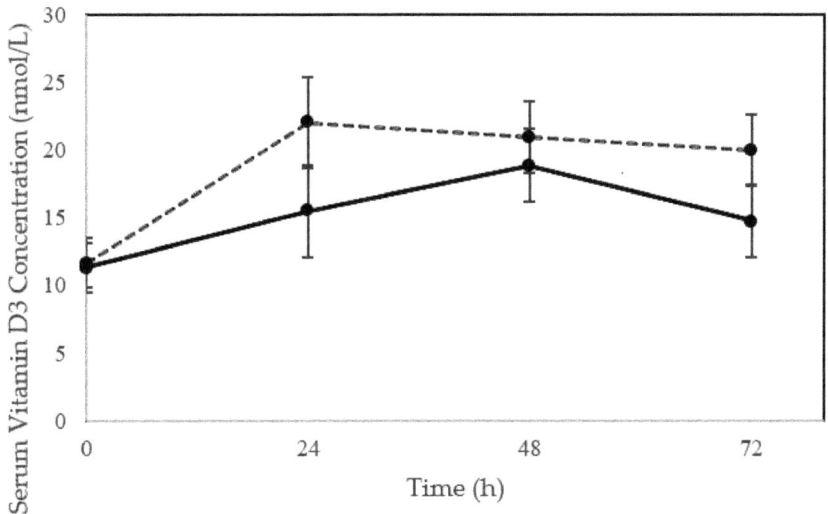

Figure 1. Vitamin D_3 concentration following a single bout of sun exposure (time 0) in older (solid line) compared to younger (dashed lines) adults. Serum vitamin D_3 concentration increased significantly post exposure (time effect; $p < 0.002$) with a trend for a difference in vitamin D_3 response between older and younger individuals (time*group; $p = 0.09$). Error bars represent ± SE.

Despite changes in serum vitamin D_3 concentration, serum 25(OH)D concentration did not change following sunlight exposure and was not different between baseline and 72 h ($p = 0.561$) or baseline and 168 h post exposure ($p = 0.237$) (Figure 2).

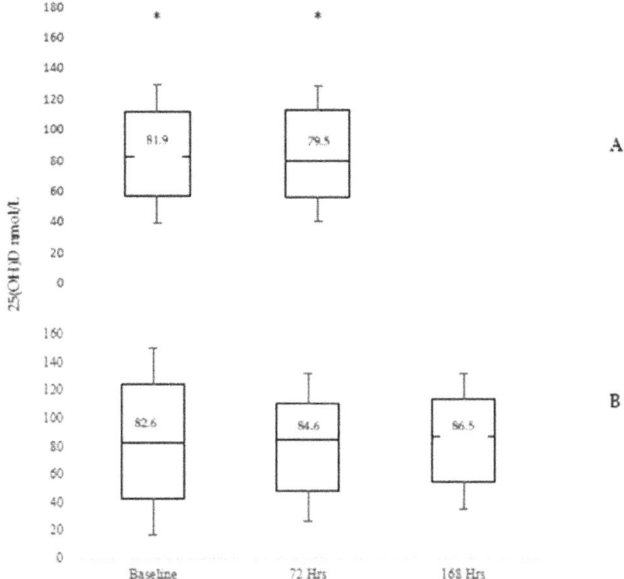

Figure 2. 25(OH)D Concentration at baseline, 72 h and 168 h post exposure to natural sunlight for a total of 30 min in the Younger (Panel A) and Older (Panel B) Adult Cohorts. * represents single data points that were greater than three times the interquartile range.

3.4. Predictors of D_3 Production

Using the best subsets method with the log of D_3 production (change from baseline to peak) as the dependent variable and age, baseline serum D_3 concentration, fat mass, lean mass, reported vitamin D intake and reported sun exposure history entered as independent variables, the single best predictor of D_3 production was age ($r^2 = 0.238$). The best pairs of predictors were age and lean body mass ($r^2 = 0.30$) and age and baseline serum D_3 concentration ($r^2 = 0.298$). Age, baseline serum D_3 concentration and lean body mass were the best triplet of predictors ($r^2 = 0.352$). Fat mass, reported time spent outside and vitamin D intake were not selected as predictors until four, five or six predictors were entered, and contributed little to the model.

3.5. Modeling of D_3 Production with Ageing

As shown in Figure 3, a linear regression model using data from both cohorts across the age spectrum (21 to 69 years) was created with age as the independent variable and log D_3 production (change from baseline to peak) as the dependent variable ($p = 0.023$). Age accounted for 20 percent of the variance in D_3 production ($r^2 = 0.206$). The regression model (Figure 4) further demonstrated that for every decade of life, there is a 13 percent decrease in mean D_3 production.

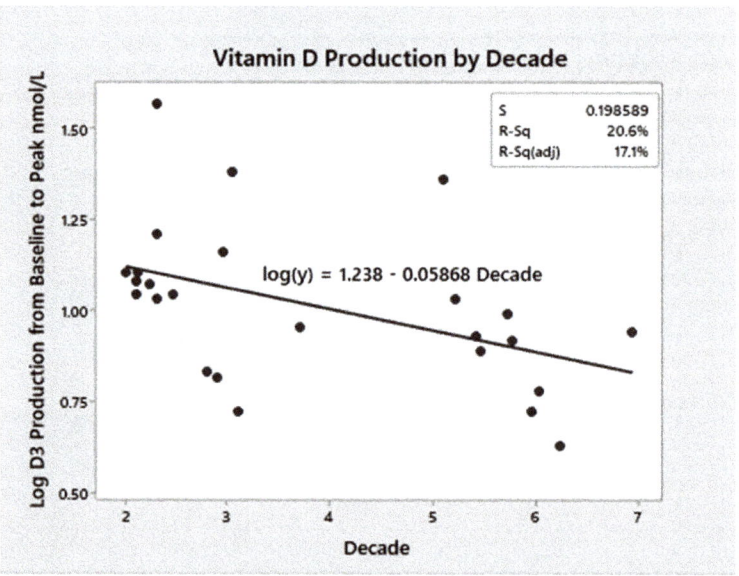

Figure 3. Vitamin D_3 Production and Age Model. The linear regression model with age as the independent variable and log D_3 production was constructed. Age accounted for 20% of the variance in D_3 production ($r^2 = 0.206$).

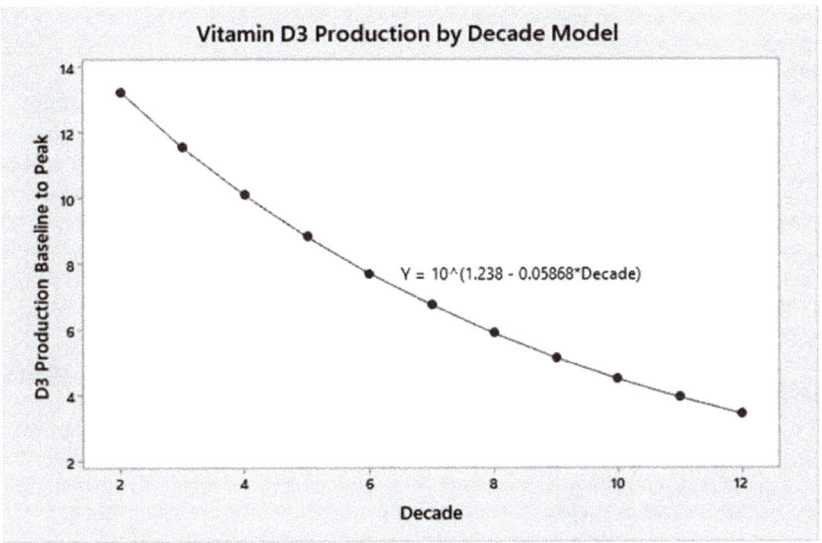

Figure 4. Vitamin D_3 Production Age Continuum Modeling. The simple linear regression model with decade as the independent variable and log D_3 production was used to demonstrate the 13% decrease in D_3 production per decade of life. D_3 production at age 70 years is approximately half that produced at age 20. The graph demonstrates that D_3 production is possible even in the later decades of life.

4. Discussion

The primary aim of the current study was to characterize the response of a single bout of sun exposure on cutaneous vitamin D synthesis in a cohort of younger and older adults, and determine if the response in older adults differed from that of a younger cohort. Overall, we found that 30 min of sun exposure (15-min to the arms, torso and legs on both the front and backsides of the body while lying in the supine and prone positions) significantly increased serum vitamin D_3 by an average of 9.8 nmol/L with no significant differences in cohorts. The peak response in D_3 concentration to a single bout of "sensible sun exposure," however, was about 1/5th the response observed following delivery of 1 MED in a photobiology laboratory [42]. A model created from continuous data on peak D_3 concentration in response to sun exposure found evidence that D_3 production in adults declines with ageing (by ~13% per decade) but is still possible at 120 years of age. To our knowledge, this is the first study to evaluate the effect of a single bout of sensible sun exposure on vitamin D_3 concentration using natural sunlight exposure of a carefully monitored duration as the sole UVB source, which is important for understanding the implication of "sensible sun exposure" guidelines in older as well as younger individuals.

Previous calculations from studies performed in a photobiology laboratory suggest that the equivalent 10,000–25,000 IUs of vitamin D can be synthesized from UVB irradiation in individuals wearing a bikini in peak July sun [43] after exposure of 1 MED, suggesting that sun exposure is the most significant source of vitamin D. While sufficient exposure to the UVB radiation from sunlight is important for cutaneous vitamin D synthesis, too much sun exposure increases the risk for photo ageing and skin cancer [33]. Guidelines for "sensible sun exposure," which are thought to promote vitamin D synthesis at minimal risk of excess exposure, were established from studies conducted within a photobiology laboratory. Only a few studies have investigated and compared (rather than modeled) the efficacy of solar and artificial UVB radiation on cutaneous synthesis [44] or estimated the outdoor exposure time necessary to achieve a serum 25(OH)D concentration equivalent to a specific oral dose (e.g., 1000 IU) of supplemental vitamin D according to season, location and skin type [45].

The most accepted guidelines established by Holick et al. [2] indicate that exposing the arms, hands and face to one-third to one-half of a MED, which is about five minutes at noon in Boston for individuals with skin type II, with a frequency of two to three times per week during the spring, summer or fall, is more than adequate to achieve sufficient vitamin D status [46]. More specific guidelines are difficult to make because of the multiple variables involved in cutaneous production of vitamin D, such as season, latitude, cloud cover, skin pigmentation and body surface area exposed. Updated guidelines suggest exposure of the arms, legs and torso (when possible) to sunlight for approximately 25% to 50% of the time it would take to develop a mild sunburn (e.g., 1 MED) for this same frequency (two–three times/week), and exemplify that if 30 min of noontime sun would cause a mild sunburn, than 10 to 15 min of exposure (followed by sun protection) should be sufficient for adequate vitamin D synthesis [30]. The present study suggests that a single session of solar exposure to both the front and back-sides of the body at the outer limits of the "sensible sun exposure" guidelines was sufficient to promote D_3 synthesis in most individuals aged 20 to 69 years who self-identified with skin types II and III, but also that some individuals may be non-responsive to a single exposure. This is of interest because UVB exposure achieved in a natural environment is likely to be more variable than that of a photobiology laboratory, where the dose of UVB delivered can be controlled and directly quantified. For example, one study at a latitude of 56° N concluded that artificial UVB exposure to the hands and face was at least eight times as effective at increasing 25(OH)D synthesis than solar UVR from early spring exposure under natural conditions [44]. Another estimated from spectral characteristics that sunbeds were ~25–30% more efficient in producing pre-vitamin D than mid-June sun at 59° N latitude [34]. Despite the variability of natural sunlight, achieving vitamin D from "sensible sun exposure" is inexpensive and freely available.

Results of the current study provide important data to help address the influence of ageing on vitamin D synthesis and the appropriate sensible sun exposure guidelines for older individuals. Previous research has demonstrated decreased cutaneous D_3 production in older adults. A classic ex vivo study of MacLaughlin and Holick found that skin samples obtained from older adults aged 77 to 82 had significantly less 7-DHC concentration compared to skin samples from young adults [12]. A two-fold decrease in pre-vitamin D_3 synthesis in skin samples from the older adults compared to those of an 8- and 18-year-old was also observed [12]. Another study in the photobiology laboratory found that older adults ages 62–80 years with type III skin produced three times less D_3 than young adults age 20–30 years with this same skin type following simulated whole-body sunlight exposure of 32 mJ/cm^2 [17]. To our knowledge, however, previous research has not firmly established a specific age at which a reduction in cutaneous D_3 occurs.

In the current study, both older and younger individuals experienced significant positive increases in circulating D_3 following sun exposure, with only a trend for a different pattern of response between cohorts. The older cohort tended to experience a peak in circulating D_3 at 48 h in contrast to the younger cohort, who experienced peak D_3 concentration nearly equally at 24 h or 48 h. While studies in the photobiology laboratory indicated that D_3 concentrations typically peak within 24 to 48 h following UVB exposure [42], the later peak time in the majority of the older cohort (nine out of 10 participants) could be explained by an age-related decline in the surface area between the dermis and epidermis that ultimately affects nutrient exchange [47,48]. Reduction in basal cell growth in keratinocytes is a major consequence of epidermal thinning [47,48], which has the potential to influence D_3 production.

Perhaps more importantly, our regression modeling conducted throughout the adult age continuum (ages 20–69) showed that alterations in cutaneous vitamin D_3 production declines throughout adulthood. Our regression modeling (Figures 3 and 4) demonstrated that for every decade of life, there is a 13 percent decrease in D_3 production (1.3% per year); by the seventh decade, vitamin D_3 production is approximately half that at age 20. The model, however, demonstrates that even at 120 years of age, vitamin D_3 production is still possible. This is in support of thinking that "... skin has a great capacity to make vitamin D even in the elderly" [2]. This also highlights that there is no specific age at which cutaneous synthesis suddenly stops but rather that it declines slowly over the years.

While not an original intent of the study, the current study also provides interesting results concerning "non-responders" that constituted approximately 17 percent of both cohorts. These non-responders did not have an increase in circulating vitamin D_3 concentration following a full 30-min of exposure. Curiously, however, there were little differences between these five individuals and the rest of the group other than their baseline serum D_3 concentration, which were on average higher than the 25 responders (34 vs. 11 nmol/L) despite reporting both limited sun exposure and no supplemental vitamin D for at least 3 months prior to study initiation. One individual in the older cohort was also the largest participant, with Class II obesity (BMI > 35.2 kg/m^2; body fat = 43.4%). These data combined with our regression models (best subset method) suggest that baseline vitamin D status may influence cutaneous vitamin D synthesis or at least its appearance in circulation. Biochemically it is well-recognized that vitamin D synthesis is regulated through control mechanisms that prohibit vitamin D intoxication through sun exposure by converting excess pre-vitamin D_3 to biologically inert molecules including tachysterol and lumisterol [33]. Baseline 25(OH)D concentration, which averaged 33.1 ± 3.0 ng/mL and were generally sufficient, could also have significantly impacted cutaneous vitamin D synthesis [32] even though D3 was more directly influential in the modeling. Other possible explanations include genetic variation [49] or the misclassification of skin type [45] in the non-responders. For example, genetic variants in close proximity genes involved in cholesterol synthesis, hydroxylation and vitamin D transport have been linked to the elevated risk of vitamin D insufficiency in individuals of European descent, and could be present in some of our non-responders [49]. Alternately, misclassification of individuals with skin types IV and V may have resulted in decreased D_3 synthesis because time of exposure was not sufficient in these skin types [32].

Additionally, while D_3 increased significantly in response to the sun exposure session, 25(OH)D did not change from baseline to 72 h post exposure in the younger and older cohorts or from baseline to 168 h in the older cohort who had data collected at this additional time point. The observed phenomenon may be a result of a combination of factors including the single exposure, sample timing and participant baseline 25(OH)D concentration and/or adiposity [13]. Although vitamin D_3 is known to quickly rise within 24–48 h after artificial UVB exposure, 25(OH)D is thought to gradually rise and peak 7 to 14 days post exposure [42]. The kinetics of 25(OH)D synthesis, appearance in circulation and sequestration in adipose tissue following sun exposure, however, has not been fully elucidated and may require several repeated exposures under natural conditions [44], perhaps to achieve a certain peak D_3 concentration. The relatively good status of our participants also may have also contributed. Bogh et al., for example, reported an inverse relationship between baseline 25(OH)D and subsequent increases in 25(OH)D concentration after UVB exposure [50]. Additionally, as previously stated, our participant's 25(OH)D levels were quite good, and under these conditions, further elevations in circulating 25(OH)D levels become refractory due to enzyme inhibition [51]. Thus, a rise of only of 9.8 nmol vitamin D_3 is simply not enough to drive product levels higher. Furthermore, adiposity in general was relatively high in some of our participants and could have diminished the appearance of 25(OH)D in circulation. This may be related to adipose tissue sequestration of D_3 and 25(OH)D following synthesis [52,53].

While to our knowledge this is the first study to evaluate the effect of a single bout of sensible sun exposure on vitamin D_3 concentration using sunlight exposure for a carefully monitored duration, the study is not without limitations. Limitations include the relatively small sample size, variable characteristics between the older and younger cohorts (the older cohort had more women), inclusion of participants with optimal baseline serum 25(OH)D, inability to study subjects all on the same exposure day and time span between measurements in the older and younger cohort. The later points, however, are an inherent reality of "sensible sun exposure" guidelines. Our exclusionary criteria limited the number of qualified participants—particularly in the older cohort—combined with the unpredictable number of warm, cloudless days and a limited sample size. The dependence on accurate self-reporting and knowledge of dietary vitamin D intake, supplement usage and sun exposure may have also allowed for inclusion of participants with optimal serum 25(OH)D that may have accounted for several non-responders. Additionally, more frequent sampling of D_3 over the first 72 h (e.g., every 6 to 12 h), a longer follow-up period for 25(OH)D sampling, serial exposures (i.e., three consecutive days) and assessment of age-related thickness differences in the epidermis and/or dermis could be employed in future studies to fully capture the relationship between peak D_3, serum 25(OHD concentration [42] and ageing to confirm a rise in 25(OH)D relative to the rise in vitamin D_3 following sun exposure. Employment of non-invasive procedures including optical coherence tomography, two-photon microscopy [10] or confocal laser scanning microscopy [11] would be particularly important to better understand the effect of age-related epidermal thickness changes in relation to vitamin D_3 production following controlled sunlight exposure.

5. Conclusions

A single 30-min bout of sun exposure during late spring at close to solar noon was sufficient to observe an increase in vitamin D_3 concentration within 24 to 48 h in a cohort of younger and older adults as has been previously observed in the photobiology laboratory with a measured dose of UVB radiation. The response, however, was ~25 to 30% of that observed with delivery of 1 MED in the photobiology laboratory. This study is one of the first to evaluate and practically apply UVB exposure from natural sunlight to examine the effect of subcutaneous vitamin D_3 synthesis in younger and older adults. Regression modeling of the appearance of D_3 in circulation suggested that age accounted for approximately 20 percent of the variance in D_3 production from baseline to peak and revealed a 13% decrease in D_3 production with every decade of life. Increases in serum 25(OH)D, however, were not observed at 3 days post-exposure in our younger cohort or at 7 days postexposure in our older cohort. Additional research is needed to better formulate sensible sun exposure guidelines that optimize vitamin D status but avert skin damage, which can lead to skin cancers and other sun associated problems [54]. Additional research is needed to determine the influence of age on timing of peak D_3 concentration, investigate the kinetics of in vivo D_3 adipose tissue sequestration to explain the relationship between cutaneous D_3 production and 25(OH)D response and better understand the specific limitations of ageing (which potentially include reduced dermal and epidermal thickness) on cutaneous vitamin D production.

Author Contributions: Conceptualization, D.E.L.-M. and B.M.A.; methodology, J.R.C., L.M.C., P.J.W. and D.E.L.-M.; software, P.J.W.; validation, P.J.W., B.W.H. and D.E.L.-M.; formal analysis, J.R.C., L.C., P.J.W., K.G.G. and D.E.L.-M.; investigation, J.R.C., L.M.C., P.J.W. and D.E.L.-M.; resources, P.J.W., B.W.H. and D.E.L.-M.; data curation, J.R.C., L.M.C., K.G.G. and D.E.L.-M.; writing—original draft preparation, J.R.C., L.M.C. and D.E.L.-M.; writing—review and editing, B.W.H., B.M.A. and J.F.K.; visualization, P.J.W., J.F.K. and D.E.L.-M.; supervision, D.E.L.-M.; project administration, J.R.C., L.M.C. and D.E.L.-M.; funding acquisition, J.R.C., L.M.C. and D.E.L.-M. All authors have read and agreed to the published version of the manuscript.

Funding: This research was funded in part graduate student grants from the Rocky Mountain Chapter of the American College of Sports Medicine (L.M.C.) and the University of Wyoming Department of Family and Consumer Sciences (L.M.C. and J.R.C.).

Acknowledgments: The authors would like to thank all participants for their time and cooperation. We would also like to thank Katelyn Zavala, RN, Susan Lescznske, RN, Megan Pankey, RN and Rebecca Munn, RN for assistance with blood drawing, Margaretha Troutman and Kelley Fischer for preparing lunches and Sarah Rich for assistance with data entry.

Data Availability: Data available upon reasonable request.

Conflicts of Interest: The authors declare no conflict of interest.

References

1. Wang, J.; Ma, J.; Cheng, G. An accident of acute hydrogen sulfide poisoning when cleaning up a salted vegetables pool. *Zhonghua Lao Dong Wei Sheng Zhi Ye Bing Za Zhi* **2015**, *33*, 918–919. [CrossRef] [PubMed]
2. Holick, M.F. Vitamin D deficiency. *N. Engl. J. Med.* **2007**, *357*, 266–281. [CrossRef] [PubMed]

3. Orces, C.H. Association between leisure-time aerobic physical activity and vitamin D concentrations among US older adults: The NHANES 2007–2012. *Aging Clin. Exp. Res.* **2019**, *31*, 685–693. [CrossRef] [PubMed]
4. Sherman, F.T. Vitamin D deficiency is rampant in older adults. *Geriatrics* **2008**, *63*, 9–11. [PubMed]
5. Ginter, J.K.; Krithika, S.; Gozdzik, A.; Hanwell, H.; Whiting, S.; Parra, E.J. Vitamin D status of older adults of diverse ancestry living in the Greater Toronto Area. *BMC Geriatr.* **2013**, *13*, 66. [CrossRef] [PubMed]
6. Carrillo-Vega, M.F.; Garcia-Pena, C.; Gutierrez-Robledo, L.M.; Perez-Zepeda, M.U. Vitamin D deficiency in older adults and its associated factors: A cross-sectional analysis of the Mexican Health and Aging Study. *Arch. Osteoporos.* **2017**, *12*, 8. [CrossRef]
7. Brouwer-Brolsma, E.M.; Vaes, A.M.M.; van der Zwaluw, N.L.; van Wijngaarden, J.P.; Swart, K.M.A.; Ham, A.C.; van Dijk, S.C.; Enneman, A.W.; Sohl, E.; van Schoor, N.M.; et al. Relative importance of summer sun exposure, vitamin D intake, and genes to vitamin D status in Dutch older adults: The B-PROOF study. *J. Steroid Biochem. Mol. Biol.* **2016**, *164*, 168–176. [CrossRef]
8. Herrick, K.A.; Storandt, R.J.; Afful, J.; Pfeiffer, C.M.; Schleicher, R.L.; Gahche, J.J.; Potischman, N. Vitamin D status in the United States, 2011-2014. *Am. J. Clin. Nutr.* **2019**, *110*, 150–157. [CrossRef]
9. Holick, M.F. *Vitamin D and Health: Evolution, Biologic Functions, and Recommended Dietary Intakes for Vitamin D. Vitamin D: Physiology, Molecular Biology, and Clinical Applications*, 2nd ed.; Springer: Totowa, NJ, USA, 2010.
10. Czekalla, C.; Schonborn, K.H.; Lademann, J.; Meinke, M.C. Noninvasive Determination of Epidermal and Stratum Corneum Thickness in vivo Using Two-Photon Microscopy and Optical Coherence Tomography: Impact of Body Area, Age, and Gender. *Skin Pharmacol. Physiol.* **2019**, *32*, 142–150. [CrossRef]
11. Sauermann, K.; Clemann, S.; Jaspers, S.; Gambichler, T.; Altmeyer, P.; Hoffmann, K.; Ennen, J. Age related changes of human skin investigated with histometric measurements by confocal laser scanning microscopy in vivo. *Skin Res. Technol.* **2002**, *8*, 52–56. [CrossRef]
12. MacLaughlin, J.; Holick, M.F. Aging decreases the capacity of human skin to produce vitamin D3. *J. Clin. Investig.* **1985**, *76*, 1536–1538. [CrossRef] [PubMed]
13. Snijder, M.B.; van Dam, R.M.; Visser, M.; Deeg, D.J.; Dekker, J.M.; Bouter, L.M.; Seidell, J.C.; Lips, P. Adiposity in relation to vitamin D status and parathyroid hormone levels: A population-based study in older men and women. *J. Clin. Endocrinol. Metab.* **2005**, *90*, 4119–4123. [CrossRef] [PubMed]
14. Hill, T.R.; Granic, A.; Aspray, T.J. Vitamin D and Ageing. *Subcell Biochem.* **2018**, *90*, 191–220. [CrossRef] [PubMed]
15. Tsai, K.S.; Heath, H., 3rd; Kumar, R.; Riggs, B.L. Impaired vitamin D metabolism with aging in women. Possible role in pathogenesis of senile osteoporosis. *J. Clin. Investig.* **1984**, *73*, 1668–1672. [CrossRef]
16. Veldurthy, V.; Wei, R.; Oz, L.; Dhawan, P.; Jeon, Y.H.; Christakos, S. Vitamin D, calcium homeostasis and aging. *Bone Res.* **2016**, *4*, 16041. [CrossRef]
17. Holick, M.F.; Matsuoka, L.Y.; Wortsman, J. Age, vitamin D, and solar ultraviolet. *Lancet* **1989**, *2*, 1104–1105. [CrossRef]
18. Meehan, M.; Penckofer, S. The Role of Vitamin D in the Aging Adult. *J. Aging Gerontol.* **2014**, *2*, 60–71. [CrossRef]
19. Orces, C.; Lorenzo, C.; Guarneros, J.E. The Prevalence and Determinants of Vitamin D Inadequacy among U.S. Older Adults: National Health and Nutrition Examination Survey 2007–2014. *Cureus* **2019**, *11*, e5300. [CrossRef]
20. Boucher, B.J. The problems of vitamin d insufficiency in older people. *Aging Dis.* **2012**, *3*, 313–329.
21. Chel, V.G.; Ooms, M.E.; Popp-Snijders, C.; Pavel, S.; Schothorst, A.A.; Meulemans, C.C.; Lips, P. Ultraviolet irradiation corrects vitamin D deficiency and suppresses secondary hyperparathyroidism in the elderly. *J. Bone Miner. Res.* **1998**, *13*, 1238–1242. [CrossRef]
22. Chel, V.G.; Ooms, M.E.; Pavel, S.; de Gruijl, F.; Brand, A.; Lips, P. Prevention and treatment of vitamin D deficiency in Dutch psychogeriatric nursing home residents by weekly half-body UVB exposure after showering: A pilot study. *Age Ageing* **2011**, *40*, 211–214. [CrossRef] [PubMed]
23. Corless, D.; Gupta, S.P.; Switala, S.; Barragry, J.M.; Boucher, B.J.; Cohen, R.D.; Diffey, B.L. Response of plasma-25-hydroxyvitamin D to ultraviolet irradiation in long-stay geriatric patients. *Lancet* **1978**, *2*, 649–651. [CrossRef]
24. Reid, I.R.; Gallagher, D.J.; Bosworth, J. Prophylaxis against vitamin D deficiency in the elderly by regular sunlight exposure. *Age Ageing* **1986**, *15*, 35–40. [CrossRef] [PubMed]

25. Baggerly, C.A.; Cuomo, R.E.; French, C.B.; Garland, C.F.; Gorham, E.D.; Grant, W.B.; Heaney, R.P.; Holick, M.F.; Hollis, B.W.; McDonnell, S.L.; et al. Sunlight and Vitamin D: Necessary for Public Health. *J. Am. Coll. Nutr.* **2015**, *34*, 359–365. [CrossRef]
26. Vainio, H.; Miller, A.B.; Bianchini, F. An international evaluation of the cancer-preventive potential of sunscreens—Meeting held at Lyon, France, 10–18, 2000. *Int. J. Cancer* **2000**, *88*, 838–842. [CrossRef]
27. American Cancer Society Skin Cancer Facts. Available online: http://www.cancer.org/cancer/cancercauses/sunanduvexposure/skin-cancer-facts (accessed on 5 February 2017).
28. (US Department of Health and Human Services). The Surgeon General's Call to Action to Prevent Skin Cancer. Available online: https://www.hhs.gov/sites/default/files/call-to-action-prevent-skin-cancer.pdf (accessed on 23 July 2020).
29. Seleh, N. MDLinx A Daily Dose of This Can Help Fight Chronic Conditions. Available online: https://www.mdlinx.com/article/a-daily-dose-of-this-can-help-fight-chronic-conditions/P5i9BWT7H9W1VJGPntebl (accessed on 29 May 2020).
30. Hossein-Nezhad, A.; Holick, M.F. Vitamin D for health: A global perspective. *Mayo Clin. Proc.* **2013**, *88*, 720–755. [CrossRef]
31. Baron, E.D.; Suggs, A.K. Introduction to photobiology. *Dermatol. Clin.* **2014**, *32*, 255–266. [CrossRef]
32. Jager, N.; Schope, J.; Wagenpfeil, S.; Bocionek, P.; Saternus, R.; Vogt, T.; Reichrath, J. The Impact of UV-dose, Body Surface Area Exposed and Other Factors on Cutaneous Vitamin D Synthesis Measured as Serum 25(OH)D Concentration: Systematic Review and Meta-analysis. *Anticancer Res.* **2018**, *38*, 1165–1171. [CrossRef]
33. Holick, M.F. Sunlight and Vitamin D for bone health and prevention of autoimmune diseases, cancers and cardioavascular disease. *Am. J. Clin. Nutr.* **2004**, *80*, 1678S–1688S. [CrossRef]
34. Lagunova, Z.; Porojnicu, A.C.; Aksnes, L.; Holick, M.F.; Iani, V.; Bruland, O.S.; Moan, J. Effect of vitamin D supplementation and ultraviolet B exposure on serum 25-hydroxyvitamin D concentrations in healthy volunteers: A randomized, crossover clinical trial. *Br. J. Dermatol.* **2013**, *169*, 434–440. [CrossRef]
35. Fitzpatrick, T.B. The validity and practicality of sun-reactive skin types I through VI. *Arch. Dermatol.* **1988**, *124*, 869–871. [CrossRef] [PubMed]
36. Mosteller, R.D. Simplified calculation of body-surface area. *N. Engl. J. Med.* **1987**, *317*, 1098. [CrossRef] [PubMed]
37. Larson-Meyer, D.E.; Douglas, C.S.; Thomas, J.J.; Johnson, E.C.; Barcal, J.N.; Heller, J.E.; Hollis, B.W.; Halliday, T.M. Validation of a Vitamin D Specific Questionnaire to Determine Vitamin D Status in Athletes. *Nutrients* **2019**, *11*, 2732. [CrossRef] [PubMed]
38. Moan, J.; Dahlback, A.; Porojnicu, A.C. At what time should one go out in the sun? *Adv. Exp. Med. Biol.* **2008**, *624*, 86–88. [CrossRef]
39. Grigalavicius, M.; Moan, J.; Dahlback, A.; Juzeniene, A. Daily, seasonal, and latitudinal variations in solar ultraviolet A and B radiation in relation to vitamin D production and risk for skin cancer. *Int. J. Dermatol.* **2016**, *55*, e23–e28. [CrossRef]
40. Helmer, A.C.; Jansen, C.H. Vitamin D precursors removed from human skin by washing. *Stud. Inst. Divi Thomae* **1937**, *1*, 207–216.
41. Kollias, N.; Ruvolo, E., Jr.; Sayre, R.M. The value of the ratio of UVA to UVB in sunlight. *Photochem. Photobiol.* **2011**, *87*, 1474–1475. [CrossRef]
42. Adams, J.S.; Clemens, T.L.; Parrish, J.A.; Holick, M.F. Vitamin-D synthesis and metabolism after ultraviolet irradiation of normal and vitamin-D-deficient subjects. *N. Engl J. Med.* **1982**, *306*, 722–725. [CrossRef]
43. Holick, M.F. Vitamin D and Health: Evolution, Biologic Functions, and Recommended Dietary Intakes for Vitamin D. *Clin. Rev. Bone Miner. Metab.* **2009**, *7*, 2–19. [CrossRef]
44. Datta, P.; Bogh, M.K.; Olsen, P.; Eriksen, P.; Schmedes, A.V.; Grage, M.M.; Philipsen, P.A.; Wulf, H.C. Increase in serum 25-hydroxyvitamin-D3 in humans after solar exposure under natural conditions compared to artificial UVB exposure of hands and face. *Photochem. Photobiol. Sci.* **2012**, *11*, 1817–1824. [CrossRef]
45. Terushkin, V.; Bender, A.; Psaty, E.L.; Engelsen, O.; Wang, S.Q.; Halpern, A.C. Estimated equivalency of vitamin D production from natural sun exposure versus oral vitamin D supplementation across seasons at two US latitudes. *J. Am. Acad. Dermatol.* **2010**, *62*, 929. e1–929. e9. [CrossRef] [PubMed]
46. Holick, M. Sunlight "D"ilemma: Risk of skin cancer or bone disease and muscle weakness. *Lancet* **2001**, *357*, 3. [CrossRef]

47. Makrantonaki, E.; Zouboulis, C.C. William J. Cunliffe Scientific Awards. Characteristics and pathomechanisms of endogenously aged skin. *Dermatology* **2007**, *214*, 352–360. [CrossRef] [PubMed]
48. Moragas, A.; Castells, C.; Sans, M. Mathematical morphologic analysis of aging-related epidermal changes. *Anal. Quant. Cytol. Histol.* **1993**, *15*, 75–82.
49. Wang, T.J.; Zhang, F.; Richards, J.B.; Kestenbaum, B.; van Meurs, J.B.; Berry, D.; Kiel, D.P.; Streeten, E.A.; Ohlsson, C.; Koller, D.L.; et al. Common genetic determinants of vitamin D insufficiency: A genome-wide association study. *Lancet* **2010**, *376*, 180–188. [CrossRef]
50. Bogh, M.K.B.; Schmedes, A.V.; Philipsen, P.A.; Thieden, E.; Wulf, H.C. Vitamin D Production after UVB Exposure Depends on Baseline Vitamin D and Total cholesterol but Not on skin Pigmentation. *J. Investig. Dermatol.* **2009**, *130*, 546–553. [CrossRef]
51. Hollis, B.W.; Johnson, D.; Hulsey, T.C.; Ebeling, M.; Wagner, C.L. Vitamin D supplementation during pregnancy: Double-blind, randomized clinical trial of safety and effectiveness. *J. Bone Miner. Res.* **2011**, *26*, 2341–2357. [CrossRef]
52. Savastano, S.; Barrea, L.; Savanelli, M.C.; Nappi, F.; Di Somma, C.; Orio, F.; Colao, A. Low vitamin D status and obesity: Role of nutritionist. *Rev. Endocr. Metab. Dis.* **2017**, *18*, 215–225. [CrossRef]
53. Abboud, M.; Rybchyn, M.S.; Rizk, R.; Fraser, D.R.; Mason, R.S. Sunlight exposure is just one of the factors which influence vitamin D status. *Photochem. Photobiol. Sci.* **2017**, *16*, 302–313. [CrossRef]
54. Girgis, C.M.; Clifton-Bligh, R.J.; Turner, N.; Lau, S.L.; Gunton, J.E. Effects of Vitamin D in Skeletal Muscle: Falls, Strength, Athletic Performance and Insulin Sensitivity. *Clin. Endocrinol. (Oxf.)* **2013**. [CrossRef] [PubMed]

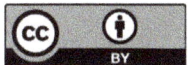

© 2020 by the authors. Licensee MDPI, Basel, Switzerland. This article is an open access article distributed under the terms and conditions of the Creative Commons Attribution (CC BY) license (http://creativecommons.org/licenses/by/4.0/).

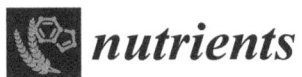 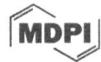

Article

Nutrihealth Study: Seasonal Variation in Vitamin D Status Among the Slovenian Adult and Elderly Population

Maša Hribar [1,2], Hristo Hristov [1], Matej Gregorič [3], Urška Blaznik [3], Katja Zaletel [4], Adrijana Oblak [4], Joško Osredkar [4,5], Anita Kušar [1], Katja Žmitek [1,6], Irena Rogelj [2] and Igor Pravst [1,2,6,*]

1. Nutrition Institute, Tržaška cesta 40, SI-1000 Ljubljana, Slovenia; masa.hribar@nutris.org (M.H.); hristo.hristov@nutris.org (H.H.); anita.kusar@nutris.org (A.K.); katja.zmitek@vist.si (K.Ž.)
2. Biotechnical Faculty, University of Ljubljana, Jamnikarjeva 101, SI-1000 Ljubljana, Slovenia; irena.rogelj@bf.uni-lj.si
3. National Institute of Public Health, Trubarjeva 2, SI-1000 Ljubljana, Slovenia; matej.gregoric@nijz.si (M.G.); urska.blaznik@nijz.si (U.B.)
4. University Medical Centre Ljubljana, Zaloška cesta 7, SI-1000 Ljubljana, Slovenia; katja.zaletel@kclj.si (K.Z.); adrijana.oblak@kclj.si (A.O.); josko.osredkar@kclj.si (J.O.)
5. Faculty of pharmacy, University of Ljubljana, Aškerčeva cesta 7, SI-1000 Ljubljana, Slovenia
6. VIST–Higher School of Applied Sciences, Gerbičeva cesta 51A, SI-1000 Ljubljana, Slovenia
* Correspondence: igor.pravst@nutris.org; Tel.: +386-590-68871; Fax: +386-310-07981

Received: 21 May 2020; Accepted: 17 June 2020; Published: 19 June 2020

Abstract: Several studies conducted around the world showed substantial vitamin D insufficiency and deficiency among different population groups. Sources of vitamin D in the human body include ultraviolet B (UVB)-light-induced biosynthesis and dietary intake, but people's diets are often poor in vitamin D. Furthermore, in many regions, sun exposure and the intensity of UVB irradiation during wintertime are not sufficient for vitamin D biosynthesis. In Slovenia, epidemiological data about vitamin D status in the population were investigated through a national Nutrihealth study—an extension to the national dietary survey SI.Menu (2017/18). The study was conducted on a representative sample of 125 adult (18–64 years) and 155 elderly (65–74 years old) subjects, enrolled in the study in different seasons. Their vitamin D status was determined by measuring the serum 25-hydroxy-vitamin D (25(OH)D) concentration. Thresholds for vitamin D deficiency and insufficiency were 25(OH)D levels below 30 and 50 nmol/L, respectively. Altogether, 24.9% of the adults and 23.5% of the elderly were found to be vitamin D deficient, while an insufficient status was found in 58.2% and 62.9%, respectively. A particularly concerning situation was observed during extended wintertime (November–April); vitamin D deficiency was found in 40.8% and 34.6%, and insufficient serum 25(OH)D levels were observed in 81.6% and 78.8%, respectively. The results of the study showed high seasonal variation in serum 25(OH)D levels in both the adult and elderly population, with deficiency being especially pronounced during wintertime. The prevalence of this deficiency in Slovenia is among the highest in Europe and poses a possible public health risk that needs to be addressed with appropriate recommendations and/or policy interventions.

Keywords: 25(OH)vitamin D; biomarkers; dietary survey; public health; EU Menu; Slovenia; Europe

1. Introduction

Research related to the epidemiology of vitamin D status in different populations is linked to public health concerns due to the high prevalence rates of vitamin D insufficiency and deficiency [1,2]. Several studies conducted in Europe and around the world have shown substantial vitamin D insufficiency and deficiency among different population groups [1–8]. Due to the many roles of vitamin D in human physiology, its low serum concentrations can pose a health risk [3,9]. Vitamin D is a fat-soluble vitamin that is involved in calcium and phosphorus homeostasis, and it therefore plays a crucial role in bone health [10]. While several epidemiological studies have also linked vitamin D deficiency with non-skeletal health outcomes, disease occurrence, immune system function, and reduced life expectancy, the cause–effect evidence from randomized controlled studies remains limited [11,12]. Vitamin D sufficiency varies among and between populations. The elderly are considered an especially vulnerable population group, with a higher prevalence of low vitamin D status and associated health risks [13].

The main sources of vitamin D are skin exposure to ultraviolet B light (UVB) radiation and dietary intake. The amount of vitamin D production via UVB radiation in the skin depends on latitude, season, and time of the day [14–16]. It was suggested that sun exposure covers most vitamin D requirements, but in many European countries, sun exposure during most of the wintertime does not lead to the production of vitamin D in the skin, since the intensity of UVB radiation in the sunlight is too low for the efficient cutaneous biosynthesis of cholecalciferol [17–19]. Examples of other factors influencing the cutaneous biosynthesis of vitamin D are skin pigmentation, age (especially an age >65 years), and the topical application of sunscreen [14]. On the other hand, the dietary intake of vitamin D with food is commonly low [1,5]. Very few foods are a rich source of vitamin D, and such foods are seldom consumed. The majority of vitamin D intake is, therefore, achieved with foods that are poorer in vitamin D but consumed more regularly [1,20]. Therefore, fortified foods and food supplements also represent an important dietary source of vitamin D [1]. Recommendations for vitamin D intake in the adult population vary widely across Europe [21]. The WHO sets the recommended vitamin D intake at 10 µg/day (400 International Units (IUs); 51–65 years) and 15 µg/day (600 IU; > 65 years) [22], and the daily recommended levels by the European Food Safety Authority (EFSA) and D-A-CH (The nutrition societies of Germany, Austria, and Switzerland) are 15 (600 IU) and 20 µg/day (800 IU) (in the absence of endogenous synthesis), respectively [23,24]. The latter recommendations include the total vitamin D supplied from food and cutaneous biosynthesis. It is estimated that the daily dietary intake of vitamin D in many European populations is well below 10 µg [25,26]. However, because vitamin D status in individuals is particularly affected by the efficiency of cutaneous biosynthesis, dietary intake is not considered a reliable predictor. Therefore, vitamin D status is mainly determined using serum 25-OH vitamin D (25(OH)D) levels [27]. Vitamin D deficiency is usually defined as serum levels below 30 nmol/L (10–12 ng/mL) [24,28–30], while serum levels below 50 nmol/L (20 ng/mL) are considered insufficient [24,28,30,31]. On the other hand, a serum 25(OH)D concentration above 75 nmol/L (30 ng/mL) is recommended by the Endocrine Society's clinical practice guidelines [29].

Slovenia is a country in Central Europe with a latitude between 45° and 46° north, with a population of approximately 2 million people. To date, only two studies have systematically investigated vitamin D deficiency in Slovenia; both were conducted among pregnant women and reported high prevalence rates of vitamin D deficiency [32,33]. Considering the results of the studies conducted in other countries in our region [1,2,5,6,8,30,34], there is a clear need for epidemiological data on the vitamin D status among the Slovenian general population.

Considering these facts, a nutritional Nutrihealth study was conducted as part of the larger research project, "Children's and adults' nutrition as a protective or health-risk factor", which was funded by the Slovenian Research Agency and the Ministry of Health. This Nutrihealth study is an extension of the national dietary SI.Menu survey with a collection of blood and urine samples, thus enabling the assessment of micronutrient status and helping policymakers engage in evidence-based policy decisions. The objective of the present study was to elucidate the seasonal variation in vitamin D status among the Slovenian adult and elderly population.

2. Experimental Section

2.1. Study Design and Data Collection

The Nutrihealth study was conducted as an upgrade to the Slovenian national dietary survey SI.Menu 2017/2018, which was carried out following the EFSA Guidance on EU Menu Methodology [35]. The complete methodology of the SI.Menu study is detailed elsewhere [36]. In short, the SI.Menu study included nationally representative (age/sex/region) samples of adolescents (10–17 years of age), adults (18–64 years), and the elderly (65–74 years). The recruitment period ran from March 2017 to February 2018, divided into quarters (Q): Q1 (March–May 2017), Q2 (June–August 2017), Q3 (September–November 2017), and Q4 (December 2017–February 2018). The survey contained a food propensity questionnaire (FPQ); two non-consecutive 24 h dietary recalls; information concerning eating habits; consumer habits; food allergies; food supplement use; lifestyle; socio-demographic and socio-economic status; body height; weight; self-evaluated health status; and percentage of fat, water, and fat-free mass measured with a bioimpedance scale. Physical activity levels were assessed using the International Physical Activity Questionnaire (IPAQ) and scored as described by Craig et al. [37]. A subsample of adult participants that completed the SI.Menu study (all participating adults (18–74 years) in Q2, Q3, and Q4) was invited to participate in the Nutrihealth study.

The Nutrihealth study protocol was approved by the Slovenian National Medical Ethics Committee (Ministry of Health, Republic of Slovenia), identification number KME 72/07/16 (approval letter ID 0120-337/2016-4, date of approval: 7 July 2017) and was registered at ClinicalTrials.gov (ID: NCT03284840). The study was performed in compliance with the requirements of the local authorities. All subjects signed a written informed consent form (ICF) before participation in the study. The Nutrihealth study included the collection of fasting blood samples, spot urine samples, and thyroid inspection/palpations and ultrasounds. The collection of biological samples was carried out in local healthcare centers from June 2017 to September 2018. Blood samples were collected on daily basis during regular working hours of the local healthcare centers and transported to a central laboratory at the University Medical Center in Ljubljana, where they were stored at −80 °C until analysis. Determination of the serum 25(OH)D was conducted at the Department of Nuclear Medicine on a complete set of samples after sample collection was completed.

2.2. Study Population

While the SI.Menu study was conducted on a nationally representative sample of adolescents, adults, and the elderly; only the adults and elderly were included in the Nutrihealth study. Altogether, 1319 participants (a 62.2% response rate) fully completed the SI.Menu study (484 adolescents, 385 adults, and 450 elderly), and 620 participants (282 adults and 338 elderly) were invited to the Nutrihealth study. Altogether, 394 subjects (183 adults and 211 elderly) signed the consent, and 280 (125 adults and 155 elderly; 68.3% and 73.5%, respectively) provided biological samples. Descriptive characteristics of the final populations are provided in Table 1.

2.3. Serum 25(OH)D Concentration

Serum 25(OH)D concentration was measured in human serum at the Department of Nuclear Medicine (University Medical Center, Ljubljana) with the chemiluminescence immunoassay vitamin D total (25-hydroxy-vitamin D) determined on an IDS-iSYS analyzer (Immunodiagnostic Systems, Boldon, UK). The correlation coefficient using the ID-LC-MS/MS method within the assay measuring interval (22.5–246.5 nmol/L) was r = 0.925. Vitamin D status was assigned with consideration of serum 25(OH)D concentration according to the literature: Deficient below 30 nmol/L (12 ng/mL) and insufficient bellow 50 nmol/L (20 ng/mL) [28].

Table 1. Descriptive characteristics of the population.

Variable		Adults (18–64 Years Old) N = 125	Elderly (65–74 Years Old) N = 155
Age (mean ± SD)		46.5 (13.2)	68.6 (2.8)
Residential area (%)	village	50.4	54.2
	town	15.2	15.5
	city	34.4	30.3
Sex (%)	male	41.6	49
	female	58.4	51
Education (%)	primary school	8.8	19.4
	high school	60	55.5
	higher education	31.2	25.1
Monthly net income (%)	≤900 €	20.3	32.2
	900–1800 €	47.8	55
	>1800 €	31.9	12.8
Season (%)	November–April	58.4	58.7
	May–October	41.6	41.3
BMI (mean ± SD)		27.6 (5.5)	27.9 (4.7)
BMI (%)	<25	39.2	29.7
	≥25	60.8	70.3
Smoking status (%)	current smoker	17.6	11.6
	ex-/non-smoker	82.4	88.4
Physical activity * (%)	low level	31.2	33.1
	moderate level	32	31.8
	high level	36.8	35.1
Vitamin D supplement use (%)	users	8.8	8.4
	non-users	91.2	91.6

Notes: SD = standard deviation; BMI = body mass index; * physical activity according to International Physical Activity Questionnaire (IPAQ).

2.4. Statistical Analysis

The statistical analysis was conducted using STATA version 13 (StataCorp, Coledge Station, TX, USA). Descriptive characteristics (means, median, and proportions), as well as the proportions of participants with different levels of 25(OH)D, are presented for all participants and per age group. Considering the sampling approach, most of the analyses were done separately for the adults and the elderly. For serum 25(OH)D levels and for the prevalence low serum 25(OH)D (levels below 30/50/75 nmol/L) we used population weighting (sex and age) separately for the sample groups of adults and elderly. As Slovenia lies at latitudes lacking sufficient sunlight to produce cutaneous vitamin D during the extended winter [19], two seasonal periods were used for the statistical analyses: May–October (extended summer) and November–April (extended winter). On the other hand, weighting of the serum 25(OH)D levels in bimonthly periods (January–February, March–April, May–June; July–August; September–October; November–December) was performed on the merged samples of the adults and elderly ($N = 280$). Weighting factors were computed using the iterative proportional fitting method with the Slovenian national census data for July 2017.

The unadjusted mean values of serum 25(OH)D were determined by sex, education, income, season, body mass index (BMI), smoking status, physical activity, and vitamin D supplement use. BMI was defined as lean or normal weight (BMI < 25) and overweight/obese (BMI ≥ 25) and was calculated as weight (kg)/height(m^2). Data on household monthly net income were used to assign the income status (≤900 €; between 900 € and 1800 €/month; and >1800 €/month). A linear logistic regression analysis was used to investigate the differences between the different sub-populations of both samples. The mean 25(OH)D levels were further adjusted for the above-mentioned variables as possible confounders. The prevalence of adults and elderly with serum 25(OH)D levels less than 30 nmol/L and 50 nmol/L was determined by sex, education, income, season, BMI, smoking status, physical activity, and vitamin D supplement use. A multivariable logistic regression analysis was undertaken with all of the above-mentioned variables per age group to determine the independent predictors of vitamin D insufficiency (serum 25(OH)D level < 50 nmol/L). In all comparisons, significance was considered at $p < 0.05$.

The aggregated data for adults and elderly participants within the extended wintertime ($n = 164$) were used to conduct a prevalence analysis (serum 25(OH)D level < 50 nmol/L) considering the consumption of the selected dietary sources of the vitamin. We used the food propensity questionnaire (FPQ) data (FPQ options: at least once per day, 4–6 times per week, 2–4 times per week, once per week, 1–3 times per month or less, or never) for seafood; saltwater fish; yogurts, sour milk, and curd; and milk to differentiate between regular consumers (a consumption frequency of at least once per week) and non-consumers (a consumption frequency of never).

3. Results

As a part of the Nutrihealth study, blood samples were collected from the 280 subjects. Considering the sampling approach, the data were analyzed separately for adults (18–64 years) and the elderly (65–74 years). The study population thus consisted of 125 adults and 155 elderly; the characteristics of both sample groups are summarized in Table 1.

The yearly population-weighted (age and sex) serum 25(OH)D levels and prevalence of serum 25(OH)D levels below 30/50/75 nmol/L for both populations are presented in Table 2. Critically low serum 25(OH)D levels (<30 nmol/L) were observed in about a quarter of both samples, while about 60% had levels below the recommended 50 nmol/L. Only around a fifth of the population had serum 25(OH)D levels above 75 nmol/L. Notably, we observed seasonal differences in the serum 25(OH)D levels in different periods of the year. Figure 1 presents the population-weighted (age, sex) mean serum 25(OH)D concentrations in two-month intervals, considering the measurements in both samples ($N = 280$). It can be observed that the serum 25(OH)D levels are notably higher between May and October (extended summer) compared to the period between November and April (extended winter).

Table 2. Yearly population-weighted (age, sex) serum 25(OH)D levels and prevalence of serum 25(OH)D levels <30, <50, and <75 nmol/L (95% CI) for adults (18–64 years) and elderly (65–74 years).

	N (%) *	Serum 25(OH)D Level (nmol/L)			Prevalence (%)		
		Mean	S.E.	Median	<30 nmol/L	<50 nmol/L	<75 nmol/L
Adults	125 (100)	50.7 (45.4–56.0)	2.7	45.3	24.9 (17.5–34.1)	58.2 (48.5–67.3)	83.3 (74.9–89.2)
-Male	52 (41.6)	55.3 (46.4–64.1)	4.5	50.7	22.8 (12.6–37.8)	50.0 (35.4–64.6)	79.6 (65.7–88.8)
-Female	73 (58.4)	46.2 (40.4–51.9)	2.9	43.8	27.0 (17.6–39.0)	66.4 (54.3–76.7)	86.9 (76.1–93.2)
Elderly	155 (100)	47.7 (43.9–51.5)	1.9	42.4	23.5 (17.4–30.9)	62.9 (54.9–70.2)	84.4 (77.8–89.4)
-Male	76 (49.0)	48.2 (43.0–53.3)	2.6	42.1	19.1 (11.8–29.5)	60.3 (48.7–70.7)	84.9 (74.7–91.5)
-Female	79 (51.0)	47.3 (41.8–52.8)	2.8	43.1	27.5 (18.6–38.5)	65.2 (54.1–74.9)	84.0 (74.2–90.5)

Notes: S.E. = Standard error.; * N = unweighted number of subjects for the whole year.

To provide further insights into the vitamin D status of the population, we calculated seasonal population-weighted serum 25(OH)D levels and prevalence of serum 25(OH)D levels below 30/50/75 nmol/L separately for the extended summer and winter periods (Table 3).

Relatively low levels of vitamin D deficiency (<30 nmol/L) were observed during the extended summer. In adults, the prevalence of deficiency was 2.6% (95%CI: 0.6, 10.2), without notable differences between males and females. On the other hand, 16.1% (95%CI: 4.9, 41.5) of males and 34.6% (19.5–53.6) of females had serum 25(OH)D levels below 50 nmol/L. Among the elderly, the prevalence of vitamin D deficiency during extended summer was somewhat higher; 7.8% of males (95%CI: 3.2, 17.5) and 40.2% of females (95%CI: 28.8, 52.7) had serum 25(OH)D levels below 50 nmol/L. The prevalence of insufficient serum 25(OH)D levels was 27.6% (95% CI: 14.3, 46.5) in males and 51.4% (95%CI: 35.1–67.5) in females.

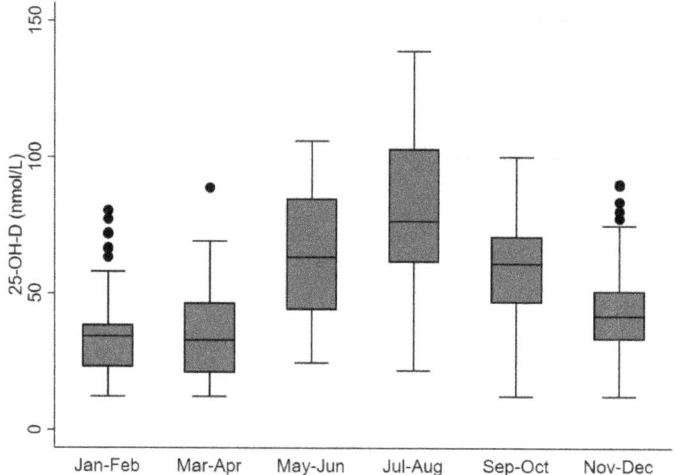

Figure 1. Box plots of the weighted (age and sex) mean serum 25(OH)D concentrations for different bi-monthly periods ($N = 280$) with presentation of outliers (·).

A notably higher prevalence of vitamin D deficiency was observed during extended winter, with 40.8% (95%CI; 29.0,53.7) of adults and 34.6% (95%CI: 25.4, 45.1) of the elderly having serum 25(OH)D levels below 30 nmol/L. Prevalence of vitamin D deficiency in females and males was 44.5% (95%CI: 29.7, 60.3) vs. 37.1% (95%CI: 20.4, 57.6) for adults and 40.9% (95%CI: 27.4, 56.0) vs. 27.7% (95%CI: 16.7, 42.2) for the elderly, respectively. During the extended winter period, about four-fifths of both populations did not meet the recommended serum 25(OH)D level of 50 nmol/L.

The reported results clearly show that serum 25(OH)D levels are affected by the season. A multivariable logistic regression analysis was done using the season, sex, residential area, education, family net income, BMI, smoking status, physical activity, and use of vitamin D supplements as possible independent predictors of the prevalence of insufficient vitamin D status. Table 4 presents a sample of serum 25(OH)D levels below 50 nmol/L and the adjusted odds ratios (ORs) for both study populations. In line with previous observations, season was identified as a significant predictor of vitamin status in both the adult and elderly populations ($p < 0.0001$). The odds ratios for insufficient vitamin D status were 34.9 for adults (95%CI: 9.2, 132.5) and 10.3 for the elderly (95%CI: 4.1, 26.1), respectively. For the elderly, only body mass index was identified as an additional significant predictor ($p = 0.014$), with subjects possessing a lower BMI having a lower odds ratio for insufficient vitamin D status (OR 0.3; 95%CI: 0.1, 0.8). On the other hand, sex ($p = 0.041$) and physical activity (0.048) were identified as significant parameters in the adult population, with a higher OR for females (OR 3.4; 95%CI: 1.1–10.7) and for those with a low level of physical activity (OR 5.6; 95%CI: 9.22–22.7; $p = 0.016$). Similar results were observed in the regression analysis of the sample mean serum 25(OH)D levels (Supplementary Materials Table S1). After adjustment for the above mentioned confounding factors, the mean serum 25(OH)D concentrations were 49.9 (95% CI: 45.3, 54.6) and 47.7 nmol/L (95% CI: 43.9, 51.4) for adults and the elderly, respectively, with higher levels in extended summer than in extended winter. It should be noted that season was again a significant parameter in both populations ($p < 0.001$), along with BMI ($p = 0.0065$) among the elderly population and sex ($p = 0.031$) among the adult population. Additionally, for adults, smoking status ($p = 0.011$) was also identified as a significant parameter, while physical activity was not significant.

Table 3. Seasonal population-weighted (age, sex) serum 25(OH)D levels and the prevalence of serum 25(OH)D levels <30, <50, and <75 nmol/L (95% CI) for the adult (18–64 years) and elderly (65–74 years) populations.

		Extended Summer: May–October							Extended Winter: November–April						
		Serum 25(OH)D Level (nmol/L)				Prevalence (%)			Serum 25(OH)D Level (nmol/L)				Prevalence (%)		
	N (%) *	Mean	S.E.	Med.	<30 nmol/L	<50 nmol/L	<75 nmol/L	N (%) *	Mean	S.E.	Med.	<30 nmol/L	<50 nmol/L	<75 nmol/L
Adults	52 (100)	70.4 (62.2–78.5)	4.1	64.0	2.6 (0.6–10.2)	25.3 (14.8–39.9)	62.6 (47.4–75.6)	73 (100)	36.7 (32.5–40.9)	2.1	34.4	40.8 (29.0–53.7)	81.6 (69.4–89.7)	98.0 (92.2–99.5)
- Male	22 (42.3)	76.2 (62.4–90.1)	6.9	71.2	2.8 (0.3–18.3)	16.1 (4.9–41.5)	56.6 (34.1–76.6)	30 (41.1)	40.3 (33.3–47.3)	3.5	37.6	37.1 (20.4–57.6)	74.2 (53.3–87.8)	96.0 (84.9–99.0)
- Female	30 (57.7)	64.5 (56.5–72.5)	4.0	63.0	2.4 (0.3–15.8)	34.6 (19.5–53.6)	68.5 (48.8–83.3)	43 (58.9)	33.1 (28.8–37.4)	2.2	32.8	44.5 (29.7–60.3)	89.1 (76.9–95.3)	100
Elderly	64 (100)	60.1 (54.0–66.2)	3.1	57.0	7.8 (3.2–17.5)	40.2 (28.8–52.7)	73.4 (61.1–82.9)	91 (100)	39.0 (35.0–43.0)	2.0	37.4	34.6 (25.4–45.1)	78.8 (69.0–86.1)	92.2 (84.4–96.3)
- Male	29 (45.3)	62.6 (54.4–70.8)	4.1	58.5	6.9 (1.7–24.1)	27.6 (14.3–46.5)	72.4 (53.5–85.7)	47 (51.7)	38.2 (33.3–43.0)	2.4	38.1	27.7 (16.7–42.2)	83.0 (69.3–91.3)	93.6 (81.8–98.0)
- Female	35 (54.7)	57.9 (49.0–66.9)	4.5	47.9	8.6 (2.7–23.8)	51.4 (35.1–67.5)	74.3 (57.2–86.2)	44 (48.3)	39.8 (33.6–46.0)	3.1	36.5	40.9 (27.4–56.0)	75.0 (60.1–85.7)	90.9 (78.0–96.6)

Notes: med. = median; * N = unweighted number of subjects per season.

Table 4. Sample prevalence of serum 25(OH)D levels below 50 nmol/L, and adjusted odds ratios (95% CI) for adult (18–64 years) and elderly (65–74 years) population.

Variable		Adults			Elderly		
		N	Prevalence N (%)	Odds Ratio	N	Prevalence N (%)	Odds Ratio
Overall		125	73 (58.4)		155	98 (63.2)	
Place of living	village	63	35 (55.6)	1.80 (0.57–5.64)	84	52 (61.9)	0.49 (0.18–1.35)
	town	19	14 (73.7)	3.77 (0.58–24.51)	24	15 (62.5)	0.87 (0.24–3.15)
	city	43	24 (55.8)	1	47	31 (66.0)	1
Sex	male	52	25 (48.1)	1	76	47 (61.8)	1
	female	73	48 (65.8)	3.36 (1.05–10.74)	79	51 (64.56)	1.94 (0.80–4.69)
Education	elementary school	11	7 (63.6)	3.23 (0.47–22.19)	30	23 (76.7)	1.16 (0.33–4.00)
	high school	75	42 (56)	1	86	53 (61.6)	1
	higher education	39	24 (61.5)	2.19 (0.58–8.23)	39	22 (56.4)	0.56 (0.21–1.54)
Family net income *	≤900 €	23	14 (60.9)	1.57 (0.34–7.34)	48	34 (70.8)	1.75 (0.65–4.76)
	900–1800 €	54	31 (57.4)	1	82	49 (59.8)	1
	>1800 €	36	21 (58.3)	1.78 (0.51–6.25)	19	13 (68.4)	1.47 (0.38–5.65)
Season	November–April	73	59 (80.8)	34.94 (9.22–132.50)	91	72 (79.1)	10.34 (4.10–26.07)
	May–October	52	14 (26.9)	1	64	26 (40.6)	1
BMI	<25	49	31 (63.3)	1.68 (0.52–5.35)	46	24 (52.2)	0.31 (0.12–0.78)
	≥25	76	22 (51.2)	1	109	34 (56.7)	1
Smoking status	current smoker	22	15 (56.3)	1	18	11 (63.5)	1
	ex-/non-smoker	103	58 (68.2)	5.01 (0.90–27.78)	137	87 (61.1)	1.40 (0.36–5.43)
Physical activity	low level	39	28 (71.8)	5.59 (1.38–22.69)	51	33 (64.7)	1.78 (0.66–4.81)
	moderate level	40	20 (50.0)	1	49	28 (57.1)	1
	high level	46	25 (54.4)	1.76 (0.44–7.05)	54	36 (66.7)	1.57 (0.59–4.22)
Vitamin D supplement use	users	11	5 (45.5)	1	13	7 (53.9)	1
	non-users	114	68 (59.7)	1.20 (0.17–8.25)	142	91 (64.1)	3.61 (0.82–15.92)

Notes: * Logistic regression analysis conducted on samples with the excluded missing data (family net income: $n = 12$ (adults) and $n = 6$ (elderly)); variables contributing significantly to the variability in the distribution between the different 25(OH)D serum levels (adults: sex ($p = 0.041$), season ($p < 0.0001$), physical activity ($p = 0.048$; low level of physical activity: $p = 0.016$); elderly: season ($p < 0.0001$); BMI ($p = 0.014$).

To gain insight into the importance of dietary habits on vitamin D status, we next studied vitamin D status in relation to the consumption frequency of important dietary sources of vitamin D. To avoid the cofounding of sun-exposure-related vitamin biosynthesis, this analysis was done with the exclusion of extended summertime measurements. We used aggregate data for the adult and elderly populations (n = 164); food consumption frequency was measured using a survey-based food propensity questionnaire. Figure 2 presents the proportion of study subjects with serum 25(OH)D concentrations above 50 nmol/L for non-consumers and regular consumers of selected dietary sources of vitamin D. While the differences did not reach statistical significance, in all selected food categories, the proportions of vitamin D sufficiency were higher for regular consumers than for non-consumers. For example, 46.2% (95%CI: 23.2, 70.9) of regular consumers of seafood had a serum 25(OH)D level above 50 nmol/L, while for non-consumers, this was the case in only 15.4% (95%CI: 6.1–33.5).

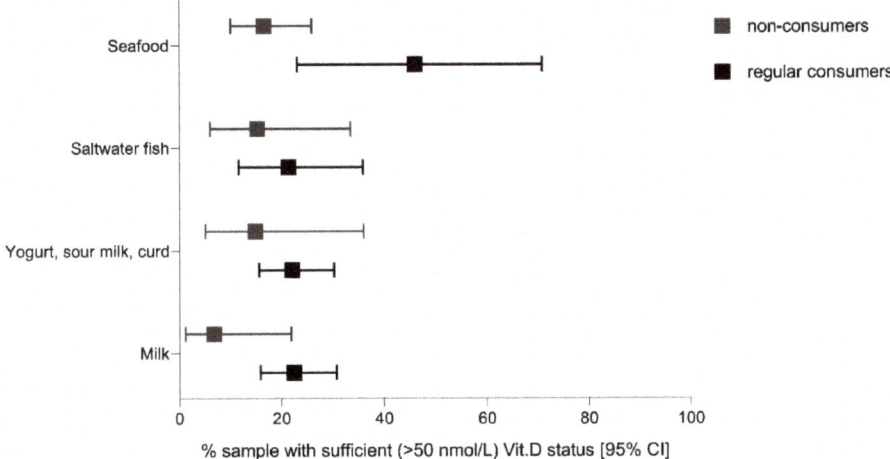

Figure 2. Proportion (%) of subjects with sufficient vitamin D status (serum 25(OH)D level >50 nmol/L) for (non)consumers of selected dietary sources of vitamin D (aggregated data for adults and the elderly during the extended winter period (November–April); n = 164).

4. Discussion

Epidemiological studies on the vitamin D status in various populations are receiving increased attention, mostly due to the various associations of vitamin D deficiency with health outcomes [1,2]. This is also the case in Europe [1–8]. In a recent ODIN study carried out among European residents living across a latitude gradient of 35° N to 69° N, about 13% of people were vitamin D deficient, and 40% were insufficient [5]. Previous research suggests that mid-latitude countries can have an even higher prevalence of deficiency than northern countries, such as Norway, Iceland, and Finland [2].

Slovenia is also a mid-latitude country (latitude 45° and 46° North) but with very limited epidemiological data on vitamin D status. Studies conducted among pregnant women showed high rates of vitamin D deficiency [32,33], indicating the need for a nationally representative study. This study was designed as an extension to the cross-sectional national dietary survey SI.Menu 2017/2018 [30].

It should be noted that the optimal serum 25(OH)D concentration remains subject to different opinions. According to the Institute of Medicine (IOM) [38], EFSA [24], and European Calcified Tissue Society [30], the recommended serum level of 25(OH)D should be above 50 nmol/L for skeletal health benefits, while the Endocrine Society [29] recommends concentrations above 75 nmol/L. In this paper, we use the term "vitamin D deficiency" for serum 25(OH)D levels below 30 nmol/L and "vitamin D insufficiency" for levels below 50 nmol/L. The reported prevalence for vitamin D deficiency in this study was 24.9% and 23.5% among the adults (18–64 years old) and elderly (65–74 years old), respectively. Insufficiency was observed in 58.2% of adults and 62.9% of the elderly population, which ranks Slovenia among the countries with the highest vitamin D insufficiency in Europe [2,5,8,30]. The prevalence of insufficiency was high even when comparing countries with similar latitudes. Germany (47–55° N; 18–79 years) reported 54.5% prevalence [2] and France (43-49° N; 18–89 years) 34.6% [39], while a >82% prevalence was reported for the Ukraine (44–52° N; 20–95 years) [40]. The vitamin D insufficiency prevalence reported here is also high when compared to some other countries across the world. A US study revealed a prevalence of 41.7% (36.0–47.6) and 41.1% (37.4–44.6) for adults (<65 years old) and the elderly (≥65 years old), respectively [41], while in China, the prevalence was 55.9% in adults [42] and 34.3% in the elderly population (>60 years old) [43]. A somewhat lower prevalence (22.7%, 95%CI: 20.5, 35.1) was observed in the Australian adult and elderly population [44]. According to the WHO, vitamin D insufficiency can be classified as a severe health problem since it affects more than 40% of the global population [45], and Slovenia, with many other countries, falls into this category.

The main source of vitamin D is dermal synthesis induced by UVB [46,47]. UVB availability varies highly during the year, and the amplitude of variation is mostly dependent on latitude [19]. Therefore, this study was also focused on investigating the seasonal variation of vitamin D status in the adult and elderly populations. We split the observation time into two periods: extended winter (November–April) and extended summer (May–October) since the winter and springtime vitamin D statuses decline and reach their nadir typically in late winter or early spring [48]. This is demonstrated in Figure 1, which shows the peak values of 25(OH)D concentrations in July and August. These values then steadily decline until late winter, with the difference of the mean values between extended winter and extended summer at almost 30 nmol/L.

The adjusted mean 25(OH)D levels were significantly lower in the extended winter period, and the odds ratios for insufficient vitamin D status were significantly lower in extended summer, both in adults and the elderly. The population weighted prevalence of vitamin D deficiency during extended winter in adults was 40.8% (95% CI: 29.0–53.7), which was more than 10 times higher than that during extended summer, when prevalence of deficiency was only 2.6% (95% CI: 0.6–10.2). At the same time, the prevalence of vitamin D insufficiency rose from 25.3% (95% CI: 14.8, 39.9) in the extended summer to 81.6% (95% CI:69.4, 89.7) in the extended winter. This means that four out of five people will be vitamin D deficient during the winter period. Such seasonal variations are common in countries at this latitude [19,43,44,47,49–52].

The literature data show that the elderly are more susceptible to lower 25(OH)D concentrations [5,13,30,34,49,53,54], likely due to their decreased cutaneous vitamin D production, sun-avoidance behaviors [55] (and consequently reduced sun exposure [56]), and lower dietary intake of vitamin D [57]. Sampling in our study was, therefore, done with a stronger focus on the elderly population. Interestingly, the prevalence of vitamin D deficiency in the summer period was notably higher than in adults (7.8% vs. 2.6%), but this was not the case during the extended wintertime. However, the elderly population in the SI.Menu study was represented by free-living individuals, excluding those living in elderly institutions. We suspect that the lower seasonal variability in vitamin D status in the elderly population is related to their sun-avoidance behavior. These findings support previous results and highlight that season is a major factor for determining vitamin D status.

The mean serum 25(OH)D levels in this study for the adult population were 50.7 nmol/L (95% CI: 45.4, 56.0) and 47.7 nmol/L (95% CI: 43.9, 51.5) for the elderly, which are lower values in comparison to most countries in the neighborhood. The reference mean values for the adult and elderly participants were 50.1 nmol/L in Germany [2], 52.3 nmol/L in Austria [34], and 60 nmol/L in France [39], while Croatian postmenopausal women had a mean value of 64.9 nmol/L [58]. In adults (but not in the elderly), we observed significant differences in the mean vitamin D values between sexes, with males having higher mean values than females at 55.3 (95% CI: 46.4, 64.1) and 46.2 (95%CI: 40.4, 51.9) nmol/L, respectively. These findings are consistent with those of some other studies [34,44,47,49,59], but there are also studies with opposite observations (India, Saudi Arabia) [60,61].

Adiposity is also a well-known risk factor for vitamin D deficiency/insufficiency [4]. The bioavailability of vitamin D from cutaneous and dietary sources decreases through its deposition in body fat compartments [62,63] and can also be lower due to reduced outdoor physical activity [50,64]. In our sample, 60.8% of adults and 70.3% of the elderly population were overweight or obese, which may have affected the high prevalence of vitamin D deficiency/insufficiency. In the elderly population, we observed a particularly high (and statistically significant; $p = 0.014$) odds ratio (OR 10.3; 95%CI: 4.10, 26.7) for vitamin D insufficiency in overweight/obese subjects in comparison to those with normal or lean BMIs. Considering our inability to observe this trend in the adult population, we should note that the sample of elderly participants (65–74 years) was much more homogenous in their age interval than the adult subjects, whose age interval was much higher (18–65 years). On the other hand, smoking was identified as a significant predictor of mean serum 25(OH)D levels, with current smokers having a lower means compared to non- or ex-smokers, which is in agreement with other studies [44,47]. Interestingly, in our study, the use of vitamin D supplements was not identified as a significant predictor of vitamin D status. While we observed higher mean serum 25(OH)D levels and a lower prevalence of vitamin D insufficiency in the group of supplement users, the proportion of vitamin D supplement users was very low (9% in adults and 8% in the elderly), and the doses of vitamin D are commonly too low to achieve sufficient vitamin D intake. For example, even within supplement (vitamin D) users, the vitamin D level in the majority of the obtained serum samples was below the recommended level of 50 nmol/L (59.7% of adults and 64.1% of the elderly).

During an extended winter period with low or no UVB-induced vitamin D biosynthesis, vitamin D becomes essential, with diet providing its only source [5,19]. In subjects (adult and elderly) whose blood samples were collected during the extended winter period, food propensity questionnaire data were used to identify some dietary habits, thus affecting vitamin D status (Figure 1). Regular consumers of seafood had a notably higher prevalence of vitamin D sufficiency compared to non-consumers of seafood, while the difference for the other food groups was less obvious.

The strengths of this study include the recruitment of a national population-based sample of Slovenian adults (18 to 64 years) and elderly (65 to 74 years) participants with a measurement of serum 25(OH)D levels, which was done centrally in one laboratory using the same methodology. However, some limitations of this study should be also noted. First, while the sample was nationally representative, the sample size limited our ability to identify additional parameters affecting vitamin D status, particularly those related to dietary habits. Secondly, this is a cross-sectional study. Thus, the causality between vitamin D deficiency and its determinants could not be determined. Third, we did not obtain data on the prevailing weather conditions, ozone, or sun exposure practices, including clothing type in summer, time spent outdoors, and sunscreen use. Therefore, specific analyses were done on the samples obtained during extended wintertime to avoid the effects of UV-B induced vitamin D biosynthesis. It should be noted, however, that even if data on sun exposure were available, any compensation for vitamin D biosynthesis would be very difficult. Our study results also showed that season is the strongest parameter affecting vitamin D status, wich seriously limits the ability to identify other predictors of vitamin D status during the extended summer, where biosynthesis presents the most important source of vitamin D. Another study limitation is that the national dietary survey SI.Menu was not conducted in a way that facilitated the reliable estimation of dietary vitamin D intake at the individual level. Therefore, the food propensity questionnaire data were used only to provide some insights about the vitamin D supply with consideration of the (non)consumption of specific food types, while the effects of total daily dietary vitamin D intake were not investigated.

5. Conclusions

Ultimately, we observed considerable seasonal variability in the vitamin D status of both the adult and elderly populations. The highest vitamin D deficiency rates were observed during extended wintertime (November–April; 40.8% of adults and 34.6% of the elderly). During that time, about 80% of the population had insufficient vitamin D levels (<50 nmol/L). In addition to season, other important factors affecting vitamin D status included sex and physical activity for adults and BMI for the elderly population. The high prevalence of vitamin D deficiency and insufficiency in Slovenia during extended wintertime poses a possible public health risk, which should be addressed with appropriate recommendations and/or policy interventions. This could be done at the national or European Union level. Considering that we observed relatively low serum 25(OH)D levels also on those reporting use of vitamin D supplements, further studies should focus into identification of existing supplementation practices, to identify usual dosages and forms of vitamin D that are being used by different populations.

Supplementary Materials: The following are available online at http://www.mdpi.com/2072-6643/12/6/1838/s1. Table S1: Sample mean (95% CI) serum 25(OH)D levels (nmol/L) for the different groups of the adult and elderly population.

Author Contributions: M.H.; performed the data analyses and wrote the manuscript. H.H.; performed statistical analyses and population weighting. J.O. was responsible for the data collection. K.Z. and A.O.; were responsible for the sample collection and laboratory analyses. M.G., U.B., A.K., K.Ž. and I.R.; critically reviewed the manuscript. I.P.; was responsible for assuring the set-up and funding of the study, preparing the study design, collaborating in the data analyses, and reviewing the manuscript. All authors have read and agreed to the published version of the manuscript.

Funding: The Nutrihealth study was part of the research project L3-8213 "Children's and adults' nutrition as a protective or health-risk factor", funded by the Slovenian Research Agency and Ministry of Health of Republic of Slovenia. This work was also supported within the research program P3-0395 (Nutrition and Public health) and project L7-1849 (Challenges in achieving adequate vitamin D status in the adult population).

Acknowledgments: We acknowledge the regional community healthcare centers and hospitals for collection of biological samples in the Nutrihealth study. We are grateful to the staff of UKC Ljubljana (Troha Poljančič Vera, Gaberšček Simona) and all medical laboratory teams across Slovenia led by Spomenka Lajtner (Community Health Center Ljubljana); Jana Žnidaršič (Community Health Center Cerknica), Katarina Furar (Community Health Center Ivančna Gorica); Tomaž Vargazon (Community Health Center Kamnik); Ljubica Štefanič (Community Health Center Kočevje); Irena Sluga (Community Health Center Litija); Jolanda Prah (Community Health Center Maribor); Jelica Štanta (Community Health Center Gornja Radgona); Ana Gruškovnjak (Community Health Center Ljutomer); Edita Ružič (Community Health Center Murska Sobota); Mojca Završnik (Hospital Ptuj); Tanja Lađić (General Hospital Slovenj Gradec); Tina Kochler (Community Health Center Slovenska Bistrica); Mojca Kozmelj (Community Health Center Celje); Maja Škerjanc (Community Health Center Velenje); Branka Svetic (Community Health Center Kranj); Sabina Nabernik (Community Health Center Jesenice); Marko Rudež (Community Health Center Škofja Loka); Vanja Pahor (General Hospital Izola); Damjana Bogataj (Community Health Center Ajdovščina); Andreja Seljak (Community Health Center Idrija); Kristina Gruden (Community Health Center Nova Gorica); Valentina Buda (Community Health Center Postojna); Polonca Stopar (Community Health Center Sežana); Zalka Murovec (Community Health Center Tolmin); Danijela Furlan (General Hospital Novo mesto); and Andreja Kerin (General hospital Brežice). This study was conducted on participants of the SI.Menu 2017/18 survey, funded by the European Food Safety Authority (EFSA contract No. OC/EFSA/DATA/2014/02-LOT2-CT03), Ministry of Health of the Republic of Slovenia, and the Slovenian Research Agency. Therefore, we also acknowledge support from all SI.Menu project partners and their researchers, particularly Nataša Defar, Metka Zaletel, Darja Lavtar, Ada Hočevar Grom, and Ivan Eržen (National Institute of Public Health, Ljubljana, Slovenia); Anita Kušar (Nutrition Institute, Ljubljana, Slovenia); Petra Golja and Katja Zdešar Kotnik (University of Ljubljana, Biotechnical Faculty, Ljubljana, Slovenia); Stojan Kostanjevec (University of Ljubljana, Faculty of Education, Ljubljana, Slovenia); Majda Pajnkihar (University of Maribor, Faculty of Health Sciences, Maribor, Slovenia); Tamara Poklar Vatovec (University of Primorska, Faculty of Health Sciences, Koper, Slovenia); Barbara Koroušić Seljak (Jožef Stefan Institute, Ljubljana, Slovenia); Nataša Fidler Mis and Evgen Benedik (University Medical Center Ljubljana, University Children's Hospital, Ljubljana, Slovenia). We also acknowledge the support of Mrs. Veronika Belec and her team and interviewers at the GfK Research Institute (Slovenia) in conducting field work for this survey.

Conflicts of Interest: The authors declare no conflicts of interest. The funders had no role in the design of the study; in the collection, analyses, or interpretation of data; in the writing of the manuscript; or in the decision to publish the results. I.P. has led and participated in various other research projects in the area of nutrition, public health, and food technology that were (co)funded by the Slovenian Research Agency, Ministry of Health of the Republic of Slovenia, the Ministry of Agriculture, Forestry and Food of the Republic of Slovenia, and, for specific applied research projects, also by food businesses. I.P., K.Ž., M.G., and U.B are members of a national workgroup responsible for the development of recommendations for assuring adequate vitamin D status among the Slovenian population.

References

1. Spiro, A.; Buttriss, J.L. Vitamin D: An overview of vitamin D status and intake in Europe. *Nutr. Bull.* **2014**, *39*, 322–350. [CrossRef] [PubMed]
2. Cashman, K.D.; Dowling, K.G.; Skrabakova, Z.; Gonzalez-Gross, M.; Valtuena, J.; De Henauw, S.; Moreno, L.; Damsgaard, C.T.; Michaelsen, K.F.; Molgaard, C.; et al. Vitamin D deficiency in Europe: Pandemic? *Am. J. Clin. Nutr.* **2016**, *103*, 1033–1044. [CrossRef] [PubMed]
3. Palacios, C.; Gonzalez, L. Is vitamin D deficiency a major global public health problem? *J. Steroid Biochem. Mol. Biol.* **2014**, *144 (Pt A)*, 138–145. [CrossRef]
4. Holick, M.F. The vitamin D deficiency pandemic: Approaches for diagnosis, treatment and prevention. *Rev. Endocr. Metab. Disord.* **2017**, *18*, 153–165. [CrossRef]
5. Kiely, M.; Cashman, K.D. Summary Outcomes of the ODIN Project on Food Fortification for Vitamin D Deficiency Prevention. *Int. J. Environ. Res. Public Health* **2018**, *15*, 2342. [CrossRef] [PubMed]
6. Lips, P. Vitamin D status and nutrition in Europe and Asia. *J. Steroid Biochem. Mol. Biol.* **2007**, *103*, 620–625. [CrossRef]
7. Pludowski, P.; Grant, W.B.; Bhattoa, H.P.; Bayer, M.; Povoroznyuk, V.; Rudenka, E.; Ramanau, H.; Varbiro, S.; Rudenka, A.; Karczmarewicz, E.; et al. Vitamin d status in central europe. *Int. J. Endocrinol.* **2014**, *2014*, 589587. [CrossRef]
8. Manios, Y.; Moschonis, G.; Lambrinou, C.P.; Tsoutsoulopoulou, K.; Binou, P.; Karachaliou, A.; Breidenassel, C.; Gonzalez-Gross, M.; Kiely, M.; Cashman, K.D. A systematic review of vitamin D status in southern European countries. *Eur. J. Nutr.* **2018**, *57*, 2001–2036. [CrossRef]
9. Holick, M.F. The vitamin D deficiency pandemic and consequences for nonskeletal health: Mechanisms of action. *Mol. Aspects Med.* **2008**, *29*, 361–368. [CrossRef]
10. Molina, P.; Carrero, J.J.; Bover, J.; Chauveau, P.; Mazzaferro, S.; Torres, P.U.; European Renal, N.; Chronic Kidney, D.-M.; Bone Disorder Working Groups of the European Renal Association-European Dialysis Transplant Association. Vitamin D, a modulator of musculoskeletal health in chronic kidney disease. *J. Cachexia Sarcopenia Muscle* **2017**, *8*, 686–701. [CrossRef]
11. Autier, P.; Mullie, P.; Macacu, A.; Dragomir, M.; Boniol, M.; Coppens, K.; Pizot, C.; Boniol, M. Effect of vitamin D supplementation on non-skeletal disorders: A systematic review of meta-analyses and randomised trials. *Lancet Diabetes Endocrinol.* **2017**, *5*, 986–1004. [CrossRef]
12. EFSA Scientific Panel NDA. Scientific Opinion on the substantiation of a health claim related to vitamin D and contribution to the normal function of the immune system pursuant to Article 14 of Regulation (EC) No. 1924/2006. *EFSA J.* **2015**, *13*, 7.
13. Lips, P. Vitamin D Deficiency and Secondary Hyperparathyroidism in the Elderly: Consequences for Bone Loss and Fractures and Therapeutic Implications. *Endocr. Rev.* **2001**, *22*, 477–501. [CrossRef] [PubMed]
14. Holick, M.F. Vitamin D and Health: Evolution, Biologic Functions, and Recommended Dietary Intakes for Vitamin D; Clinic. *Rev. Bone. Miner. Metab.* **2009**, *7*, 2–19. [CrossRef]
15. O'Connor, A.; Benelam, B. An update on UK Vitamin D intakes and status, and issues for food fortification and supplementation. *Nutr. Bull.* **2011**, *36*, 390–396. [CrossRef]
16. Bleizgys, A.; Kurovskij, J. Vitamin D Levels of Out-Patients in Lithuania: Deficiency and Hypervitaminosis. *Medicina* **2018**, *54*, 25. [CrossRef]
17. Holick, M.F. Sunlight and vitamin D for bone health and prevention of autoimmune diseases, cancers, and cardiovascular disease. *Am. J. Clin. Nutr.* **2004**, *80*, 1678S–1688S. [CrossRef]
18. Kimlin, M.G. Geographic location and vitamin D synthesis. *Mol. Aspects Med.* **2008**, *29*, 453–461. [CrossRef]
19. O'Neill, C.M.; Kazantzidis, A.; Ryan, M.J.; Barber, N.; Sempos, C.T.; Durazo-Arvizu, R.A.; Jorde, R.; Grimnes, G.; Eiriksdottir, G.; Gudnason, V.; et al. Seasonal Changes in Vitamin D-Effective UVB Availability in Europe and Associations with Population Serum 25-Hydroxyvitamin D. *Nutrients* **2016**, *8*, 533. [CrossRef]
20. Roseland, J.M.; Phillips, K.M.; Patterson, K.Y.; Pehrsson, P.R.; Taylor, C.L. Chapter 60–Vitamin D in Foods: An Evolution of Knowledge. In *Vitamin D*, 4th ed.; Feldman, D., Ed.; Academic Press: Cambridge, MA, USA, 2018; pp. 41–77.
21. Bouillon, R. Comparative analysis of nutritional guidelines for vitamin D. *Nat. Rev. Endocrinol.* **2017**, *13*, 466–479. [CrossRef]

22. World Health Organization; Food and Agriculture Organization of the United Nations. *Vitamin and Mineral Requirements in Human Nutrition: Report of a Joint FAO/WHO Expert Consultation, Bangkok, Thailand, 21–30 September 1998*, 2nd ed.; World Health Organization: Geneva, Switzerland; FAO: Rome, Italy, 2004; p. xix, 341p.
23. German Nutrition Society. New reference values for vitamin D. *Ann. Nutr. Metab.* **2012**, *60*, 241–246. [CrossRef] [PubMed]
24. EFSA Panel on Dietetic Products, N.a.A.N. Dietary reference values for vitamin D. *EFSA J.* **2016**, *14*, e04547. [CrossRef]
25. Roman Vinas, B.; Ribas Barba, L.; Ngo, J.; Gurinovic, M.; Novakovic, R.; Cavelaars, A.; de Groot, L.C.; van't Veer, P.; Matthys, C.; Serra Majem, L. Projected prevalence of inadequate nutrient intakes in Europe. *Ann. Nutr. Metab.* **2011**, *59*, 84–95. [CrossRef] [PubMed]
26. Lichthammer, A.; Nagy, B.; Orbán, C.; Tóth, T.; Csajbók, R.; Molnár, S.; Tátrai-Nèmeth, K.; Bálint, M.V. A comparative study of eating habits, calcium and vitamin D intakes in the population of Central-Eastern European countries. *New Med.* **2015**, *2*, 66–70.
27. Seamans, K.M.; Cashman, K.D. Existing and potentially novel functional markers of vitamin D status: A systematic review. *Am. J. Clin. Nutr.* **2009**, *89*, 1997S–2008S. [CrossRef]
28. Institute of Medicine Committee to Review Dietary Reference Intakes for Vitamin D and Calcium. The National Academies Collection: Reports funded by National Institutes of Health. In *Dietary Reference Intakes for Calcium and Vitamin D*; Ross, A.C., Taylor, C.L., Yaktine, A.L., Del Valle, H.B., Eds.; National Academies Press (US), National Academy of Sciences: Washington, DC, USA, 2011.
29. Holick, M.F.; Binkley, N.C.; Bischoff-Ferrari, H.A.; Gordon, C.M.; Hanley, D.A.; Heaney, R.P.; Murad, M.H.; Weaver, C.M.; Endocrine, S. Evaluation, treatment, and prevention of vitamin D deficiency: An Endocrine Society clinical practice guideline. *J. Clin. Endocrinol. Metab.* **2011**, *96*, 1911–1930. [CrossRef]
30. Lips, P.; Cashman, K.D.; Lamberg-Allardt, C.; Bischoff-Ferrari, H.A.; Obermayer-Pietsch, B.; Bianchi, M.L.; Stepan, J.; El-Hajj Fuleihan, G.; Bouillon, R. Current vitamin D status in European and Middle East countries and strategies to prevent vitamin D deficiency: A position statement of the European Calcified Tissue Society. *Eur. J. Endocrinol.* **2019**, *180*, P23–P54. [CrossRef]
31. Cesareo, R.; Attanasio, R.; Caputo, M.; Castello, R.; Chiodini, I.; Falchetti, A.; Guglielmi, R.; Papini, E.; Santonati, A.; Scillitani, A.; et al. Italian Association of Clinical Endocrinologists (AME) and Italian Chapter of the American Association of Clinical Endocrinologists (AACE) Position Statement: Clinical Management of Vitamin D Deficiency in Adults. *Nutrients* **2018**, *10*, 546. [CrossRef]
32. Dovnik, A.; Mujezinović, F.; Treiber, M.; Pečovnik Balon, B.; Gorenjak, M.; Maver, U.; Takač, I. Seasonal variations of vitamin D concentrations in pregnant women and neonates in Slovenia. *Eur. J. Obstet. Gynecol. Reprod. Biol.* **2014**, *181*, 6–9. [CrossRef]
33. Soltirovska Salamon, A.; Benedik, E.; Bratanic, B.; Velkavrh, M.; Rogelj, I.; Fidler Mis, N.; Bogovic Matijasic, B.; Paro-Panjan, D. Vitamin D Status and Its Determinants in Healthy Slovenian Pregnant Women. *Ann. Nutr. Metab.* **2015**, *67*, 96–103. [CrossRef]
34. Kudlacek, S.; Schneider, B.; Peterlik, M.; Leb, G.; Klaushofer, K.; Weber, K.; Woloszczuk, W.; Willvonseder, R. Assessment of vitamin D and calcium status in healthy adult Austrians. *Eur. J. Clin. Investig.* **2003**, *33*, 323–331. [CrossRef] [PubMed]
35. European Food Safety Authority. Guidance on the EU Menu methodology. *EFSA J.* **2014**, *15*, 3944.
36. Gregorič, M.; Blaznik, U.; Delfar, N.; Zaletel, M.; Lavtar, D.; Koroušić Seljak, B.; Golja, P.; Zdešar Kotnik, K.; Pravst, I.; Fidler Mis, N.; et al. Slovenian national food consumption survey in adolescents, adults and elderly. *EFSA Supporting Publ.* **2019**, *EN-1729*, 28.
37. Craig, C.L.; Marshall, A.L.; Sjostrom, M.; Bauman, A.E.; Booth, M.L.; Ainsworth, B.E.; Pratt, M.; Ekelund, U.; Yngve, A.; Sallis, J.F.; et al. International physical activity questionnaire: 12-country reliability and validity. *Med. Sci. Sports Exerc.* **2003**, *35*, 1381–1395. [CrossRef] [PubMed]
38. Ross, A.C.; Manson, J.E.; Abrams, S.A.; Aloia, J.F.; Brannon, P.M.; Clinton, S.K.; Durazo-Arvizu, R.A.; Gallagher, J.C.; Gallo, R.L.; Jones, G.; et al. The 2011 report on dietary reference intakes for calcium and vitamin D from the Institute of Medicine: What clinicians need to know. *J. Clin. Endocrinol. Metab.* **2011**, *96*, 53–58. [CrossRef] [PubMed]

39. Souberbielle, J.-C.; Massart, C.; Brailly-Tabard, S.; Cavalier, E.; Chanson, P. Prevalence and determinants of vitamin D deficiency in healthy French adults: The VARIETE study. *Endocrine* **2016**, *53*, 543–550. [CrossRef] [PubMed]
40. Povoroznyuk, V.V.; Balatska, N.I.; Muts, V.Y.; Klymovytsky, F.V.; Synenky, O.V. Vitamin D deficiency in Ukraine: A demographic and seasonal analysis. *Gerontologija* **2012**, *13*, 191–198.
41. Forrest, K.Y.; Stuhldreher, W.L. Prevalence and correlates of vitamin D deficiency in US adults. *Nutr. Res.* **2011**, *31*, 48–54. [CrossRef]
42. Yu, S.; Fang, H.; Han, J.; Cheng, X.; Xia, L.; Li, S.; Liu, M.; Tao, Z.; Wang, L.; Hou, L.; et al. The high prevalence of hypovitaminosis D in China: A multicenter vitamin D status survey. *Medicine* **2015**, *94*, e585. [CrossRef]
43. Chen, J.; Yun, C.; He, Y.; Piao, J.; Yang, L.; Yang, X. Vitamin D status among the elderly Chinese population: A cross-sectional analysis of the 2010-2013 China national nutrition and health survey (CNNHS). *Nutr. J.* **2017**, *16*, 3. [CrossRef]
44. Gill, T.K.; Hill, C.L.; Shanahan, E.M.; Taylor, A.W.; Appleton, S.L.; Grant, J.F.; Shi, Z.; Dal Grande, E.; Price, K.; Adams, R.J. Vitamin D levels in an Australian population. *BMC Public Health* **2014**, *14*, 1001. [CrossRef] [PubMed]
45. World Health Organization. *Worldwide Prevalence of Anaemia 1993–2005: WHO Global Database on Anaemia*; World Health Organization: Geneva, Switzerland, 2008.
46. Antonucci, R.; Locci, C.; Clemente, M.G.; Chicconi, E.; Antonucci, L. Vitamin D deficiency in childhood: Old lessons and current challenges. *J. Pediatr. Endocrinol. Metab.* **2018**, *31*, 247–260. [CrossRef] [PubMed]
47. Duarte, C.; Carvalheiro, H.; Rodrigues, A.M.; Dias, S.S.; Marques, A.; Santiago, T.; Canhao, H.; Branco, J.C.; da Silva, J.A.P. Prevalence of vitamin D deficiency and its predictors in the Portuguese population: A nationwide population-based study. *Arch. Osteoporos.* **2020**, *15*, 36. [CrossRef]
48. Webb, A.R.; Kline, L.; Holick, M.F. Influence of season and latitude on the cutaneous synthesis of vitamin D3: Exposure to winter sunlight in Boston and Edmonton will not promote vitamin D3 synthesis in human skin. *J. Clin. Endocrinol. Metab.* **1988**, *67*, 373–378. [CrossRef]
49. Daly, R.M.; Gagnon, C.; Lu, Z.X.; Magliano, D.J.; Dunstan, D.W.; Sikaris, K.A.; Zimmet, P.Z.; Ebeling, P.R.; Shaw, J.E. Prevalence of vitamin D deficiency and its determinants in Australian adults aged 25 years and older: A national, population-based study. *Clin. Endocrinol.* **2012**, *77*, 26–35. [CrossRef]
50. Bolland, M.J.; Chiu, W.W.; Davidson, J.S.; Grey, A.; Bacon, C.; Gamble, G.D.; Reid, I.R. The effects of seasonal variation of 25-hydroxyvitamin D and fat mass on diagnosis of vitamin D insufficiency. *N. Z. Med. J.* **2008**, *121*, 63–74.
51. Chang, S.W.; Lee, H.C. Vitamin D and health—The missing vitamin in humans. *Pediatr. Neonatol.* **2019**, *60*, 237–244. [CrossRef] [PubMed]
52. Osredkar, J.; Marc, J. Vitamin D and metabolites: Physiology, pathophisiology and reference values. *Med. Razgl.* **1996**, *35*, 543–565.
53. McKenna, M.J. Differences in vitamin D status between countries in young adults and the elderly. *Am. J. Med.* **1992**, *93*, 69–77. [CrossRef]
54. Brouwer-Brolsma, E.M.; Vaes, A.M.M.; van der Zwaluw, N.L.; van Wijngaarden, J.P.; Swart, K.M.A.; Ham, A.C.; van Dijk, S.C.; Enneman, A.W.; Sohl, E.; van Schoor, N.M.; et al. Relative importance of summer sun exposure, vitamin D intake, and genes to vitamin D status in Dutch older adults: The B-PROOF study. *J. Steroid Biochem. Mol. Biol.* **2016**, *164*, 168–176. [CrossRef]
55. MacLaughlin, J.; Holick, M.F. Aging decreases the capacity of human skin to produce vitamin D3. *J. Clin. Investig.* **1985**, *76*, 1536–1538. [CrossRef] [PubMed]
56. Santos, A.; Amaral, T.F.; Guerra, R.S.; Sousa, A.S.; Alvares, L.; Moreira, P.; Padrao, P.; Afonso, C.; Borges, N. Vitamin D status and associated factors among Portuguese older adults: Results from the Nutrition UP 65 cross-sectional study. *BMJ Open* **2017**, *7*, e016123. [CrossRef]
57. Ter Borg, S.; Verlaan, S.; Hemsworth, J.; Mijnarends, D.M.; Schols, J.M.; Luiking, Y.C.; de Groot, L.C. Micronutrient intakes and potential inadequacies of community-dwelling older adults: A systematic review. *Br. J. Nutr.* **2015**, *113*, 1195–1206. [CrossRef]
58. Laktasic-Zerjavic, N.; Korsic, M.; Crncevic-Orlic, Z.; Kovac, Z.; Polasek, O.; Soldo-Juresa, D. Vitamin D status, dependence on age, and seasonal variations in the concentration of vitamin D in Croatian postmenopausal women initially screened for osteoporosis. *Clin. Rheumatol.* **2010**, *29*, 861–867. [CrossRef] [PubMed]

59. Touvier, M.; Deschasaux, M.; Montourcy, M.; Sutton, A.; Charnaux, N.; Kesse-Guyot, E.; Assmann, K.E.; Fezeu, L.; Latino-Martel, P.; Druesne-Pecollo, N.; et al. Determinants of vitamin D status in Caucasian adults: Influence of sun exposure, dietary intake, sociodemographic, lifestyle, anthropometric, and genetic factors. *J. Investig. Dermatol.* **2015**, *135*, 378–388. [CrossRef]
60. Sanghera, D.K.; Sapkota, B.R.; Aston, C.E.; Blackett, P.R. Vitamin D Status, Gender Differences, and Cardiometabolic Health Disparities. *Ann. Nutr. Metab.* **2017**, *70*, 79–87. [CrossRef] [PubMed]
61. AlQuaiz, A.M.; Kazi, A.; Fouda, M.; Alyousefi, N. Age and gender differences in the prevalence and correlates of vitamin D deficiency. *Arch. Osteoporos.* **2018**, *13*, 49. [CrossRef]
62. Wortsman, J.; Matsuoka, L.Y.; Chen, T.C.; Lu, Z.; Holick, M.F. Decreased bioavailability of vitamin D in obesity. *Am. J. Clin. Nutr.* **2000**, *72*, 690–693. [CrossRef]
63. Zmitek, K.; Hribar, M.; Hristov, H.; Pravst, I. Efficiency of Vitamin D Supplementation in Healthy Adults is Associated with Body Mass Index and Baseline Serum 25-Hydroxyvitamin D Level. *Nutrients* **2020**, *12*, 1268. [CrossRef]
64. Scragg, R.; Camargo, C.A., Jr. Frequency of leisure-time physical activity and serum 25-hydroxyvitamin D levels in the US population: Results from the Third National Health and Nutrition Examination Survey. *Am. J. Epidemiol.* **2008**, *168*, 577–586. [CrossRef]

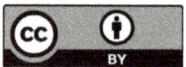

© 2020 by the authors. Licensee MDPI, Basel, Switzerland. This article is an open access article distributed under the terms and conditions of the Creative Commons Attribution (CC BY) license (http://creativecommons.org/licenses/by/4.0/).

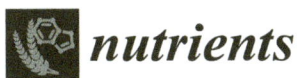

Article

Long-Term Effects of Vitamin D Supplementation in Obese Children During Integrated Weight–Loss Programme—A Double Blind Randomized Placebo–Controlled Trial

Michał Brzeziński [1,2,*], Agnieszka Jankowska [1], Magdalena Słomińska-Frączek [3], Paulina Metelska [2,4], Piotr Wiśniewski [5], Piotr Socha [6] and Agnieszka Szlagatys-Sidorkiewicz [1]

1. Department of Paediatrics, Gastroenterology, Allergology and Paediatric Nutrition, Medical University of Gdańsk, 80–803 Gdańsk, Poland; ajankowska@gumed.edu.pl (A.J.); agnieszka.szlagatys-sidorkiewicz@gumed.edu.pl (A.S.-S.)
2. Department of Public Health and Social Medicine, Medical University of Gdansk, 80–210 Gdańsk, Poland; metelska.paulina@gumed.edu.pl
3. Department of Paediatrics, Copernicus Medical Center, 80-462 Gdańsk, Poland; madds@wp.pl
4. "6–10–14 for Health"–University Clinical Center, 80-952 Gdańsk, Poland
5. Department of Endocrinology and Internal Medicine, Medical University of Gdansk, 80–952 Gdańsk, Poland; piotr.wisniewski@gumed.edu.pl
6. Department of Gastroenterology, Hepatology and Feeding Disorders, The Children's Memorial Health Institute, 04–730 Warszawa, Poland; p.socha@ipczd.pl
* Correspondence: brzezinski@gumed.edu.pl; Tel.: +48-501-762-172

Received: 24 March 2020; Accepted: 13 April 2020; Published: 15 April 2020

Abstract: Background: Vitamin D was studied in regards to its possible impact on body mass reduction and metabolic changes in adults and children with obesity yet there were no studies assessing the impact of vitamin D supplementation during a weight management program in children and adolescence. The aim of our study was to assess the influence of 26 weeks of vitamin D supplementation in overweight and obese children undergoing an integrated 12–months' long weight loss program on body mass reduction, body composition and bone mineral density. Methods: A double–blind randomized placebo–controlled trial. Vitamin D deficient patients (<30 ng/ml level of vitamin D) aged 6–14, participating in multidisciplinary weight management program were randomly allocated to receiving vitamin D (1200 IU) or placebo for the first 26 weeks of the intervention. Results: Out of the 152 qualified patients, 109 (72%) completed a full cycle of four visits scheduled in the program. There were no difference in the level of BMI (body mass index) change – both raw BMI and BMI centiles. Although the reduction of BMI centiles was greater in the vitamin D vs. placebo group (-4.28 ± 8.43 vs. -2.53 ± 6.10) the difference was not statistically significant ($p = 0.319$). Similarly the reduction in fat mass—assessed both using bioimpedance and DEXa was achieved, yet the differences between the groups were not statistically significant. Conclusions: Our study ads substantial results to support the thesis on no effect of vitamin D supplementation on body weight reduction in children and adolescents with vitamin D insufficiency undergoing a weight management program.

Keywords: vitamin D; obesity; weight–loss; body composition

1. Introduction

Worldwide prevalence of overweight and obesity is increasing both in adults and children [1,2]. It is observed on all continents, with the highest burden in those from lower socioeconomic and educational groups [1,3]. Obesity among others is associated with a wide range of metabolic disorders, such as insulin resistance, hyperinsulinemia, and impaired tolerance of glucose, abnormal fasting plasma glucose, symptomatic diabetes mellitus, lipid disorders and cardiovascular disorders, namely arterial hypertension [4–6]. Obesity alone is responsible for a significant increase in the risk of mortality in general population with [7]. In view of high risk of complications resulting from childhood obesity, early implementation of intervention programs seems to be vitally important, as in children and adolescents it is the first–choice intervention, although with limited effectiveness [8]. Several previous studies showed that integrated multidisciplinary weight–loss programs, which include the child's family as well, are the most effective [9–11]. Reduction of fat mass is associated with normalization of metabolic parameters, such as inflammatory markers, lipid profile, insulin resistance and arterial blood pressure [12–14]. Therefore, early and efficient intervention increases likelihood of staying healthy in the future. As pharmacological and surgical interventions in children are limited [15–17], trials looking for substances supporting lifestyle interventions were run, looking at several different dietary supplements, hers (green tea, yerba mate), DHA (docosahexaenoic acid) among others [18–22]. Vitamin D was also studied in regards to its possible impact on body mass reduction and metabolic changes in adults and children with obesity [23,24].

The role of vitamin D in energetic metabolism has been emphasized recently. Obese children frequently present with low blood concentrations of vitamin D [25–27]. This probably results from lower dietary intake of this vitamin by obese individuals on the one hand, and less outdoor physical activity on the other [28–30]. Moreover, a higher percentage of fat mass is associated with a lower blood concentration of vitamin D, which may, at least partially, result from its sequestration in adipose tissue [31]. Animal experiments with labelled vitamin D showed that this vitamin is accumulated in adipose tissue and slowly released to blood [32].

Consequently, a vitamin D deficiency in obese children seems to be associated with a significant increase of risk of many metabolic disorders associated with obesity, such as insulin resistance, hyperinsulinemia, impaired tolerance of glucose, abnormal fasting plasma glucose, symptomatic diabetes mellitus, lipid disorders and cardiovascular morbidity, namely arterial hypertension [5,6]. There is a number of observational studies which demonstrate the substantial role of vitamin D deficiency in developing metabolic syndrome and other complications of obesity [33–35]. However, we lack interventional studies to link these observations to demonstrate a causal relationship.

In this study we wanted to assess the influence of 26 weeks of vitamin D supplementation in overweight and obese children undergoing an integrated 12–months' long weight loss program on body mass reduction, body composition and bone mineral density [36].

2. Materials and Methods

Detailed information about the study protocol, participants and design of the interventional program has been previously published [36]. All study participants were recruited from "6–10–14 for Health" program run by University Clinical Center in Gdansk, Poland. The program is a multidisciplinary, interventional program dedicated to children aged 6–15 and their parents. All school children in Gdansk aged 6–15 are screened in a 3–4–year–interval by dedicated teams (pediatrician and or nurses). All children with BMI centile above 85th centile are invited to the "6–10–14 for Health" program. All participants of the "6–10–14 for Health" program and their family members (parents/caregivers) were offered 12–month integrated intervention, including individual medical (pediatric), dietetic, physical activity and psychological counselling, during one meeting (4 x 20–25min). This intervention was offered to all the participants in a 0–3–6–12 month scheme.

2.1. Trial Design

A double–blind placebo–controlled trial. Vitamin D deficient patients (<30 ng/ml level of vitamin D) participating in multidisciplinary weight program were randomized to two arms (1:1 ratio): receiving vitamin D (1200 IU) or placebo for the first 26 weeks of the intervention.

We hypothesized that the supplementation with vitamin D in obese children showing low serum 25(OH)D3 during weight–loss program could positively influence body mass index (BMI), muscle mass, bone mass and mineral density and biochemical markers of metabolic complications related to obesity compared to placebo.

The study was conducted at the Department of Paediatrics, Paediatric Gastroenterology, Allergology and Children Nutrition, the Medical University of Gdansk and within the framework of "6–10–14 for Health" Interventional Programme, University Clinical Centre in Gdansk.

2.2. Participants

Eligible participants were children aged 6, 9–11 and 14, according to the "6–10–14 for Health" program protocol:

Inclusion criteria: overweight (BMI ≥ 85th < 95th percentile) or obesity (BMI ≥ 95th percentile), identified on the basis of anthropometric parameters using Polish reference centile charts—OLAF project [37]; blood concentration of 25(OH)D3 < 30 ng/ml; written informed consent of legal caregivers.

Exclusion criteria: Chronic conditions (asthma or allergies, inflammatory diseases of connective tissue, gastrointestinal disorders, diseases of kidneys and liver, disorders of bone metabolism); contraindications to administration of vitamin D; administration of any preparation containing vitamin D, calcium, or steroid hormones during three months preceding the study.

2.3. Ethics Approval and Consent to Participate

The study is approved by Independent Bioethics Committee for Scientific Research at Medical University of Gdansk, Poland, [NKBBN/130–206/2015] dated 25.05.2015. The parents/caregivers gave their written consent before the start of any study procedure. The study protocol was peer reviewed by financial supporter (Fundacja Nutricia) independent commission, during the grant application process. Trial registration no: NCT 02828228; trial registration date: 8 June 2016 registered in: ClinicalTrials.gov.

2.4. Study Procedure

The study period covered four appointments within the "6–10–14 for Health" obesity management program at the 0, 3, 6 and 12 month mark. All visits included individual meetings with a pediatrician, dietician, physical activity specialist and psychologist. All child/parent dyads had individual meetings with all 4 specialists—one directly after other. Detailed information about the program can be found in previous publications [36]. During the first appointment, the caregivers of all children were asked to provide written consent to the child taking part in the trial. Refusal to participate in the trial did not influence participation in the interventional obesity management program. Children with low blood concentration of 25(OH)D3 (<30 ng/ml) were referred for DXA (dual–energy x–ray absorptiometry) within two weeks from the starting visit.

The enrolled subjects were randomly assigned to one of the two groups using computer generated randomization tables. Then participants were randomly assigned to one of the two trial groups:

- GROUP I (Vitamin D group): medical intervention, intervention of dietician, psychologist and physical education specialist, parental education + oral administration of vitamin D3 (1200 i.u. daily) for 26 weeks
- GROUP II (Placebo group): medical intervention, intervention of dietician, psychologist and physical education specialist, parental education + daily oral administration of placebo for 26 weeks.

Study time line chart is shown in Figure 1.

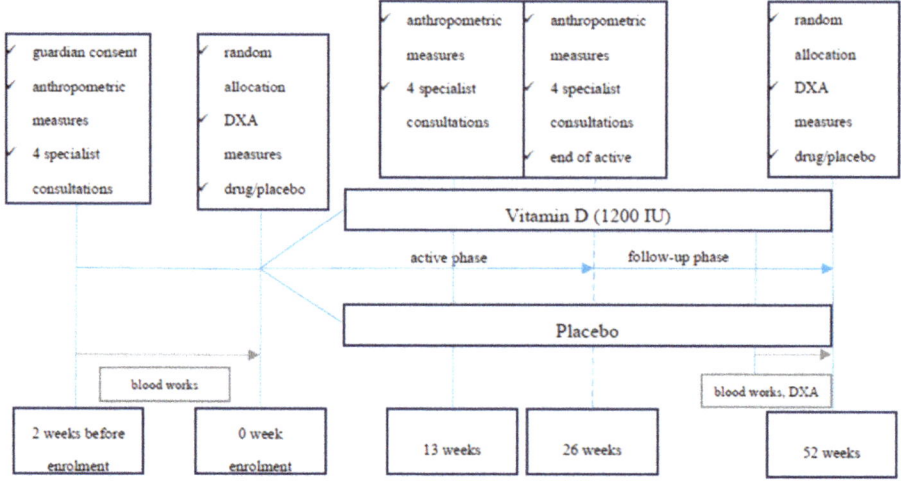

Figure 1. Patients' time line in the study.

2.5. Randomization and Blinding

The randomization list was generated by Office of Clinical and Scientific Research, University Clinical Centre (OCSR UCK), with no clinical involvement in the trial, via a computer program (StatsDirect) with an allocation ratio of 1:1 and with a block of 6. The allocation sequence was concealed from the researchers responsible for enrolling and assessing participants. Throughout the duration of the study, all investigators, participants, outcome assessors, and data analysts were blinded to the assigned treatment. Allocation to groups and drug/placebo distribution was performed by an independent researcher (M.S–F) not directly involved in the interventional program.

2.6. Treatment Dispensing and Assessment of Compliance

Both of the study treatments: vitamin D (1200 IU) and placebo were provided by the company (Sequoia) in identical capsules and packages (5 capsules in one blister, 6 blisters in a box). The sets of 7 boxes (6 months treatment) were prepared and blinded by Office of Clinical and Scientific Research, University Clinical Centre. Study treatment was dispensed by the investigator at the enrolment visit. At the final visit the sets of blisters and boxes were retrieved from the patient. The number of remaining capsules were documented to assess the compliance.

2.7. Outcome Measures

Primary endpoint: Change in BMI, BMI centile after 26 weeks of vitamin D supplementation. Secondary endpoints: change in body composition and bone mineral density and vitamin D level after 26 weeks of vitamin D supplementation. Additionally, we assessed changes in blood level of vitamin D.

2.8. Sample Size

Assuming probability of the event (at least 10% reduction in baseline BMI over the follow–up period) at 0.85 and 0.6 for the experimental and control group, respectively, minimum sample size providing 0.9 statistical power for alpha equal 0.05 or lower and beta equal 0.1 or lower was estimated at 130 (65 per group).

2.9. Statistical Analysis

Normal distribution of continuous variables was verified with the Shapiro–Wilk test. Descriptive statistics are presented as the mean or median and standard deviation from the mean. Between groups comparisons were carried out using the Mann–Whitney U test. Nonparametric tests were chosen because of the large number of significant Shapiro tests, which were used for normality assumption assessment. All statistical tests were two–tailed and performed at the 5% level of significance. All analyses were performed on the intention–to–treat basis, in which all of the participants in a trial are analyzed according to the intervention to which they were assigned, analyzing only participants who completed the whole weight management intervention program. Statistical analyses were performed with the Statistica 13 (TIBCO Software Inc., Tulsa, USA 2017).

3. Results

After obtaining and verifying the correctness of the recorded data (cross-checked with source data of 30% of patients), the data was decoded according to the protocol received from OCSR UCK in Gdansk.

After decoding, a full analysis of available anthropometric data and the results of densitometric examination was performed for patients divided into groups—receiving placebo and vitamin D.

A total of 170 patients were eligible for enrolment in the study during the enrolment period. A total of 152 patients were eventually included in the study ($n = 8$—no parental consent, $n = 10$—vitamin D intake during three months before the study). Subsequently the patients were randomly assigned to groups: 67 to the placebo group and 85 to the Vitamin D group. Out of the 152 qualified patients, 109 (72%) completed a full cycle of four visits scheduled in the program. In the placebo group, 64 patients completed the active phase of 26 weeks of supplementation, 53 completed the comprehensive treatment program (52 week duration).

The patient flow is shown in Figure 2.

Basic demographic and clinical data for both groups are presented in Table 1.

Table 1. Basic anthropometric and clinical data of studied groups (vitamin D and placebo) at visit 1.

	vitamin D ($n = 85$)		placebo ($n = 67$)		p
	Mean ± SD	(95% CI)	Mean ± SD	CI (−95%)	
age (years)	11.10 ± 2.84	10.49–11.72	10.70 ± 3.13	9.92–11.47	0.389
body mass (kg)	59.01 ± 21.04	54.47–63.55	56.89 ± 20.08	52.00–61.9	0.706
height (cm)	150.79 ± 16.69	147.19–154.39	149.31 ± 18.29	144.85–153.77	0.660
BMI	24.97 ± 4.12	24.08–25.86	24.53 ± 3.57	23.66–25.41	0.759
BMI centile	95.18 ± 3.24	94.49–95.88	95.23 ±3.43	94.41–96.06	0.812
no. of girls at visit 1	46		38		0.827
% of girls at visit 1	54.12%		56.72%		

$p < 0.05$ Mann–Whitney U test analysis.

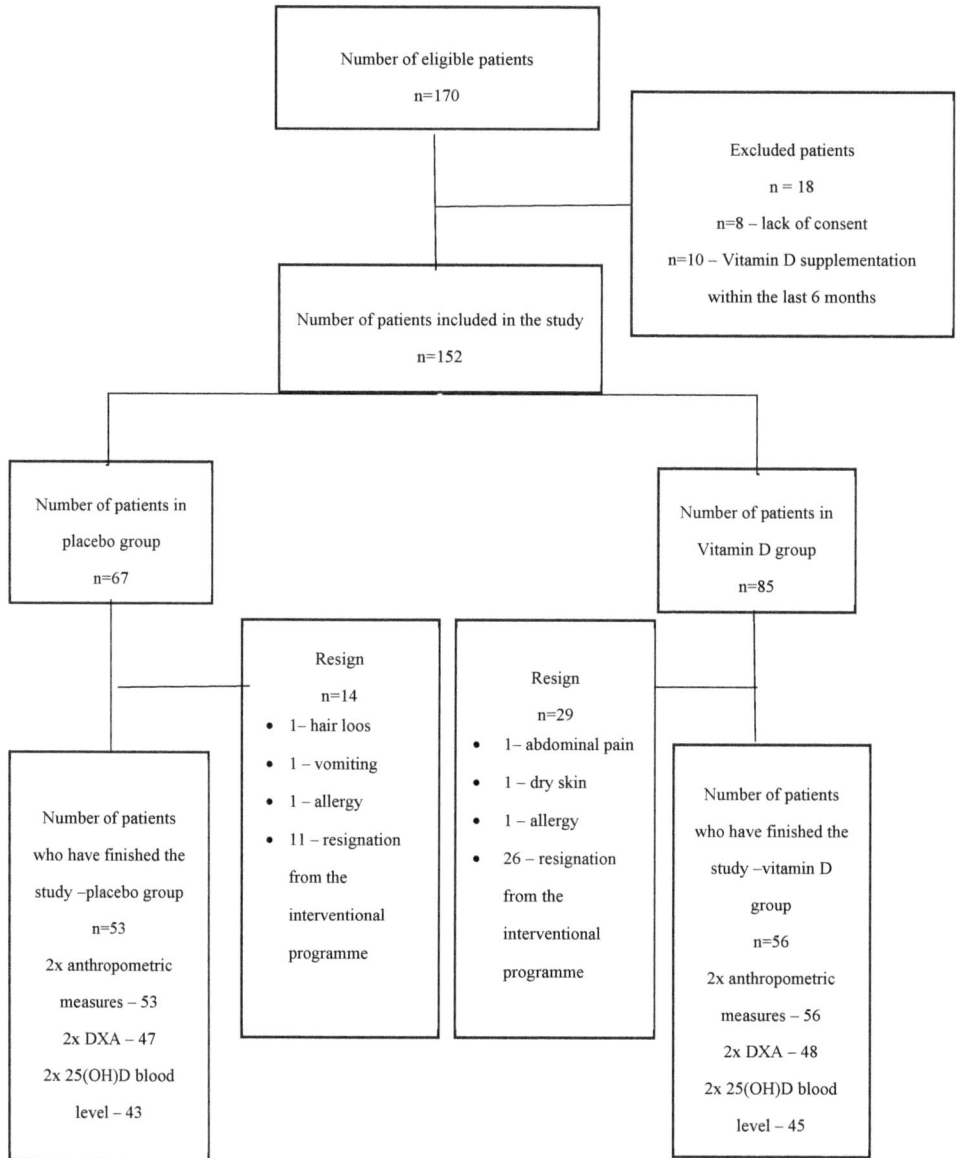

Figure 2. Patient flowchart in the study

There were no statistically significant differences between the vitamin D and placebo groups at the start of the study.

The differences between the groups in terms of main endpoints were subsequently assessed. The results of basic anthropometric and 25(OH)D concentration tests are shown in Table 2.

Table 2. Results of basic anthropometric and 25(OH)D concentration tests in studied groups.

Variable		vitamin D			placebo		
	No	Mean ± SD	95% CI	No	Mean ±	95% CI	p
BMI visit 1	85	24.97 ± 4.12	24.08–25.86	67	24.53 ± 3.58	23.66–25.41	0.759
BMI visit 4	56	24.33 ± 3.97	23.27–25.39	53	24.68 ± 3.46	23.73–25.64	0.479
ΔBMI visit 4–1	56	−0.46 ± 1.80	−0.94–0.03	53	0.11 ±1.84	−0.40–0.61	0.203
BMI centile 1 visit	85	95.18 ± 3.22	94.49–95.88	67	95.23 ± 3.39	94.41–96.06	0.812
BMI centile 4 visit	56	90.91 ± 9.40	88.39–93.43	53	92.64 ± 7.53	90.56–94.71	0.303
Δ in BMI centiles visit 4–1	56	−4.28 ± 8.43	−6.54–−2.03	53	−2.53 ± 6.10	−4.21–−0.85	0.319
25 (OH) D level visit 1	85	19.35 ± 5.46	18.16–20.55	66	19.79 ± 5.15	18.52–21.06	0.622 *
25 (OH) D level visit 4	45	24.99 ± 5.54	23.33–26.66	43	18.3 ± 6.70	16.25–20.37	0.000 *
Δ 25 (OH) level visit 4–1	45	6.06 ± 5.80	4.32–7.81	43	−2.40 ± 5.97	−4.24–−0.57	0.000 *

$p < 0.05$ Mann–Whitney U test, * t–student test for independent samples.

The results of bioelectric impedance measurements are shown in Table 3.

Table 3. Results of bioelectric impedance measurements in studied groups.

Variable		vitamin D			placebo		
	No	Mean	CI (–95%)	No	Mean	CI (–95%)	p
BI_FM (kg) visit 1	82	18.32 ± 8.01	16.56–20.08	64	17.80 ± 7.30	15.97–19.62	0.820
BI_FM (kg) visit 4	55	18.29 ± 8.07	16.11–20.47	53	18.13 ± 7.18	16.15–20.11	0.907
Δ BI_FM (kg) visit 4–1	54	−0.11 ± 4.09	−1.23–1.00	51	0.01 ± 4.01	−1.11–1.14	0.890
BI_FM (%) visit 1	54	31.15 ± 4.90	29.81–32.48	51	31.23 ± 5.91	29.57–32.89	0.741
BI_FM (%) visit 4	54	29.57 ± 6.03	27.92–31.21	51	29.39 ± 6.95	27.44–31.35	0.889*
Δ BI_FM (%) visit 4–1	54	−1.58 ± 4.04	−2.68–0.47	51	−1.83 ± 4.56	−3.12–−0.55	0.951
BI_MM (kg) visit 1	82	38.46 ± 14.00	35.39–41.54	64	37.10 ± 13.65	33.69–40.51	0.586
BI_MM (kg) visit 4	56	40.12 ± 12.85	36.68–43.56	53	40.80 ± 12.92	37.24–44.36	0.886
Δ BI_MM (kg) visit 4–1	55	2.45 ±2.57	1.75–3.14	51	3.33 ± 2.75	2.56–4.10	0.091 *
BI_MM (%) visit 1	82	65.69 ±5.39	64.50–66.87	64	65.48 ± 5.03	64.22–66.73	0.350
BI_MM (%) visit 4	56	66.63 ±5.68	65.11–68.16	53	66.81 ± 6.52	65.01–68.61	0.896
Δ BI_MM (%) visit 4–1	55	1.42 ±4.02	0.33–2.51	51	1.48 ± 3.72	0.43–2.53	0.949

$p < 0.05$ Mann–Whitney U test, * t–student test for independent samples. BI—bioimpedance, FM—fat mass, Δ –delta–difference, MM—muscle mass.

The results of the dual X–ray absorptiometry (DXA) measurements are presented in Table 4.

Table 4. Results of dual X–ray absorptiometry (DXA) measurements in studied groups.

		Vitamin D			Placebo		
	No	Mean	CI (–95%)	No	Mean	CI (–95%)	p
Sp BMD visit 1	83	0.76 ± 0.18	0.72–0.80	67	0.74 ± 0.18	0.70–0.79	0.447
Sp BMD visit 4	47	0.82 ± 0.19	0.76–0.87	47	0.80 ± 0.19	0.75–0.86	0.623
Δ in Sp BMD visit 4–1	47	0.04 ± 0.04	0.03–0.06	47	0.06 ± 0.04	0.05–0.08	0.025 *
TBLH BMD visit 1	83	0.87 ± 0.14	0.84–0.90	67	0.86 ± 0.15	0.82–0.89	0.672
TBLH BMD visit 4	48	0.91 ± 0.14	0.87–0.95	47	0.90 ± 0.15	0.86–0.94	0.740
Δ in TBLH BMD visit 4–1	48	0.04± 0.03	0.04–0.05	47	0.04 ± 0.03	0.03–0.05	0.504*
TFM (kg) visit 1	83	25.18 ± 9.76	23.05–27.31	67	24.29 ± 9.08	22.08–26.51	0.652
TFM (kg) visit 4	48	25.17 ± 8.72	22.63–27.70	47	25.07 ± 8.96	22.44–27.70	0.959*
Δ in TFM visit 4–1	48	0.73 ±4.55	−0.59–2.05	47	0.68 ± 4.96	−0.77–2.14	0.734
TLM (kg) visit 1	83	32.52 ± 4.55	30.04–34.99	67	31.83 ± 10.94	29.16–34.50	0.823
TLM (kg) visit 4	48	34.41 ± 10.33	31.41–37.42	47	34.48 ± 12.19	30.90–38.06	0.976 *
TFM (%) visit 1	48	43.46 ± 3.82	42.35–44.57	47	43.30 ± 4.42	42.00–44.60	0.847
TFM (%) visit 4	48	41.89 ± 5.29	40.35–43.43	47	42.32 ± 5.50	40.71–43.94	0.695
Δ in TFM (%) visit 4–1	48	−1.57 ± 4.12	−2.77–0.38	47	−0.98 ± 3.97	−2.14–0.19	0.472 *
TLM (%) visit 1	48	56.54 ± 3.82	55.43–57.65	47	56.70 ± 4.42	55.40–58.00	0.847
TLM (%) visit 4	48	58.11 ± 5.29	56.57–59.65	47	57.68 ± 5.50	56.06–59.29	0.695
Δ in TLM (%) visit 4–1	48	1.57 ± 4.12	0.38–2.77	47	0.98 ± 3.97	−0.19–2.14	0.472

$p < 0.05$ Mann–Whitney U test, * t–student test for independent samples. Sp—spine, BMD—bone mineral density, Δ—delta–difference, TBLH—total body less head, TFM—total fat mass, TLM—total lean mass.

Both groups had a reduction in BMI centiles. Although the reduction was greater in the vitamin D vs. placebo group (−4.28 ± 8.43 vs. −2.53 ±6.10) the difference was not statistically significant ($p = 0.319$). Similarly the reduction in fat mass—assessed both using bioimpedance and DEXa was achieved, yet the differences between the groups were not statistically significant, as shown in Tables 3 and 4.

The analysis showed statistically significant differences between the groups only in 25(OH) D3 concentration in the measurements taken after the supplementation period (24.99 vs. 16.25; $p = 0.000$) and in the difference between second and first measurement of vitamin D levels (6.06 vs. −4.24; $p = 0.000$), and in the difference between second and first measurement of bone mineral density in the spine (Sp BMD) (0.04 vs. 0.06; $p < 0.0256$). The difference was higher in the placebo group.

There was no difference between the placebo group and the vitamin D group in BMI reduction, BMI centile, fat tissue in kg, % of fat tissue (assessed both by performing BIA and densitometry analysis).

Additionally, we have performed an analysis of correlations (Spearman rank correlation coefficient) between vitamin D levels at Visit 1 and 4 and changes of vitamin D level between the visits dependent on several anthropometric variables. Results are presented in Table 5.

Table 5. Correlation between vitamin D levels and anthropometric variables.

	25 (OH) D Level Visit 1	25 (OH) D Level Visit 4	Δ 25 (OH) Level Visit 4–1
BMI centile 1 visit	−0.088910	**−0.232998**	−0.066400
BMI centile 4 visit	−0.128452	**−0.297140**	−0.147392
Δ in BMI centiles visit 4–1	−0.059634	−0.141315	−0.138827
BI_FM (%) visit 1	**−0.248164**	**−0.238226**	−0.020100
BI_FM (%) visit 4	**−0.213330**	**−0.226632**	−0.019981
Δ BI_FM (%) visit 4–1	0.073786	−0.013645	−0.058235
BI_MM (%) visit 1	**0.214256**	0.202164	−0.005444
BI_MM (%) visit 4	**0.204376**	**0.233062**	0.045692
Δ BI_MM (%) visit 4–1	−0.077210	0.057706	0.107305
25 (OH) D level visit 1	1.000000	**0.322476**	**−0.426874**
25 (OH) D level visit 4	**0.322476**	1.000000	**0.692743**
Δ 25 (OH) level visit 4–1	**−0.426874**	**0.692743**	1.000000
TBLH BMD visit 1	**−0.357821**	−0.164349	0.102925
TBLH BMD visit 4	**−0.377036**	−0.222562	0.012532
Δ in TBLH BMD visit 4–1	0.079692	0.007924	−0.047583
TFM (%) visit 1	−0.177243	−0.206046	−0.111781
TFM (%) visit 4	−0.035164	−0.122583	−0.069020
Δ in TFM (%) visit 2–1	0.174996	−0.008749	−0.047612
TLM (%) visit 1	0.177243	0.206046	0.111781
TLM (%) visit 4	0.035164	0.122583	0.069020
Δ in TLM (%) visit 4–1	−0.174996	0.008749	0.047612

Spearman rank correlation coefficient; bolded when $p < 0.05$, BI—bioimpedance, FM—fat mass, Δ—delta–difference, MM—muscle mass, BMD—bone mineral density, TBLH—total body less head, TFM—total fat mass, TLM—total lean mass.

The results show that there were no important correlation between the initial BMI centile and vitamin D level at the first visit. Additionally the correlation did not show any significant influence of BMI changes on changes in vitamin D level after the supplementation period. There were significant negative correlations ($p < 0.05$) between fat mass % and levels of vitamin D during both visits—which can confirm the relation between the fat mass and blood level of vitamin D. Yet this was a rather weak correlation (−0.25 to −0.21). Further, it was not confirmed in DXA measurements.

4. Discussion

4.1. Effect of Vitamin D Supplementation on Body Mass Reduction

Presented study is the first randomized trial to assess potential effects of vitamin D supplementation in body mass reduction in overweight and obese children. Results of present study show that supplementation of vitamin D did not have a statistically significant, put potentially clinically important, influence on body mass (BMI, BMI centile) body composition or bone mineral density comparing to placebo groups during an organized obesity management program in children.

Biological role of vitamin D in etiopathogenesis of metabolic syndrome represents an interesting issue. Previous studies conducted among children revealed inverse relationship between blood concentration of vitamin D and waist circumference, systolic blood pressure, insulin resistance, fasting glucose, total cholesterol, triglycerides and LDL cholesterol, as well as positive association between the concentration of vitamin D and HDL cholesterol [25,38,39]. It seems that vitamin D can interfere with secretion of insulin both directly—binding to its receptors [VDR] on pancreatic β cells, and indirectly by modulating concentration of calcium in extracellular space [40].

Importantly, a positive association between the concentration of vitamin D and sensitivity to insulin was observed in obese children, along with an inverse relationship between the level of this vitamin and concentration of glycated hemoglobin (HbA1c) [41]. Supplementation with vitamin D in obese adolescents resulted in decrease of insulin resistance, while levels of inflammatory markers [CRP, TNF–α, IL–6] remained unchanged [42]. Till now, to the best of our knowledge, no studies were carried out in children or adolescents regarding the effects of vitamin D supplementation on body mass reduction during an organized lifestyle modification program. As we presented, adding a 1200 IU/day dose of vitamin D did not lead to higher changes in BMI (BMI centile) or fat mass as well as fat free mass changes in children aged 6–14. It needs to be stated that the results presented show that although there was a reduction in BMI in vitamin D group compared to placebo group (–0.46 ± 1.80 vs. 0.11 ±1.84) and BMI centiles also showed higher reduction in children supplemented with vitamin D (–4.28 ± 8.43 vs. –2.53 ±6.10) none of those results was statistically significant ($p = 0.203$ and $p = 0.319$ respectively). Similar results can be found in bioimpedance measurements, but not DXA assessment. Presented results would be presented as clinically valid. Although this 26-week long supplementation had an influence on blood concentration level of 25(OH) D in the active treatment group, only 6 out of all patients reached a level above 30 ng/ml in the final assessment (2 in the placebo group) 52 weeks after the start of the intervention. This shows that vitamin D can potentially have an impact on weight loss level but possibly due to resignation ratio or sample size we were not able to show that effect.

As previous studies in adolescents and adults showed, low (~1000 IU/daily) or high doses (up to 300,000 IU/month) of vitamin D supplementation have a very mixed results in influencing changes in fat mass, free fat mass or muscle mass [43–45]. Data regarding effect of vitamin D supplementation on body mass/body fat changes are limited to studies and meta–analyses/ reviews regarding adults with wide range of interventions (medical weight loss, bariatric surgery, low–caloric diet) were used together with vitamin D supplementation. Additionally those studies were focused on finding the optimal dose of supplementation to reach the optimal (>30 ng/l) level of vitamin D [44] or assessing the association of vitamin level and body fat. Meta-analysis of studies in obese adults showed that although there was an impact of vitamin D supplementation on body fat, the results were not statistically significant [43]. This study also acknowledges that the impact of vitamin D supplementation on body fat reduction has a linear effect up to 2000 IU/d, with no benefits in increasing the dose in adults. The only review regarding impact of vitamin D supplementation on bone mineral density was focused on general population—as no studies was directly focused on overweight/obese children. In addition, no sub–analysis was performed to show the effect depending on body mass. Winzenberg states that the impact of vitamin D supplementation can be higher in vitamin D deficient children, but the effect is small—in most studies standardized mean difference between groups was small (<0,3) [45]. Yet all of these measures are only proxy measures to changes in body weight as a primary outcome of supplementation of vitamin D in obese children/adolescents. As for now, no studies have demonstrated effectiveness of such a strategy for supporting body fat reduction throughout a long–term interventional process.

4.2. Effect of Vitamin D Supplementation on Bone Mineral Density During Weight Loss

Metabolic effects of obesity on growth and maturation of bones are still not fully understood. Moreover, the results of previous studies analyzing bone mass and density in obese individuals are highly inconclusive. While some authors claimed a decrease in bone mass relative to body weight [46], others did not document significant differences in bone mineral density [47] or showed an increase in body mass and bone size in obese children, adolescents and adults. Increased bone mass and density observed in obese individuals is postulated to be a response to greater mechanical load, direct influence of leptin or enhanced enzymatic activity of aromatase [48,49]. Nevertheless, obesity markedly increases the risk of bone fractures in children [50]. Vitamin D plays important biological role in the process of bone maturation and mineralization. Previous studies documented an inverse relationship between blood concentration of vitamin D and bone mineral density [51,52]. One meta–analysis revealed that supplementation of vitamin D can improve both bone mineral density and bone mass in individuals with low blood levels of this vitamin [45]. The effects of supplementation are particularly favorable in premenarcheal girls with normal body weight, in whom administration of vitamin D resulted in increases of both bone mass and fat–free mass [53]. An analysis of 58 morbidly obese teenagers showed that individuals with physiological blood concentration of PTH (parathyroid hormone) have normal bone mineral density, irrespectively of their vitamin D levels [54]. In contrast, a recently published study involving a small group of adolescents with obesity ($n = 24$) and normal body weight ($n = 25$) showed that obese people present with higher bone mineral density, irrespectively their blood concentration of vitamin D and despite lower level of physical activity than their normal-weight peers. Moreover, the differences in bone mineral density turned out to be independent from fat-free mass content. Furthermore, bone mineral density was associated with blood concentrations of leptin and insulin [55]. Our study shows clearly that we can observe an increase of bone mineral density both spinal and subtotal BMD with body mass reduction. Yet there is no impact of vitamin D supplementation on the level of bone density assessed using DXA. This shows that the body mass reduction itself impacts the bone mineralization the most.

Apart from many unquestioned favorable health effects of losing excessive weight, this process may also be associated with enhanced bone turnover and decrease in bone mineral density. In recently published systemic review, the decrease of bone mass was reported following calorie-restricting diet but not in exercise–induced weight-loss [56]. However, this evidence originates mostly from studies conducted among adults [57–59], and to the best of our knowledge, the issue in question was a subject of only one study of adolescents after bariatric surgeries [60]. The results from previous intervention studies suggest that a low-calorie albeit high-protein (ca. 30%) diet, containing high amounts of dairy products, can prevent the loss of bone mass and a decrease in bone mineralization [61]. Yet supplementation with high doses of vitamin D can have a negative effect on bone mineralization in adults—as a recent study by Burt et al. showed [62].

Study limitations:

This study has some limitations that need to be taken into account when assessing the usefulness of the results:

– Children aged 6–14 years old were included in the study—this is not a homogenic group when it comes to maturation/puberty status—and this has an impact on both the ability to decrease body mass and bone turnover and mineralization;

– We were giving one dose of vitamin D (1200 IU) to all participants independent the body mass and age, which could have result in less effective increase of 25(OH)D level, which in turn could have impacted the changes in body mass or bone mineral density;

– 26 weeks may be too short to establish the effects of vitamin D supplementation on the rate of skeletal mineralization

– There was an almost 30% drop–out, seen especially in the second part of the program—after finishing the active supplementation with vitamin D/placebo period. This was unlikely to be due to the treatment itself (as there were no important side effects registered). The level of lost to follow-up patients in the interventional program is similar to other such programs seen in Poland and other European countries [63,64].

– Finally, the sample sizes were smaller than anticipated and there is a possibility that with the estimated reduction of 10% of BMI reduction the study sample is underestimated. It is possible that the study was underpowered to detect smaller changes in BMI/BMI centiles as well as other parameters.

5. Conclusions

Available data on the efficacy of vitamin supplementation during weight loss are inconclusive and mostly limited to adults. Our study shows that there is a limited or no effect of vitamin D supplementation on body weight reduction in children and adolescents with vitamin D insufficiency. Being aware and understanding the potential limitation of our study—wide age group, one dose of vitamin D, small sample of the study we believe that further research in this field is needed.

Author Contributions: M.B. participated in the study design and coordination of the study, performed the statistical data analysis, drafted the paper and revised and approved the manuscript; A.J., M.S.-F., P.M., and P.W. participated in the study design, patient recruitment, data collection, revised and approved the manuscript; P.S. participated in the study design and revised and approved the manuscript; A.S.-S. participated in the study design and coordination of the study, data analysis, drafted, revised and approved the manuscript. All authors have read and agreed to the published version of the manuscript.

Funding: The study was awarded a financial grant from a charitable foundation (Fundacja Nutricia) Grant no RG–1/2015. The Fundacja Nutricia did not take part in any element of study design or study realization such as the study design or; collection, management, analysis, and interpretation of data; writing of the report; and the decision to submit the report for publication.

Acknowledgments: All authors would like to sincerely thank all participant, parents and members of the "6–10–14 for Health" team for their input into the study. Authors would also like to thank University Clinical Centre administration for help in performing the study.

Conflicts of Interest: The authors declare no conflicts of interest.

References

1. Bentham, J.; Di Cesare, M.; Bilano, V.; Bixby, H.; Zhou, B.; Stevens, G.A.; Riley, L.M.; Taddei, C.; Hajifathalian, K.; Lu, Y.; et al. Worldwide trends in body-mass index, underweight, overweight, and obesity from 1975 to 2016: A pooled analysis of 2416 population-based measurement studies in 128·9 million children, adolescents, and adults. *Lancet* **2017**, *390*, 2627–2642.
2. Ng, M.; Fleming, T.; Robinson, M.; Thomson, B.; Graetz, N.; Margono, C.; Mullany, E.C.; Biryukov, S.; Abbafati, C.; Abera, S.F.; et al. Global, regional, and national prevalence of overweight and obesity in children and adults during 1980–2013: A systematic analysis for the Global Burden of Disease Study 2013. *Lancet* **2014**, *384*, 766–781. [CrossRef]
3. Bann, D.; Johnson, W.; Li, L.; Kuh, D.; Hardy, R. Socioeconomic inequalities in childhood and adolescent body-mass index, weight, and height from 1953 to 2015: An analysis of four longitudinal, observational, British birth cohort studies. *Lancet Public Health* **2018**, *3*, e194–e203. [CrossRef]
4. Kumar, S.; Kelly, A.S. Review of Childhood Obesity: From Epidemiology, Etiology, and Comorbidities to Clinical Assessment and Treatment. *Mayo Clin. Proc.* **2017**, *92*, 251–265. [CrossRef] [PubMed]
5. Kelly, A.S.; Barlow, S.E.; Rao, G.; Inge, T.H.; Hayman, L.L.; Steinberger, J.; Urbina, E.M.; Ewing, L.J.; Daniels, S.R. Severe obesity in children and adolescents: Identification, associated health risks, and treatment approaches: A scientific statement from the American Heart Association. *Circulation* **2013**, *128*, 1689–1712. [CrossRef] [PubMed]
6. Kinlen, D.; Cody, D.; O'Shea, D. Complications of obesity. *QJM An Int. J. Med.* **2018**, *111*, 437–443. [CrossRef]
7. Di Angelantonio, E.; Bhupathiraju, S.; Wormser, D.; Gao, P.; Kaptoge, S.; Berrington de Gonzalez, A.; Cairns, B.; Huxley, R.; Jackson, C.; et al.; Global BMI Mortality Collaboration Body-mass index and all-cause mortality: Individual-participant-data meta-analysis of 239 prospective studies in four continents. *Lancet* **2016**, *388*, 776–786. [CrossRef]

8. Brown, T.; Moore, T.H.; Hooper, L.; Gao, Y.; Zayegh, A.; Ijaz, S.; Elwenspoek, M.; Foxen, S.C.; Magee, L.; O'Malley, C.; et al. Interventions for preventing obesity in children. *Cochrane Database Syst. Rev.* **2019**, *2019*. [CrossRef]
9. Nemet, D.; Levi, L.; Pantanowitz, M.; Eliakim, A. A combined nutritional-behavioral-physical activity intervention for the treatment of childhood obesity—A 7-year summary. *J. Pediatr. Endocrinol. Metab.* **2014**, *27*, 445–451. [CrossRef]
10. Oude Luttikhuis, H.; Baur, L.; Jansen, H.; Shrewsbury, V.A.; O'Malley, C.; Stolk, R.P.; Summerbell, C.D. Interventions for treating obesity in children. *Cochrane Database Syst. Rev.* **2019**, *3*, CD001872. [CrossRef]
11. Masquio, D.C.L.; De Piano, A.; Campos, R.M.S.; Sanches, P.L.; Carnier, J.; Corgosinho, F.C.; Netto, B.D.M.; Carvalho-Ferreira, J.P.; Oyama, L.M.; Nascimento, C.M.O.; et al. The role of multicomponent therapy in the metabolic syndrome, inflammation and cardiovascular risk in obese adolescents. *Br. J. Nutr.* **2015**, *113*, 1920–1930. [CrossRef] [PubMed]
12. Ferreira, Y.A.M.; Kravchychyn, A.C.P.; Vicente, S.d.C.F.; Campos, R.M.d.S.; Tock, L.; Oyama, L.M.; Boldarine, V.T.; Masquio, D.C.L.; Thivel, D.; Shivappa, N.; et al. An interdisciplinary weight loss program improves body composition and metabolic profile in adolescents with obesity: Associations with the dietary inflammatory index. *Front. Nutr.* **2019**, *6*, 77. [CrossRef] [PubMed]
13. Reinehr, T. Calculating cardiac risk in obese adolescents before and after onset of lifestyle intervention. *Expert Rev. Cardiovasc. Ther.* **2013**, *11*, 297–306. [CrossRef] [PubMed]
14. Masquio, D.C.L.; De Piano, A.; Sanches, P.L.; Corgosinho, F.C.; Campos, R.M.S.; Carnier, J.; Da Silva, P.L.; Caranti, D.A.; Tock, L.; Oyama, L.M.; et al. The effect of weight loss magnitude on pro-/anti-inflammatory adipokines and carotid intima-media thickness in obese adolescents engaged in interdisciplinary weight loss therapy. *Clin. Endocrinol.* **2013**, *79*, 55–64. [CrossRef]
15. Cuda, S.E.; Censani, M. Pediatric Obesity Algorithm: A Practical Approach to Obesity Diagnosis and Management. *Front. Pediatr.* **2019**, *6*, 431. [CrossRef]
16. Boland, C.L.; Harris, J.B.; Harris, K.B. Pharmacological Management of Obesity in Pediatric Patients. *Ann. Pharmacother.* **2015**, *49*, 220–232. [CrossRef]
17. Domecq, J.P.; Prutsky, G.; Leppin, A.; Sonbol, M.B.; Altayar, O.; Undavalli, C.; Wang, Z.; Elraiyah, T.; Brito, J.P.; Mauck, K.F.; et al. Drugs commonly associated with weight change: A systematic review and meta-analysis. *J. Clin. Endocrinol. Metab.* **2015**, *100*, 363–370. [CrossRef]
18. Pooyandjoo, M.; Nouhi, M.; Shab-Bidar, S.; Djafarian, K.; Olyaeemanesh, A. The effect of (L-)carnitine on weight loss in adults: A systematic review and meta-analysis of randomized controlled trials. *Obes. Rev.* **2016**, *17*, 970–976. [CrossRef]
19. Huang, J.; Wang, Y.; Xie, Z.; Zhou, Y.; Zhang, Y.; Wan, X. The anti-obesity effects of green tea in human intervention and basic molecular studies. *Eur. J. Clin. Nutr.* **2014**, *68*, 1075–1087. [CrossRef]
20. Kim, S.Y.; Oh, M.R.; Kim, M.G.; Chae, H.J.; Chae, S.W. Anti-obesity effects of Yerba Mate (Ilex Paraguariensis): A randomized, double-blind, placebo-controlled clinical trial. *BMC Complement. Altern. Med.* **2015**, *15*, 338. [CrossRef]
21. Zalewski, B.M.; Szajewska, H. No Effect of Glucomannan on Body Weight Reduction in Children and Adolescents with Overweight and Obesity: A Randomized Controlled Trial. *J. Pediatr.* **2019**, *211*, 85–91. [CrossRef] [PubMed]
22. De Luis, D.; Domingo, J.C.; Izaola, O.; Casanueva, F.F.; Bellido, D.; Sajoux, I. Effect of DHA supplementation in a very low-calorie ketogenic diet in the treatment of obesity: A randomized clinical trial. *Endocrine* **2016**, *54*, 111–122. [CrossRef] [PubMed]
23. Lerchbaum, E.; Trummer, C.; Theiler-Schwetz, V.; Kollmann, M.; Wölfler, M.; Pilz, S.; Obermayer-Pietsch, B. Effects of vitamin D supplementation on body composition and metabolic risk factors in men: A randomized controlled trial. *Nutrients* **2019**, *11*, 1894. [CrossRef] [PubMed]
24. Al-Daghri, N.M.; Amer, O.E.; Khattak, M.N.K.; Sabico, S.; Ghouse Ahmed Ansari, M.; Al-Saleh, Y.; Aljohani, N.; Alfawaz, H.; Alokail, M.S. Effects of different vitamin D supplementation strategies in reversing metabolic syndrome and its component risk factors in adolescents. *J. Steroid Biochem. Mol. Biol.* **2019**, *191*, 105378. [CrossRef] [PubMed]
25. Aypak, C.; Türedi, Ö.; Yüce, A. The association of vitamin D status with cardiometabolic risk factors, obesity and puberty in children. *Eur. J. Pediatr.* **2014**, *173*, 367–373. [CrossRef]

26. Lee, D.Y.; Kwon, A.R.; Ahn, J.M.; Kim, Y.J.; Chae, H.W.; Kim, D.H.; Kim, H.-S. Relationship between serum 25-hydroxyvitamin D concentration and risks of metabolic syndrome in children and adolescents from Korean National Health and Nutrition Examination survey 2008–2010. *Ann. Pediatr. Endocrinol. Metab.* **2015**, *20*, 46. [CrossRef]
27. Voortman, T.; van den Hooven, E.H.; Heijboer, A.C.; Hofman, A.; Jaddoe, V.W.; Franco, O.H. Vitamin D Deficiency in School-Age Children Is Associated with Sociodemographic and Lifestyle Factors. *J. Nutr.* **2015**, *145*, 791–798. [CrossRef]
28. Kamycheva, E.; Joakimsen, R.M.; Jorde, R. Intakes of Calcium and Vitamin D Predict Body Mass Index in the Population of Northern Norway. *J. Nutr.* **2003**, *133*, 102–106. [CrossRef]
29. Pourshahidi, L.K. Vitamin D and obesity: Current perspectives and future directions. In Proceedings of the Nutrition Society; Cambridge University Press: Cambridge, UK, 2015; Volume 74, pp. 115–124.
30. Engberg, E.; Figueiredo, R.A.O.; Rounge, T.B.; Weiderpass, E.; Viljakainen, H. Heavy screen users are the heaviest among 10,000 children. *Sci. Rep.* **2019**, *9*, 11158. [CrossRef]
31. Pacifico, L.; Anania, C.; Osborn, J.F.; Ferraro, F.; Bonci, E.; Olivero, E.; Chiesa, C. Low 25(OH)D3 levels are associated with total adiposity, metabolic syndrome, and hypertension in Caucasian children and adolescents. *Eur. J. Endocrinol.* **2011**, *165*, 603–611. [CrossRef]
32. Rosenstreich, S.J.; Rich, C.; Volwiler, W. Deposition in and release of vitamin D3 from body fat: Evidence for a storage site in the rat. *J. Clin. Invest.* **1971**, *50*, 679–687. [CrossRef] [PubMed]
33. Fu, J.; Han, L.; Zhao, Y.; Li, G.; Zhu, Y.; Li, Y.; Li, M.; Gao, S.; Willi, S.M. Vitamin D levels are associated with metabolic syndrome in adolescents and young adults: The BCAMS study. *Clin. Nutr.* **2019**, *38*, 2161–2167. [CrossRef] [PubMed]
34. Denova-Gutiérrez, E.; Muñoz-Aguirre, P.; López, D.; Flores, M.; Medeiros, M.; Tamborrel, N.; Clark, P. Low serum vitamin D concentrations are associated with insulin resistance in Mexican children and adolescents. *Nutrients* **2019**, *11*, 2109. [CrossRef] [PubMed]
35. Mitri, J.; Nelson, J.; Ruthazer, R.; Garganta, C.; Nathan, D.M.; Hu, F.B.; Dawson-Hughes, B.; Pittas, A.G. Plasma 25-hydroxyvitamin D and risk of metabolic syndrome: An ancillary analysis in the Diabetes Prevention Program. *Eur. J. Clin. Nutr.* **2014**, *68*, 376–383. [CrossRef]
36. Szlagatys-Sidorkiewicz, A.; Brzeziński, M.; Jankowska, A.; Metelska, P.; Słomińska-Fraczek, M.; Socha, P. Long-term effects of vitamin D supplementation in vitamin D deficient obese children participating in an integrated weight-loss programme (a double-blind placebo-controlled study)—Rationale for the study design. *BMC Pediatr.* **2017**, *17*, 97. [CrossRef]
37. Kułaga, Z.; Litwin, M.; Tkaczyk, M.; Palczewska, I.; Zajączkowska, M.; Zwolińska, D.; Krynicki, T.; Wasilewska, A.; Moczulska, A.; Morawiec-Knysak, A.; et al. Polish 2010 growth references for school-aged children and adolescents. *Eur. J. Pediatr.* **2011**, *170*, 599–609. [CrossRef]
38. Reyman, M.; Verrijn Stuart, A.A.; Van Summeren, M.; Rakhshandehroo, M.; Nuboer, R.; De Boer, F.K.; Van Den Ham, H.J.; Kalkhoven, E.; Prakken, B.; Schipper, H.S. Vitamin D deficiency in childhood obesity is associated with high levels of circulating inflammatory mediators, and low insulin sensitivity. *Int. J. Obes.* **2014**, *38*, 46–52. [CrossRef]
39. Ganji, V.; Zhang, X.; Shaikh, N.; Tangpricha, V. Serum 25-hydroxyvitamin D concentrations are associated with prevalence of metabolic syndrome and various cardiometabolic risk factors in US children and adolescents based on assay-adjusted serum 25-hydroxyvitamin D data from NHANES 2001-2006. *Am. J. Clin. Nutr.* **2011**, *94*, 225–233. [CrossRef]
40. Song, Y.; Wang, L.; Pittas, A.G.; Del Gobbo, L.C.; Zhang, C.; Manson, J.E.; Hu, F.B. Blood 25-Hydroxy Vitamin D Levels and Incident Type 2 Diabetes. *Diabetes Care* **2013**, *36*, 1422–1428. [CrossRef]
41. Alemzadeh, R.; Kichler, J.; Babar, G.; Calhoun, M. Hypovitaminosis D in obese children and adolescents: Relationship with adiposity, insulin sensitivity, ethnicity, and season. *Metabolism* **2008**, *57*, 183–191. [CrossRef]
42. Belenchia, A.M.; Tosh, A.K.; Hillman, L.S.; Peterson, C.A. Correcting vitamin D insufficiency improves insulin sensitivity in obese adolescents: A randomized controlled trial. *Am. J. Clin. Nutr.* **2013**, *97*, 774–781. [CrossRef] [PubMed]
43. Golzarand, M.; Hollis, B.W.; Mirmiran, P.; Wagner, C.L.; Shab-Bidar, S. Vitamin D supplementation and body fat mass: A systematic review and meta-analysis. *Eur. J. Clin. Nutr.* **2018**, *72*, 1345–1357. [CrossRef]
44. Bassatne, A.; Chakhtoura, M.; Saad, R.; Fuleihan, G.E.H. Vitamin D supplementation in obesity and during weight loss: A review of randomized controlled trials. *Metabolism* **2019**, *92*, 193–205. [CrossRef] [PubMed]

45. Winzenberg, T.; Powell, S.; Shaw, K.A.; Jones, G. Effects of vitamin D supplementation on bone density in healthy children: Systematic review and meta-analysis. *BMJ* **2011**, *342*, 267. [CrossRef] [PubMed]
46. Goulding, A.; Taylor, R.W.; Jones, I.E.; McAuley, K.A.; Manning, P.J.; Williams, S.M. Overweight and obese children have low bone mass and area for their weight. *Int. J. Obes.* **2000**, *24*, 627–632. [CrossRef] [PubMed]
47. El Hage, R.; El Hage, Z.; Jacob, C.; Moussa, E.; Theunynck, D.; Baddoura, R. Bone Mineral Content and Density in Overweight and Control Adolescent Boys. *J. Clin. Densitom.* **2011**, *14*, 122–128. [CrossRef]
48. McVey, M.K.; Geraghty, A.A.; O'Brien, E.C.; McKenna, M.J.; Kilbane, M.T.; Crowley, R.K.; Twomey, P.J.; McAuliffe, F.M. The impact of diet, body composition, and physical activity on child bone mineral density at five years of age—Findings from the ROLO Kids Study. *Eur. J. Pediatr.* **2020**, *179*, 121–131. [CrossRef]
49. Rønne, M.S.; Heidemann, M.; Lylloff, L.; Schou, A.J.; Tarp, J.; Laursen, J.O.; Jørgensen, N.R.; Husby, S.; Wedderkopp, N.; Mølgaard, C. Bone Mass Development in Childhood and Its Association with Physical Activity and Vitamin D Levels. The CHAMPS-Study DK. *Calcif. Tissue Int.* **2019**, *104*, 1–13. [CrossRef]
50. Kessler, J.; Koebnick, C.; Smith, N.; Adams, A. Childhood obesity is associated with increased risk of most lower extremity fractures pediatrics. *Clin. Orthop. Relat. Res.* **2013**, *471*, 1199–1207. [CrossRef]
51. Cashman, K.D.; Hill, T.R.; Cotter, A.A.; Boreham, C.A.; Dubitzky, W.; Murray, L.; Strain, J.J.; Flynn, A.; Robson, P.J.; Wallace, J.M.; et al. Low vitamin D status adversely affects bone health parameters in adolescents 1-3. *Am. J. Clin. Nutr.* **2008**, *87*, 1039–1044. [CrossRef]
52. Pekkinen, M.; Viljakainen, H.; Saarnio, E.; Lamberg-Allardt, C.; Mäkitie, O. Vitamin D is a major determinant of bone mineral density at school age. *PLoS ONE* **2012**, *7*, e40090. [CrossRef] [PubMed]
53. Fuleihan, G.E.H.; Nabulsi, M.; Tamim, H.; Maalouf, J.; Salamoun, M.; Khalife, H.; Choucair, M.; Arabi, A.; Vieth, R. Effect of vitamin D replacement on musculoskeletal parameters in school children: A randomized controlled trial. *J. Clin. Endocrinol. Metab.* **2006**, *91*, 405–412. [CrossRef] [PubMed]
54. Lenders, C.M.; Feldman, H.A.; Von Scheven, E.; Merewood, A.; Sweeney, C.; Wilson, D.M.; Lee, P.D.K.; Abrams, S.H.; Gitelman, S.E.; Wertz, M.S.; et al. Relation of body fat indexes to vitamin D status and deficiency among obese adolescents. *Am. J. Clin. Nutr.* **2009**, *90*, 459–467. [PubMed]
55. Maggio, A.B.R.; Belli, D.C.; Puigdefabregas, J.W.B.; Rizzoli, R.; Farpour-Lambert, N.J.; Beghetti, M.; McLin, V.A. High bone density in adolescents with obesity is related to fat mass and serum leptin concentrations. *J. Pediatr. Gastroenterol. Nutr.* **2014**, *58*, 723–728. [PubMed]
56. Soltani, S.; Hunter, G.R.; Kazemi, A.; Shab-Bidar, S. The effects of weight loss approaches on bone mineral density in adults: A systematic review and meta-analysis of randomized controlled trials. *Osteoporos. Int.* **2016**, *27*, 2655–2671. [CrossRef]
57. Rector, R.S.; Loethen, J.; Ruebel, M.; Thomas, T.R.; Hinton, P.S. Serum markers of bone turnover are increased by modest weight loss with or without weight-bearing exercise in overweight premenopausal women. *Appl. Physiol. Nutr. Metab.* **2009**, *34*, 933–941. [CrossRef]
58. Lindeman, K.G.; Greenblatt, L.B.; Rourke, C.; Bouxsein, M.L.; Finkelstein, J.S.; Yu, E.W. Longitudinal 5-year evaluation of bone density and microarchitecture after Roux-en-Y gastric bypass surgery. *J. Clin. Endocrinol. Metab.* **2018**, *103*, 4104–4112. [CrossRef]
59. Elaine, W.Y.; Bouxsein, M.L.; Putman, M.S.; Monis, E.L.; Roy, A.E.; Pratt, J.S.A.; Butsch, W.S.; Finkelstein, J.S. Two-year changes in bone density after Roux-en-Y gastric bypass surgery. *J. Clin. Endocrinol. Metab.* **2015**, *100*, 1452–1459.
60. Kaulfers, A.M.D.; Bean, J.A.; Inge, T.H.; Dolan, L.M.; Kalkwarf, H.J. Bone loss in adolescents after bariatric surgery. *Pediatrics* **2011**, *127*, e956–e961. [CrossRef]
61. Labouesse, M.A.; Gertz, E.R.; Piccolo, B.D.; Souza, E.C.; Schuster, G.U.; Witbracht, M.G.; Woodhouse, L.R.; Adams, S.H.; Keim, N.L.; Van Loan, M.D. Associations among endocrine, inflammatory, and bone markers, body composition and weight loss induced bone loss. *Bone* **2014**, *64*, 138–146. [CrossRef]
62. Burt, L.A.; Billington, E.O.; Rose, M.S.; Raymond, D.A.; Hanley, D.A.; Boyd, S.K. Effect of high-dose vitamin D supplementation on volumetric bone density and bone strength: A randomized clinical trial. *JAMA J. Am. Med. Assoc.* **2019**, *322*, 736–745. [CrossRef] [PubMed]

63. Inelmen, E.M.; Toffanello, E.D.; Enzi, G.; Gasparini, G.; Miotto, F.; Sergi, G.; Busetto, L. Predictors of drop-out in overweight and obese outpatients. *Int. J. Obes.* **2005**, *29*, 122–128. [CrossRef] [PubMed]
64. Ortner Hadžiabdić, M.; Mucalo, I.; Hrabač, P.; Matić, T.; Rahelić, D.; Božikov, V. Factors predictive of drop-out and weight loss success in weight management of obese patients. *J. Hum. Nutr. Diet.* **2015**, *28*, 24–32. [CrossRef] [PubMed]

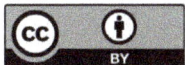

© 2020 by the authors. Licensee MDPI, Basel, Switzerland. This article is an open access article distributed under the terms and conditions of the Creative Commons Attribution (CC BY) license (http://creativecommons.org/licenses/by/4.0/).

MDPI
St. Alban-Anlage 66
4052 Basel
Switzerland
Tel. +41 61 683 77 34
Fax +41 61 302 89 18
www.mdpi.com

Nutrients Editorial Office
E-mail: nutrients@mdpi.com
www.mdpi.com/journal/nutrients

www.ingramcontent.com/pod-product-compliance
Lightning Source LLC
LaVergne TN
LVHW070630100526
838202LV00012B/773